Following a healthy detoxification program a few times a year is one of the best ways to stay well in the modern world. Every day, Americans are exposed to synthetic, often toxic chemicals on an unprecedented scale. Industrial chemicals and their pollutant run-offs in our water, pesticides, food additives, heavy metals, drug residues, and environmental hormones are trapped within the human body in greater concentrations than at any other point in history. More than 25,000 new toxins enter our environment each year.

We are all affected by the environmental toxins and stresses present in our world, and we all make unhealthy life choices now and again. Over periods of time, the toxic burden catches up to us. A detox program helps clean out the chemical toxins, drug residues, and collected waste matter trapped in our bodies.

"*Healthy Healing's Detoxification* highlights the critical importance of body cleansing in today's world. However, detoxification should not be undertaken haphazardly. Dr. Linda Page, America's foremost expert on natural health, offers safe body cleansing choices for anyone who is interested in living a healthier life."

*- Ellen Tart-Jensen, Ph.D., D.Sc., author of* Health is Your Birthright: How to Create the Health You Deserve.

"Another Dr. Linda Page health winner you can trust! Very few people can match her years of experience and expertise."

*- Patricia Bragg, N.D., Ph.D., health pioneer and author of* Bragg Vegetarian Health Recipes.

# other books by Dr. Linda Page

## Healthy Healing, 12th edition

In its first edition nearly 20 years ago, this book was the only one of its kind. Constantly updated and expanded, Healthy Healing is still the easiest to use bestselling natural health reference book on the market. Customize your own personal healing program using natural therapies for more than 300 ailments through diet, whole herb supplements and exercise.

*12th Edition, 664 Pages, Illustrated, 1884334-92-X  SRP: $32.95*      *Spiral Bound Edition - 1884334-93-8  SRP: $35.95*

## Diets for Healthy Healing

Food is powerful medicine. Sometimes it's your best medicine… even for difficult diseases. Dr. Linda Page, America's foremost nutrition and herb expert, has worked with this healing principle for over two decades and has written this book as your primary guide to using food as your best medicine.

*1st Edition, 256 Pages, Illustrated, 1884334-83-0  SRP: $18.95*

## Healthy Healing's Herbal Pharmacist

Herbs may be our most powerful 21st Century Medicines. Learn how to use whole herbs to heal your whole body. Features whole herb healing programs for over 150 ailments!

*3rd Edition, 256 Pages, Illustrated, 8 1/2 x 11  SRP: $18.95*

## Do You Want to Have a Baby? by Sarah Abernathy and Dr. Linda Page

Millions of Americans struggle with fertility problems. Most can overcome them with simple lifestyle changes and natural therapies. Written by two experts in the field of natural health, this book covers optimal nutrition for conception, the best fertility-enhancing supplements, and the documented success of bodywork therapies.

*1st Edition, 176 Pages, Illustrated 1884334-39-3  SRP: $14.95*

# dedication

This book is dedicated to all those who are
on the journey to renewed health through the
ancient practice of body purification.

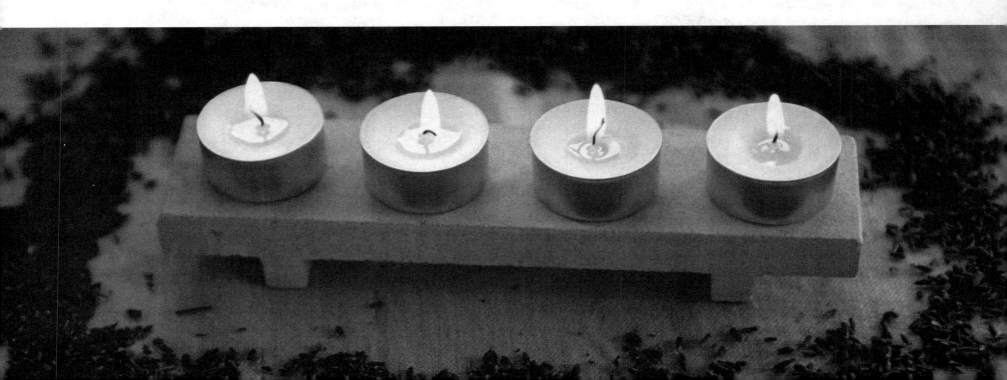

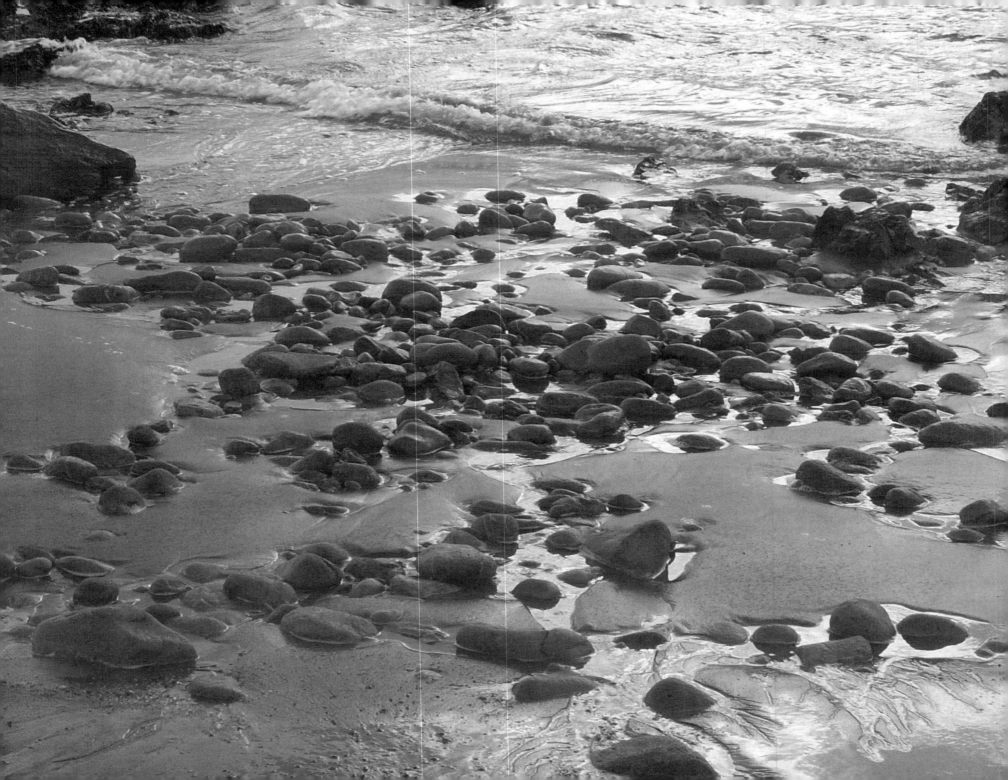

# HEALTHY HEALING'S
# DETOXIFICATION

## PROGRAMS TO CLEANSE, PURIFY & RENEW

### LINDA PAGE, Ph.D.,
#### TRADITIONAL NATUROPATH

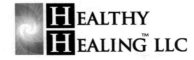

**H**EALTHY **H**EALING™ LLC

*This reference is to be used for educational information. It is not a claim for cure or mitigation of disease, but rather an adjunctive approach, supplying individual nutritional needs that otherwise might be lacking in today's lifestyle.*

First Edition, September 2008

**Publisher's Cataloging-in-Publication**
  *(Provided by Quality Books, Inc.)*

Rector-Page, Linda G.
    Healthy Healing's detoxification : programs to cleanse, purify & renew / Linda Page.
    p. cm.
    Includes bibliographical references and index.
    ISBN-13: 978-1-888-334-55-5
    ISBN-10: 1-888-334-55-X

    1. Detoxification (Health)  2. Herbs--Therapeutic use.  3. Diet therapy.    I. Title.  II. Title:
Detoxification : programs to cleanse purify & renew.

RA784.5.R43 2008            613
                           QBI08-600176

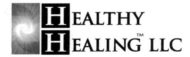

Copyright © September 2008 by Linda Page.
Published by Healthy Healing Enterprises LLC
www.HealthyHealing.com

Cover and book design by Michael Kohler

# table of contents

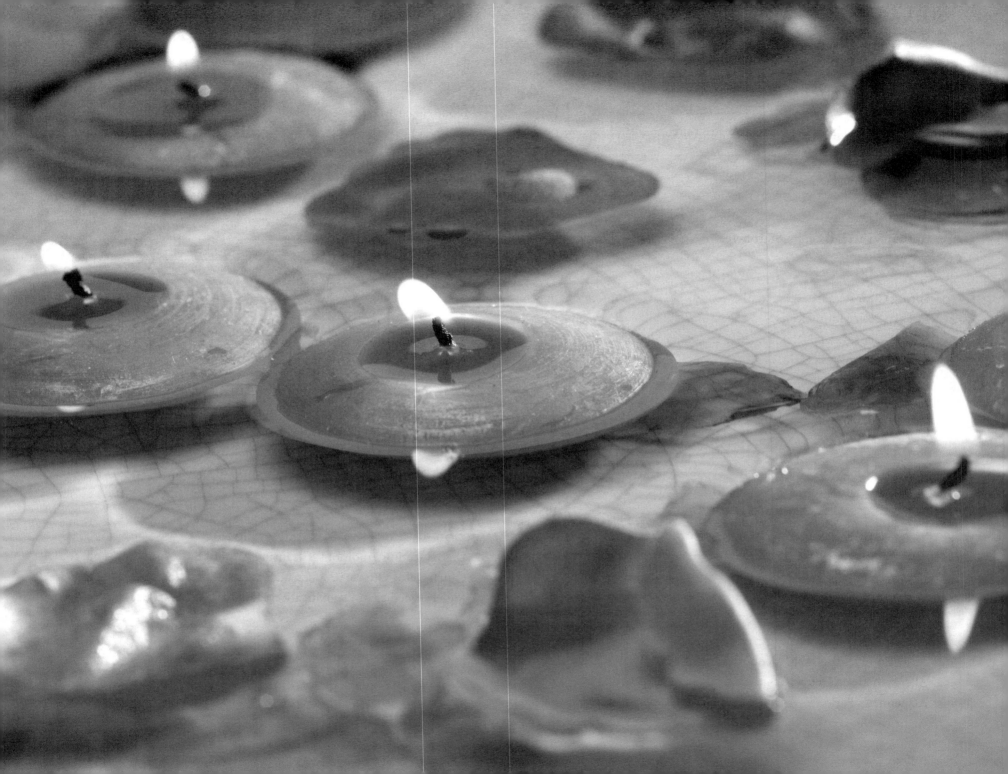

# do you need to detox?
## what is detoxification?

**OUR BODIES DO IT NATURALLY EVERY DAY.** Detoxification is a normal body process of eliminating or neutralizing toxins through the colon, liver, kidneys, lungs, lymph and skin. In fact, internal detoxification is one of our body's most basic automatic functions. Just as our hearts beat nonstop and our lungs breathe continuously, so our metabolic processes continuously dispose of accumulated toxic matter. But in our world today, body systems and organs that were once capable of cleaning out unwanted substances are now completely overloaded; thus many unwanted substances stay in our tissues. Our bodies try to protect us from dangerous material by setting it aside, surrounding it with mucous or fat so it won't cause imbalance or trigger an immune reaction. (Your body stores foreign substances in its fatty deposits—a significant reason to keep your diet and body fat low. Some people carry around up to 15 extra pounds of mucous that harbors this waste!)

Ideally, we should live in a pollution-free environment, eat untainted foods and drink pure water. But, since humans are born with a "self-cleaning system," we know this has probably never been possible. Today, it isn't even practical, so the next best thing is to keep pollutants to a minimum and to periodically get rid of them through a detoxification program.

## Detoxification the *Healthy Healing* way

Detoxification through special cleansing diets may be the missing link to disease prevention, especially for immune-compromised diseases like cancer, arthritis, diabetes and fatigue syndromes like candida albicans. Naturopaths have used detoxification therapies to achieve health and wellness for over 100 years! In Europe, detoxification has long been an integral part of the flourishing spa industry. Our chemicalized-food diet, with too much animal protein, too much fat, too much caffeine and alcohol radically alters our internal ecosystems. Research shows that about 20% of the U.S. food supply is contaminated by toxic pesticide residues, and Americans have up to 68 exposures to these substances every day! Further, the average person consumes over 4 pounds of food additives a year! Even if your diet is good, a cleanse can restore immune strength against toxins that pave the way for disease-bearing bacteria, viruses and parasites.

A detox program aims to remove the cause of disease before we ever get sick. It's a time-honored way to keep immune response high, elimination regular, circulation sound, and stress under control, so your body can handle the daily toxins it encounters. In the past, detoxification was used either clinically for recovering alcoholics and drug addicts, or individually, as a once-a-year mild "spring cleaning" for general health maintenance. Today, a regular detox program two or three times a year makes a big difference not only for health, but for the quality of our lives.

Are detoxification and body cleansing the same thing? After a detox, is my body purified? There is sometimes confusion about these terms because cleansing rituals are so ancient. In Native American cultures, cleansing was regarded first as a religious practice, purifying the body as a living temple to God. In others, such as Chinese medicine, cleansing was part of preventive health care. Today, and in this book, the terms are used interchangeably.

## Why should you detoxify?

Environmental chemicals are so widespread that we are unaware of them. But they have worked their way into our bodies faster than they can be eliminated, and are causing allergies and addictions in record numbers. More than 2 million synthetic substances are known, 25,000 are added each year, and over 30,000 are produced on a commercial scale. Only a small number are ever tested for toxicity. Many come to us from developing countries that have few safeguards in place. This doesn't even take into account the second-hand smoke, caffeine and alcohol overload, or daily stresses that are an increasing part of our lives.

The molecular structure of many chemical carcinogens interacts with human DNA, so long term exposure may result in metabolic and genetic alteration that affects cell growth, and behavior. World Health Organization research implicates environmental chemicals in 60 to 80% of all cancers. Hormone-disrupting pesticides and pollutants are linked to hormone problems, psychological disorders, birth defects, still births and now breast cancer.

As toxic matter saturates our tissues, antioxidants and minerals in vital body fluids are reduced, so immune defenses are thrown out of balance. Circumstances like this are the prime factor in today's immune compromised diseases like candidiasis, lupus, fibromyalgia, and chronic fatigue syndrome. Because their vital organs and immune systems are still developing, children are even more affected by toxic chemicals. Early tests show their chemical exposure is seven times higher than their parents! Chemical oxidation is the other process that allows disease. The oxygen that "rusts" and ages us also triggers free radical activity, a destructive cascade of incomplete molecules that damages DNA and other cell components. And if you didn't have a reason to reduce your animal fat intake before, here is a critical one: oxygen combines with animal fat in body storage cells and speeds up the free radical process.

Almost everyone can benefit from a cleanse. It's one of the best ways to remain healthy in a destructive environment. Not one of us is immune to environmental toxins, and most of us can't escape to a remote, unpolluted habitat. In the last few decades, we have become dangerously able to harm the health of our entire planet, even to the point of making it uninhabitable for life. We must develop further and take even larger steps… those of cooperation and support. We must work together—to save the environment for us all and for future generations. It starts with us. We can also take positive steps to keep our own body systems in good working order so that toxins are eliminated quickly.

We need to take a closer look at our own air, water and food, and keep an ever watchful eye on the politics that control our environment. Legislation on health and the environment follows two pathways in America today… the influence of business and profits, and the demands of the people for a healthy environment and responsible stewardship of the Earth.

## Is your body becoming toxic?

Chemicals are polluting the earth's environment faster than the human organism can adapt to them. Toxins are building up and our bodies are becoming filters trapping the pollutants. The current level of chemicals in our air, food and water supply alters us at the most basic level—our enzymes, then spreads throughout every body function to lower our threshold of resistance to disease.

Besides environmental toxins coming into our bodies, prolonged mental stress and negative emotions can create internal poisons. A lack of exercise contributes to toxicity, too. The body's natural cleansing cycle of oxygen and vital nutrients depends upon exercise. A stagnant system encourages toxic build-up.

## Are you ready for a detox?

- Do you feel congested from eating too much food or the wrong kinds of food?
- Do you feel lethargic and tired, like you need a good spring cleaning?
- Do you need to eliminate drug residues, or normalize your body after illness or hospital stay?
- Do you need a jump start for a healing program?
- Do you need a specific detox program for a serious health problem?
- Do you want to streamline your body processes for more energy?
- Do you need to remove toxins causing a health problem?
- Do you want to prevent illness, or rest and rejuvenate your whole body?
- Do you want to assist weight loss? Do you want to clear up your skin?
- Do you want to slow aging and improve body flexibility?
- Do you want to improve fertility?

**Note:** Laboratory tests like stool, urine, blood or liver function, and hair analysis can also shed light on the need for detoxification.

## What benefits can you expect from a good detox?

A detox cleans out body waste deposits, so you aren't running with a dirty engine or driving with the brakes on.

1. Your digestive tract is cleansed of accumulated waste and fermenting bacteria.
2. Excess mucous and congestion is cleared from the body.
3. Liver, kidney and blood are purified, impossible under ordinary eating patterns.
4. Mental clarity is enhanced, impossible under chemical overload.
5. Dependency on habit-formers like sugar, caffeine, nicotine, alcohol or drugs is less.
6. Bad eating habits are often turned around; the stomach has a chance to flatten to normal size for weight control.

## What are the steps in a good detox program?

You've decided your body needs a cleanse. How long can you give out of your busy life to focus on a cleansing program so that all the processes can be completed? 24 hours, 2 or 3 days, or up to ten days? The time factor is important—you'll want to allot your cleansing time in advance, and prepare both your mind and your body for the experience ahead.

## A good detox program is in 3 steps: cleansing, rebuilding and maintaining

First of all, severely restricting foods for long periods of time is not a good cleansing choice. Years of experience with detoxification have convinced me that if you have a serious health problem, a brief 3 to 7 day juice cleanse is the best way to release toxins from the system. Shorter cleanses can't get to the root of a chronic problem. Longer cleanses upset body equilibrium more than most people are ready to deal with except in a controlled, clinical environment. A 3 to 7 day cleanse can "clean your pipes" of excess mucous, old fecal matter, trapped cellular and non-food wastes, or inorganic mineral deposits that are part of arthritis.

An all-liquid diet is traditionally called a fast. It's not absolutely necessary to take only liquids, but a few days without solid food can be an enlightening experience about your lifestyle. A juice fast increases awareness and energy available for elimination. Fresh juices literally pick up dead matter from the body and carry it away. Your body becomes easier to "hear," telling you what foods and diet are right for your needs via cravings—a desire for protein foods, or B vitamins or minerals, for example. This is natural biofeedback.

Fasting works by self-digestion. During a cleanse, the body decomposes and burns only the substances and tissues that are damaged, diseased or unneeded, such as abscesses, tumors, excess fat deposits, and congestive wastes. Even a relatively short fast accelerates elimination, often causing dramatic changes as masses of accumulated waste are expelled.

You will know your body is detoxing if you experience the short period of headaches, fatigue, body odor, bad breath, diarrhea or mouth sores that commonly accompany accelerated elimination. However, digestion usually improves right away as do many gland and nerve functions. Cleansing also helps release hormone secretions that stimulate immune response and encourages a disease-preventing environment.

## Unsafe detox programs to avoid

### What about a water fast? I don't recommend it.

Leading nutritionists and detoxification experts agree that fresh vegetable and fruit juice cleansing is superior to water fasting. Indeed, juice cleansing is an evolution in detoxification methods. Fresh juices, broths and herb teas help deeply cleanse the body, rejuvenate the tissues and guide you to a faster recovery from health problems than water fasting.

A traditional water fast is harsh and demanding on your body, even in times before huge amounts of food and environmental toxins were part of the picture. Today, it can even be dangerous. Deeply buried pollutants and chemicals from our tissues are released into elimination channels too rapidly during a water fast. Your body is essentially "re-poisoned" as the chemicals move through the bloodstream all at once. Sometimes, the physical and emotional stress of a water fast even overrides the healing benefits.

Vegetable and fruit juices are alkalizing, so they neutralize uric acid and other inorganic acids, better than water, and increase the healing effects. Juices support better metabolic activity for fasting, too. Metabolic activity slows down during a water fast as the body attempts to conserve dwindling energy resources that further reduce productive cleansing. Juices are very easy on digestion, and easily assimilated into the bloodstream. They don't disturb the detoxification process.

### Overdoing purgatives and laxatives

This is another place where detoxification can go wrong. Using purgatives like magnesium salts, bentonite clay or even large amounts of aloe vera juice for long periods of time (for instance to cleanse the colon) can be too harsh.

Further, increasing the dosage on certain herbs (especially standardized and potentiated herbs) can cause some unwanted effects. Concentrated aloe vera juice is a good example. Aloe vera juice supports multiple body systems and can be used with success for a wide range of health problems. Diabetics can use it to balance their blood sugar; ulcers patients can use it to induce rapid internal healing. Some bowel disorders can even be reversed with it. It is truly of Nature's "superfoods" when used properly.

But using too much of it magnifies its laxative effects. Drinking lots of concentrated aloe vera juice (glasses of it a day) can lead to intense intestinal cramping, diarrhea, even hemorrhoids as the colon begins eliminating at a much faster rate than it's used to.

## Detoxification: the journey to health

The first step of your cleanse is elimination. For a short time, you'll be cleaning out mucous and toxins from the intestinal tract and major organs. Everything functions more effectively when toxins, obstructions and wastes are removed. Try to drink 8 glasses of water each day of your fast in addition to your juices.

The second step is rebuilding healthy tissue and restoring energy. With obstacles removed, your body can rebuild to optimum levels. Eat only fresh and simply prepared foods during the rebuilding step. Your diet should be very low in fat, with little dairy (cottage cheese and yogurt are okay), and no fried foods. Avoid alcohol, caffeine, tobacco, and sugars. Avoid meat except fish and sea foods. Include supplements and herbal aids for your specific needs.

The final step is keeping your body clean and toxin-free—very important after all the hard work of detoxification. Modifying lifestyle habits is the key to a strong resistant body. A diet for health maintenance relies heavily on fresh fruits and vegetables for fiber, cooked vegetables, grains and seeds for strength and alkalinity, sea foods, soy foods, eggs and low fat cheeses as sources of protein, and lightly cooked sea foods and vegetables with a little dinner wine for circulatory health. A personalized group of supplements and herbal aids, as well as exercise and relaxation techniques, should be included. Whole herb formulas are a wonderful cleansing choice because they are broad spectrum and gentle, encouraging the body to bring itself back into balance naturally.

# how detoxification can go wrong

**DEAR READER, LET ME TELL YOU A TRUE STORY** about how detoxification can go wrong… When I first heard about a cleansing diet in the '70s I thought it sounded like just the thing for me. I had fought my weight all my life. I was tired all the time (probably from all the crazy diets I went on to lose weight), and I felt "toxic," constantly getting fever blisters, bladder infections and yeast infections. I had dull hair, poor skin texture, peeling feet and breaking nails. Detoxification seemed like it would solve of lot of health problems.

The trouble was, I had almost no idea how to go about it. But I had some enthusiastic friends who were detoxing, too, so I started on what was essentially a 5 food diet—cabbage, lettuce with a little salad dressing, apples, oranges, peanut butter (for protein), and a few whole wheat crackers occasionally.

I was delighted with my weight loss (I averaged about 90 pounds for my 5 foot frame). I decided to keep detoxing, even though my friends had long since stopped. I rarely ate other things; and this went on for several years. My detox had gone too far… to the point that I was becoming anorexic. I honestly didn't realize it, but my body was going into major malnutrition decline.

Today with everything I know about nutrition, I know this type of diet is not a cleansing diet. It's a prescription for terrible health.  All I saw was that I was finally thin, but I was too thin. At one of my lowest points after being released from the hospital for a life threatening infection, I weighed only 69 pounds! I finally saw it was time for a major change or I wasn't going to make it. I was blessed to have the support of caring family and friends to help carry me through the process.

I read everything I could find on natural healing and herbal remedies. I got serious about healthy eating and started formulating herbal formulas to bring my body back to health. It took many many months for me to recover, put on weight, regain strength and learn new healthy eating habits. But it slowly began to happen. I could see a new me emerging, with curly hair, and a better skin tone and texture than I had before the illness. My circulation returned; my energy levels grew stronger than ever before. The healing and the experience changed my life, and I made the decision to dedicate my career to the study and practice of natural health.

One of the reasons I wanted to write this book was to pass along all I've learned about how healthy detoxification really works. A healthy detox program is a targeted diet that both cleanses the body and infuses it with essential nutrients. This book contains over 28 healthy detox programs. I've designed and refined the programs over many years and each plan has years of success behind it. You can have every confidence that the recommendations outlined in this book have been used and found to be safe and effective, in some cases by thousands of people.

To your best health,

*Linda Page*

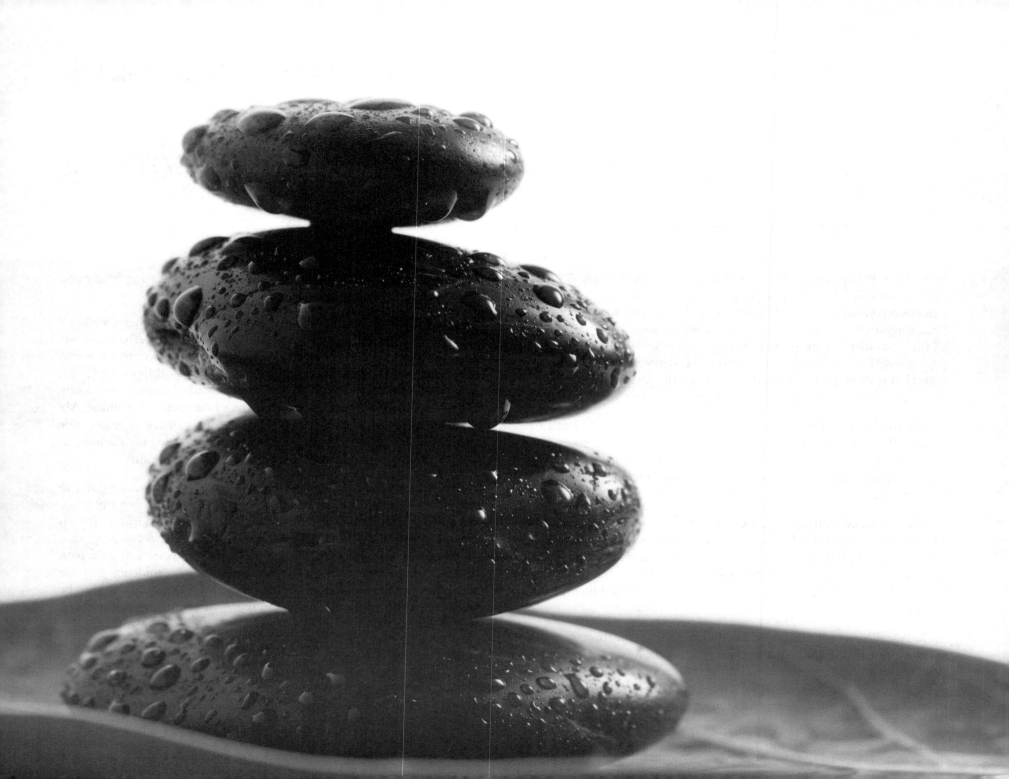

# Healthy Healing
# detoxification programs

**D**ECIDING ON THE RIGHT DETOX PROGRAM CAN be a challenge. In my thirty years of experience in natural health, I have found that most people are not prepared physically, emotionally or mentally to handle the stress of many of the popular, extended detox programs that are on the market today.

My own hard won early experience with detoxification taught me without question that there are right and wrong ways to cleanse the body (To learn more about my dangerous "detox" experience, please see page 13). A healthy detox will rejuvenate your body's systems, and clear wastes that are preventing you from achieving your best health. A poorly designed detox program could make you sicker than you were before you started.

My goal as a natural healer is to help you to stay healthy naturally and safely. I have spent years creating Healthy Healing detox programs that are livable for today's men and women. My detox programs infuse your body with essential nutrients and help you cleanse, thrive and heal naturally and safely.

After a detox, the body starts rebalancing. Energy levels often rise physically, mentally and sexually. Creativity may even begin to expand. You will look and feel like a new person, because you are. Your outlook and attitude change because through cleansing and improved diet, your actual cell make-up has changed.

## Self-test: do you need to detoxify?

*A yes answer to two or more of these questions should alert you that your body could benefit from a detox.*

- Do you have frequent body odor, bad breath or a coated tongue?
- If you're a woman, are you experiencing frequent vaginal yeast infections or UTIs (Urinary Tract Infections)?
- If you're a man, are you experiencing frequent jock itch (a sign of candida) or prostatitis?
- Is your immune response low? Are you catching frequent colds, flus or intestinal bugs?
- Have you gained weight even though your diet hasn't changed?
- Do you have unexplained headaches, back or joint pain, or arthritis?
- Do you suffer from chronic respiratory problems or sinus problems?
- Do you have food sensitivities, poor digestion or chronic constipation with intestinal bloating or gas?
- Do you have chronic fatigue or environmental sensitivities, especially to odors?

- Are you unusually tired? Are you relying on stimulant pick-me-ups like sugar and caffeine to get through the day?
- Do you have brittle, breaking nails or dull, dry, damaged hair?
- Do you have a hard to treat skin problem like psoriasis or adult acne?
- Do you have an unusually poor memory or insomnia?

# spring cleanse

Cleanses come in all shapes and sizes. You can easily tailor a cleanse to your individual needs. Unless you require a specific detox for a serious illness, or recovery from a long course of drugs or chemical therapy, I recommend a short cleanse twice a year, especially in the spring, summer or early autumn when sunshine and natural vitamin D can help the process along.

## A "spring cleaning" detox is a wonderful breath of fresh air for your body after a long, closed-in winter.

A mild spring cleanse is an important, yearly vitality technique no matter how healthy you are. Even though you may exercise during the winter to keep trim, most people still feel at an energy low during the cold seasons. Our bodies still reflect the ancient seasonal need to harbor more fat for warmth and survival. In the days when people were closer to nature than we are today, the great majority farmed the land from spring to fall, and lived lives of demanding physical labor. Winter was a time of inactivity, with a natural tendency towards rest. Harvested food supplies stored in the autumn lost much of their nutrition value through the winter, so people had to eat denser foods and more of them to receive the same nutrients. Even in modern times, many days without sunshine and vitamin D mean that our bodies are less able to utilize nutrients properly.

Cold weather prompts people to consume heavier, fattier, comfort foods. Old winter "hibernation" patterns also mean that metabolism slows, sometimes by as much as 10%. So, much to the dismay of many of us, fall and winter are the most difficult times of the year to control body weight.

Winter weather illnesses like colds and flu leave us with accumulated toxins, too. Heavy winter clothing, especially thick waterproof coats, hinders normal breathing and perspiration of the skin, and, in this way, contributes to impaired body functions. When spring finally arrives, our metabolism livens up. New green foods, with their metabolism-stimulating effects, abound from the first tender leafy vegetable shoots. Cleansing, antioxidant-rich herbs promote a feeling of new life and restored well-being. Warmer weather tends to lower our appetite needs; it prompts more activity and movement, and stimulates cleansing processes. Nature has designed the perfect time for a spring cleanse.

A "spring cleaning" is actually a very light diet, focusing on digestion and the intestines to help eliminate accumulated wastes, and improve body functions. A good length for a spring or summer cleanse is 2 or 3 days or a long weekend. A weekend is enough time to fit comfortably into most people's lives, and it doesn't become too stressful on the body. The best way is to start on Friday night with a pre-cleansing salad, then follow with a cleansing diet like the one in this book, and end with a light Monday morning fruit bowl. Amplify the purifying effect with a stimulating, circulation bath or sauna and steam baths.

## What are the body signs that you need a spring cleanse?

- Do you feel bloated, constipated and congested? (a sign that your diet has been heavier and richer than usual)
- Have you gained some unwanted pounds even though you aren't eating more food? (a sign of winter fat storage)
- Do you feel slow and low energy most of the time? (a sign of cold weather body slowdown)
- Has your digestion worsened? (a sign your body isn't using nutrients well)
- Do your chest and lungs feel clogged and swollen? (a sign of slower, shallower breathing, and perhaps a resident colony of low-grade infective microbes)

## What benefits can you expect from a spring cleanse?

- Your digestive tract will be "washed and brushed" of accumulated waste and putrefactive bacteria.

- Your liver, kidney and blood can be purified, impossible under ordinary eating patterns and habits.
- Your mental clarity will receive a boost, not possible under the constant overload of chemicals and food additives.
- Possible dependency on habit-forming refined sugars, caffeine, nicotine, alcohol or drugs is relieved as body chemistry normalizes.
- Bad eating habits get a break… with a new chance for you to reform better diet patterns.
- Your stomach has a chance to reduce to normal size for weight loss and better weight control.

## Spring cleanse nutritional plan

*Start with this 3 to 5 day nutritional plan*

Your nutrition should focus on fresh plant foods:

1. High chlorophyll plants for enzymes
2. Fruits and vegetables for fiber
3. Cultured foods for probiotics
4. Eight glasses of water a day.

## The evening before your spring cleanse…

1. Take your choice of gentle herbal laxatives.
2. Have a light salad with plenty of greens.

## The next 3 – 5 days…

**On rising:** take a cleansing and flushing booster product, or 1 heaping teaspoon of a fiber drink in juice or water. Add 1000mg vitamin C with bioflavonoids 3x a day to raise body glutathione levels, an important detox compound.

**Breakfast:** take your choice of fruit juices.

**Mid-morning:** take a small glass of potassium broth (pg. 101), or 2 tbsp. aloe juice concentrate in juice or water, or a superfood green drink (see next column); or a cup of green tea.

**Lunch:** a fresh carrot juice; or raw sauerkraut or a seaweed salad (in natural or asian food stores)

**Mid-afternoon:** take a glass of fresh apple juice; or an herbal cleansing tea.

**About 5pm:** take another small potassium broth, a fresh carrot or vegetable juice (page 106), or a superfood green drink (see next column).

**Supper:** take miso soup with 2 tbsp. dried sea vegetables (dulse, nori, etc.) chopped over the top.

**Before Bed:** repeat the herbal cleansers that you took on rising, and take a cup of mint tea.

## On the last night of your cleanse…

Finish your cleanse with a small green salad with fresh sprouts on the last night.

## Herbs & supplements

*Choose two to three cleansing boosters*

**Gentle herbal laxatives:** Crystal Star Herbal Laxa Caps, AloeLife Aloe Gold. After your initial juice detox, Zand Herbals Quick Cleanse Kit for the intestinal tract and the liver.

**Cleansing boosters:** Crystal Star Blood Detox caps; Planetary Formulas River Of Life, clears accumulations of a long inactive winter.

**Cleansing and flushing boosters:** Crystal Star Cleansing & Purifying tea; Nature's Secret Supercleanse tabs; Crystal Star Herbal Laxa Caps.

**Chlorophyll-rich plants—spring's great gift to us:** Sun Wellness Sun Chlorella; Futurebiotics Colon Green caps; Green Foods Green Essence; Crystal Star Energy Green Drink Mix; Barleans Greens; Nature's Secret Ultimate Green.

**Enzyme support:** Crystal Star Dr. Enzyme; **Full spectrum enzymes:** Herbal Products Development Power-Plus Enzymes; Transformation Digestzyme.

**Electrolyte boosters help detoxify cells:** Nature's Path Trace-Lyte Minerals; Arise & Shine Alkalizer; Trace Mineral Research Concentrace.

17

**Probiotics replenish healthy bacteria:** American Health Acidophilus liquid; UAS DDS- Plus with Fos; Wakunaga Kyo-Dophilus.

**Antioxidants defeat pollutants:** Crystal Star Green Tea Cleanser; Country Life Super 10 Antioxidant; NutriCology Antiox Formula II; Biotec Food Cell Guard; Source Naturals Astaxanthin; Now Super Antioxidant.

**Fiber:** All One Whole Fiber Complex; AloeLife FiberMate.

**High-potency multiple support:** Pure Essence Labs One-n-Only multi; vitamin C 1,000mg daily.

## Bodywork techniques

*Pick bodywork and relaxation therapies to accelerate and round out your cleanse.*

**Irrigate:** Take an enema the first, second and the last day of your spring cleansing program to help release toxins out of the body.

**Exercise:** take a walk for ten minutes the first day of your cleanse. Each day increase your exercise by five minutes.

**Sauna:** Take a hot sauna or a long warm bath with a rubdown, to stimulate circulation. Dry brush your body before your sauna to help release toxins coming out through the skin.

**Massage therapy:** get one good lower back massage during your cleanse

**Aromatherapy supports detoxification. Stress-reducing flower remedies:** Aromaland Relaxing blend; Nelson Bach Rescue Remedy; or try lemon, grapefruit or juniper essential oils to speed up your detox.

**Aromatherapy bath:** add 8 to 10 drops of essential oil to a bath. Stir water briskly to disperse. Lavender and chamomile are good choices. Or try Masada Dead Sea Salts Detox blend with essential oils, herbs and ancient sea minerals.

**Deep Breathing Exercise:** Do this deep, relaxed breathing exercise often during your cleanse to remove stress, compose your mind, improve your mood and increase your energy: Take a deep, full breath. Exhale it slowly… slowly. Take another deep, full breath. Release slowly. And again. Maintain a quiet rhythm, try to exhale more slowly than you inhale. Close your eyes. As you exhale, visualize toxins dislodging and leaving your body. As you inhale, visualize pure nutrients rebuilding your vibrancy.

## For your continuing diet

After the initial cleanse above, the second part of a general health system is rebuilding healthy tissue and body energy. This stage takes 1 to 2 months for best results. It emphasizes high fiber from fresh vegetables and fruits, cultured foods to replenish healthy intestinal flora, and green foods for enzyme production, and alkalizing foods to prevent irritation while healing. Avoid refined foods, saturated fats, fried foods, red meats, caffeine and pasteurized dairy foods.

# twenty-four hour cleanse

This cleanse is a special little jewel. It's an invaluable healing tool to put into action as soon as you realize that you are not feeling well. It can swiftly be "pulled out of your pocket" at the first signs of unexplained low energy, poor skin or congestion. It's one of the best ways I know to turn around (and get quick recovery) from a cold or flu.  It's also an easy first step before making a significant diet improvement or change. A twenty-four hour cleanse can be a good answer if you need a cleanse, but your busy life won't allow you to set aside even a few days. People always tell me how busy their lives are. Sometimes, even a short cleanse seems like too much time.

"Beginning" is usually the hardest part of a cleanse. You have to set aside a block of time, gather all the ingredients for a detox diet, alter your eating times and patterns; in essence change your lifestyle and that of those you live with for a while. This is very difficult to do for many people, and can delay a needed program.

A twenty-four hour detox is a juice and herbal tea cleanse that lets you go on with your normal activities, and "jump start" a healing program. Even though it's quick, without the depth of vegetable juices needed for a major or chronic problem, it's often enough, is definitely better than no cleanse at all, and it will make a difference in the speed of healing. Even if your program is only going to consist of lifestyle changes aimed at better health, a twenty-four hour cleanse can point you in the right direction.

## Is your body showing signs that it needs a twenty-four hour cleanse?

- Do you feel "toxic"? Are you getting unusual allergy reactions?
- Are you tired a lot for no reason?
- Are you starting to feel congested? Do you have the first signs of a cold or flu? (Go right into this cleanse.)
- Is your skin dry or flaky? Is your skin tone sallow? Is your hair dull, dry and brittle?
- Are the soles of your feet or your palms often peeling?
- Do you frequently get mouth herpes?
- Do you get frequent yeast infections?
- Do you get frequent urinary tract infections?

## Pointers for best results from your twenty-four hour cleanse:

- Drink 8 to 10 glasses of water a day to hydrate and flush wastes and toxins from all cells.
- Focus on chlorophyll-rich foods (leafy greens, sea vegetables) and juices (super green foods like chlorella, barley grass or spirulina) during this cleanse. Chlorophyll is the most powerful cleansing agent found in nature. It also has a rapid tonic effect.

## Twenty-four hour cleanse nutrition plan

**The evening before you begin:** have a green leafy salad to give your bowels a good sweeping. Dry brush your skin before you go to bed to open your pores for the night's cleansing eliminations.

**The next day:** the next 24 hours take fresh juices, herbal drinks, water, and a long walk.

**On rising:** take 2 tbsp. fresh lemon or lime juice, 1 tbsp. maple syrup and 1 pinch cayenne in water.

**Breakfast:** make a fresh fruit juice with 1 pear, 2 apples, 4 oranges and 1 grapefruit; or a glass of cranberry juice.

**Mid-morning:** have a Zippy Juice: 1 handful dandelion greens, 3 fresh pineapple rings and 3 radishes; or a cleansing, energizing tea with antioxidants like Crystal Star Green Tea Cleanser.

**Lunch:** juice 4 parsley sprigs (or a handful of dandelion greens), 3 tomatoes, ½ green bell pepper, ½ cucumber, 1 scallion, 1 lemon wedge; or have a glass of fresh apple juice with 1 packet chlorella or Green Foods Green Magma granules dissolved.

**Mid-afternoon:** take a cup of Crystal Star Cleansing & Purifying Tea.

**Dinner:** take a glass of papaya/pineapple juice to enhance enzyme production; or try this high mineral broth: 7 carrots with tops, 7 celery stalks with tops, beet tops from 1 bunch, 2 potatoes, 1 onion, 4 cloves of garlic, 3 zucchini, 1 handful of parsley. Place in a large soup pot, cover with water, bring to a boil and simmer for thirty minutes. Remove and discard veggies.

**Before Bed:** have a cup of mint tea, or 1 tsp. Red Star Nutritional Yeast Broth or miso soup.

## Herbs & supplements:

*Choose two to three cleansing boosters.*

**Gentle herbal laxatives:** The night before your cleanse take an herbal laxative such as Crystal Star Herbal Laxa Caps; M. D. Labs Daily Detox Tea or Traditional Medicinals Smooth Move.

**Cleansing boosters:** Crystal Star Cleansing & Purifying Tea helps cleanse and detoxify the system while providing strength and nourishment or Crystal Star Liver Renew—a cleansing formula to re-establish an alkaline environment, which is very useful at the beginning of a cleansing program.

**Enzyme/nutrient support:** Crystal Star Dr. Enzyme with proteolytic enzymes and blend of immune enhancing herbs.

**Electrolyte boosters:** These aid in efficient removal of toxic body acids

& boost energy: Nature's Path Trace-Lyte Minerals; Alacer Emergen-C; Trace Mineral Research Concentrace; Arise & Shine Alkalizer.

**Probiotics:** Have detoxifying properties, and maintain the body's vital chemical and hormone balance. Wakunaga of America Kyo-Dophilus; Jarrow Jarro-Dophilus; American Health Acidophilus liquid.

**Chlorella:** Green algae are the highest sources of chlorophyll in the plant world; and of all the green algae, chlorella is the highest. Sun Wellness Sun Chlorella or Pure Planet Chlorella.

**Vitamin C:** Take 1,000mg of vitamin C 3x per day. (complex with bioflavonoids) vitamin C raises the body's glutathione levels (an important detox compound).

## Bodywork techniques

*Pick bodywork and relaxation therapies to accelerate and round out your cleanse*

**Dry brush:** The night before your cleanse, dry brush your skin before you go to bed to open your pores for the night's cleansing eliminations.

**Enema:** Take an enema the night before or the morning of your cleanse. After an enema there may be a heightened sense of physical well-being.

**Exercise:** Take a long, brisk walk during the day.

**Bathe:** Take a seaweed or mineral bath in the morning and one before you go to bed. (See seaweed bath, page 148) Mineral bath: add 1 cup Dead Sea salts, 1 cup Epsom salts, ½ cup regular sea salt and ¼ cup baking soda to a tub; swish in 3 drops lavender oil, 2 drops chamomile oil, 2 drops marjoram oil and 1 drop ylang-ylang oil.

**Pamper yourself:** Add some favorite beauty and skin cleansing treatments like a facial, a pedicure, or deep hair conditioning during your bath.

**Rest:** Get a full eight hours of rest the night before your cleanse. Add a nap during the day to allow your body's energies to focus on healing.

**Essential oils:** Aromatherapy can support detoxification and healing, Bach Flower Crab Apple.

**Visualize your detox:** Close your eyes and inhale and exhale long and slowly.

As you exhale, visualize toxins dislodging and leaving your body. As you inhale, visualize oxygen and nutrients renewing each cell.

## For your continuing diet

The next morning: have a cup of green tea or mint tea, or Crystal Star Green Tea Cleanser. Then break your fast with a bowl of fresh fruits. Eat fresh foods during the day—have a mixed vegetable salad for lunch with a little lemon/flax oil dressing. Have another salad for dinner with a little brown rice and tamari sauce. Before bed, have a warming Miso Broth (page 119).

# stress cleanse

You change the oil in your car because you believe it will make it run smoother and last longer. You plunge into spring cleaning, determined to make your living environment free of dirt and germs that might threaten your health. You buy air and water filters which promise to rid your environment of toxins. You sink into a hot bath, convinced that cleansing your body's exterior will keep you healthy.

How disconcerting to realize that you've left an important part of the cleansing job unattended. Cleansing on the inside improves everything on the outside. A whole body stress detox is the key to revitalizing your body, mind and spirit. A stress cleanse focuses on your entire body… eliminating toxins and rebuilding your tissues with cleansing juices and stress-relieving foods. Rather than targeting a specific body system or problem, this cleanse reflects broad spectrum, mild body refreshment. It clears the "junk" out of body pathways so that wholesome nutrients can get in quickly to rebuild energy and strength.

You may have been struggling with the low nutrition of a Standard American Diet (SAD) for decades. Many people do not recognize that much of the "food" in America's supermarkets doesn't really have much nutrition that the body can translate into usable nutrients. Some of the "foods" like designer fake fats may even ultimately contribute to ill health. One of the best ways to keep excess fat and sugar out of your life is to keep in mind what a really healthy diet is.

- It's fresh fruit and vegetable juices several times a week.
- It's fresh fruits and vegetables every day. At least once a day, have a fresh salad. Have steamed, stir-fried or baked veggies for at least one other meal.
- It's adding sea vegetables to a meal at least once a week for their packed, superior nutrition. (Six pieces of sushi are just fine.)
- It's cultured foods for friendly digestive flora (like raw sauerkraut, yogurt, kefir, kefir cheese). Raw sauerkraut, rich in acidophilus, is especially good at deterring harmful bacteria.
- It's plenty of water—at least eight 8 oz. glasses a day.
- It's whole grains, nuts, seeds and beans for protein and essential fatty acids.
- It's healthy fats, like omega-3 oils and EFAs from cold water fish, flax, perilla oil and seafood that enhance thyroid and metabolic balance; and EFAs from sea vegetables, spinach and herbs like evening primrose oil. It's just as important to include healthy fats as it is to eliminate unhealthy fats, like hydrogenated and partially hydrogenated fats.
- It's superfoods like bee pollen, royal jelly and aloe vera; or green superfoods like chlorella, spirulina or barley grass with concentrated nutrition, and they're becoming more and more popular as anti-aging factors, energy boosters, and highly supportive when dealing with a health problem, weight problem and of course detoxification.
- A healthy diet is also less meat and dairy foods. You'll feel better if you eat them in moderation. You'll feel a lot better if you avoid fried foods and chemically processed foods altogether.

## Is your body showing signs that it needs an overall body stress cleanse?

- Is your immune response low? Are you catching every bug that comes down the pike?
- Are you unusually tired? Do you feel like you need a pick-me-up?
- Have you had unusual body odor or bad breath lately?
- Do you feel mentally dull?
- Have you gained weight even though your diet hasn't changed? (A cleanse is a healthy way to lose weight.)

## Pointers for best results from your body stress cleanse

- Drink eight 8 oz. glasses of bottled water each day of your cleanse (herbal teas can be part of this).
- Add 1 tbsp. of a superfood or green superfood mix to at least one of the juices you take per day. For the best results in energy and nourishment I like to add 1 tbsp. of a green superfood to all the veggie or fruit drinks.
- Alkalize the whole body. Foods which are alkalizing should be used in a ratio of at least 4:1 to foods which are acidifying. Plenty of pure water and fresh fruit or vegetable juices are especially useful. Acidifying foods tend to aggravate any health problems.

## Benefits that you may notice as your body responds to a body stress cleanse

- Your digestion will noticeably improve as your digestive tract is cleansed of accumulated waste and fermenting bacteria.
- You'll feel lighter (most people lose about 5 pounds on this cleanse) and more energized.
- You'll feel less dependent on habit-forming substances like sugar, caffeine, nicotine, alcohol and drugs as your bloodstream purifies.
- You'll feel healthier. Most people have noticeably better resistance to common colds and flu.
- You'll feel more mentally alert, less space-y, more emotionally balanced. Creativity begins to expand.
- You'll feel more energized as your body starts rebalancing. Energy levels rise physically, psychologically and sexually.

## Stress cleanse nutrition plan

*Start with this 3 to 7 day nutrition plan. Begin with this 3 day juice/liquid diet and follow with 1 to 4 days of a diet of all fresh foods.*

**On rising:** take a glass of 2 fresh squeezed lemons, 1 tbsp. maple syrup and 8 oz. of pure water.

**Breakfast:** have a nutrient-dense Kick-Off Cleansing Cocktail: juice 1 handful fresh wheat grass or parsley—extremely rich in chlorophyll and antioxidants, 4 carrots, 1 apple, 2 celery stalks with leaves, ½ beet with top.

**Mid-morning:** have a glass of fresh carrot juice or fresh apple juice. Add 1 tbsp. of a green superfood like Crystal Star Energy Green drink mix; Green Kamut Green Kamut; Vibrant Health Green Vibrance.

**Lunch:** have a Salad-In-A-Glass: juice 4 parsley sprigs, 3 quartered tomatoes, ½ green or red pepper, ½ cucumber, 1 scallion, 1 lemon wedge.

**Mid-afternoon:** have a cup of Crystal Star Cleansing & Purifying Tea, green tea or mint tea.

**Dinner:** have a warm Potassium Essence Broth (page 101), for mineral electrolytes. Or try Super Soup, with antioxidants, antibiotic properties and immune boosters: 1 cup broccoli florets, 1 leek (white parts, a little green), 2 cups fresh peas, ½ cup sliced scallions, 4 cups chard leaves, ½ cup diced fennel bulb, ½ cup fresh parsley, 6 garlic minced cloves, 2 tsp. astragalus extract (or ¼ cup broken pieces astragalus bark), 6 cups vegetable stock, a pinch of cayenne, 1 cup diced green cabbage, ¼ cup chopped sea vegetables. Bring all ingredients bring to a boil, then simmer for 10 min. Let sit for 20 minutes. Strain and use broth only for a cleanse. (Use unstrained as a soup recipe when not on a liquid diet.)

## Herbs & supplements

*Choose two to three cleansing boosters.*

**Use alongside the liquid juice cleanse:** Crystal Star Blood Detox caps stimulate the body to eliminate wastes rapidly; or Planetary River of Life formula; or Crystal Star Cleansing & Purifying tea.

**Deep cleansing:** When solid food is again introduced, use Nature's Secret Ultimate Cleanse.

**Cleansing support formulas:** New Chapter Life Shield; Pure Essence Labs Antioxidant caps for protection against free radicals.

**Enzyme support:** Crystal Star Dr. Enzyme; Enzyme Essentials Excellzyme.

**Antioxidants help remove toxins:** Biotec Food Cell Guard; Alpha Lipoic Acid; Jarrow Coenzyme Q10.

**Probiotics support detoxification in numerous ways:** UAS DDS-Plus with FOS; Wakunaga Kyo-Dophilus; Nutricology Symbiotics.

**Electrolytes dramatically boosts energy levels:** Alacer Emergen-C; Arise & Shine Alkalizer; Nature's Path, Trace-Lyte Liquid Minerals.

**Green Superfoods:** Crystal Star Energy Green drink mix; Green Kamut Green Kamut; Wakunaga Harvest Blend.

**Detoxing gentle flower remedies:** Nelson Bach Rescue Remedy.

## Bodywork techniques

*Pick bodywork and relaxation therapies to accelerate and round out your cleanse.*

**Enema:** Enemas can be a best friend to your cleansing program. Flushing your colon on the first, the second and the last day of your stress detox program gives your body a giant step forward in releasing toxins from your body.

**Exercise:** Do this body stretch daily during your cleanse. Repeat this at least 5 times.

• Stand tall—raise your hands above your head.

• Stretch your arms and fingers to reach for the sky—move your hands and fingers as if you are trying to climb up into the sky.

• As you reach, inhale deeply through your nostrils while rising on your toes.

• Exhale slowly; gradually return to your starting position, arms hanging loosely at your sides.

• Follow your stretch with a brisk walk.

**Deep Breathing Exercise:** Deep, relaxed breathing takes away stress, induces relaxation, composes the mind, improves mood & increases energy levels. 1. Take a deep, full breath. Exhale it, slowly. Slowly. 2. Take another deep, full breath. Release slowly. 3. And again. 4. Maintain a quiet rhythm, exhaling more slowly than you inhale.

**Sauna or bath:** Take a hot sauna or a long warm bath, with a rubdown to stimulate circulation. In your bath try: Masada Dead Sea Salts; or use a relaxing essential oil like lavender (10 drops in your bath water).

**Massage:** Have a massage therapy treatment to further remove toxins and stimulate circulation.

## For your continuing diet

Eat plenty of fresh vegetables and fruits for the rest of the month. Choose foods high in fiber like whole grains and beans. Especially avoid unhealthy fats, like partially hydrogenated oils. But make a point to get plenty of EFAs from sea vegetables, herbs like evening primrose oil. Avoid refined sugars, sodas and caffeine-containing foods for the rest of the month. Don't forget to drink plenty of daily water.

# mucous cleanse

Your body needs some mucous. We tend to think of body mucous as a bad thing because it obstructs our breathing during a sinus infection, asthma or a cold. But that same mucous is also a needed body lubricant, and an important body safeguard. Human beings take about 22,000 breaths a day, and along with the oxygen, we take in dirt, pollen, disease germs, smoke and other pollutants. Mucous gathers up these irritants as they enter the nose and throat, protecting the mucous membranes that line the upper respiratory system. Mucous build-up may be a sign that your body is trying to bring itself to health. The problems start when your body holds on to too much. Some of us carry around as much as 10 to 15 pounds of excess mucous!

Your body systems work together, of course. It only seems, as we address its different parts and processes, that everything isn't wholly related. But, extra pressure of disease or heavy elimination on one body part puts extra stress on another. Support for the kidneys, for example, takes part of the waste elimination load off the lungs so they can recover faster. Similarly, promoting respiratory health also helps digestive and skin cleansing problems. The lungs, though, are on the front line of toxic intake from viruses, allergies, pollutants, and mucous-forming congestives. (The world's rainforests are also a critical part of the Earth's front lines for detoxification. It's easy to see through our own need to keep our lungs healthy, that we must care for the vital lungs of the earth through rainforest preservation.)

A program to overcome any chronic respiratory problem is usually more successful when begun with a short mucous elimination diet. A cleanse allows your body to rid itself first of toxins and accumulations that cause congestion before an attempt is made to change eating habits.

Foods that putrefy quickly inside your body are the same foods that spoil easily outside in the air—like meat, fish, eggs and dairy products. These same foods are the ones most likely to produce excess mucous, too, which in turn slows down transit time through your gastrointestinal tract and colon. Mucous also tends to form extra heavy protection pockets around foreign dietary substances that it deems harmful... like preservatives, additives, and especially food colorants. Excess mucus is especially harmful to respiratory system, digestive ability, and colon activities. This is the time to do a mucous cleanse.

## Is your body showing signs that it needs a mucous cleanse?

Any signs of respiratory system congestion may be thought of as sure signs of excess mucous in the body, especially in the colon and intestinal tract. The common cold and flu are usually accompanied by congestion and phlegm. A mucous cleanse helps to release excess mucous in the respiratory system and in the colon.

## Pointers for best results from your mucous cleanse

• Herbal supplements are a good choice during a mucous and congestion cleanse. They act as premier broncho-dilators and anti-spasmodics to open congested airspaces. They can soothe bronchial inflammation and

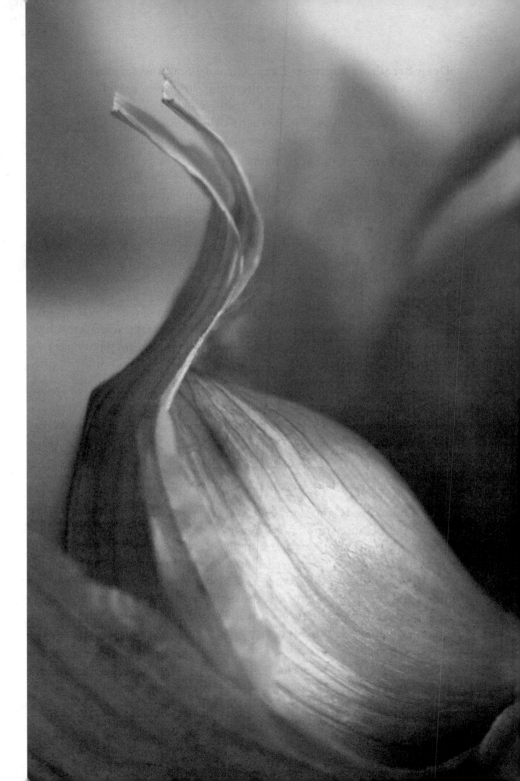

cough. They have the ability to break up mucous. They are expectorants to remove mucous from the lungs and throat.

- Drink eight to ten glasses of water daily to thin mucous.
- Take 10,000mg ascorbate vitamin C crystals with bioflavonoids daily the first three days; just dissolve ¼ tsp. in water or juice throughout the day, until the stool turns soupy, and tissues are flushed. Take 5,000mg daily for the next four days.
- Take a brisk, daily walk. Breathe deep to help lungs eliminate mucous.
- Take an enema the first and last day of your fasting diet to thoroughly clean out excess mucous.
- Apply wet ginger/cayenne compresses to the chest to increase circulation and loosen mucous.
- Take a hot sauna or a long warm bath with a rubdown, to stimulate circulation.

## Benefits that you may notice as your body responds to a mucous congestion cleanse

- The cleansing diet with supportive supplements will begin to clear any congestion in the body.
- If there is bronchial inflammation and/or cough, it will calm as the cleanse progresses.
- Mucous from the lungs and throat will break up and be eliminated from the body.
- Mucous from the colon may also be expelled from the body.

## Mucous cleanse nutrition plan

*Start with this 3 to 7 day nutrition plan.*

## The night before your mucous cleanse…

Mash 4 garlic cloves and a large slice of onion in a bowl. Stir in 3 tbsp. honey. Cover, let macerate for 24 hours; remove garlic and onion and take only the honey/syrup infusion—1 tsp. 3x daily.

## The next 3 – 7 days…

**On rising:** take 2 squeezed lemons in water with 1 tbsp. maple syrup.

**Breakfast:** take a glass of grapefruit, pineapple, or cranberry-apple juice.

**Mid-morning:** have a glass of fresh carrot juice with 1 tsp. Bragg's Liquid Aminos added; or a cup of congestion clearing extract, like Crystal Star D-Congest, an expectorant to aid mucous release, or Jiaogulan tea, an aid in oxygen uptake.

**Lunch:** have a vegetable juice like V-8, or a potassium broth (page 101); or make this Mucous Cleansing Tonic by juicing: 4 carrots, 2 celery stalks, 2 – 3 sprigs parsley, 1 radish and 1 garlic clove.

**Mid-afternoon:** have a veggie drink (page 106), or chlorella or spirulina granules in water; or a greens and sea vegetable drink like Crystal Star Energy Green drink.

**Dinner:** apple or papaya/pineapple juice.

**Before Bed:** take a hot vegetable broth (page 120), add in 1 tbsp. nutritional yeast. Have a small fresh salad on the last night of the cleanse.

**To break the fast…** begin with small simple meals. Have toasted muesli or whole grain granola for your first morning of solid food, with a little yogurt or apple juice; a small fresh salad for lunch with lemon/oil dressing; a fresh fruit smoothie during the day; a baked potato with butter and a light soup or salad for dinner.

## Herbs & supplements

*Choose two to three cleansing boosters.*

**Deep body cleanser for intestinal tract and lungs:** Use Nature's Way Thisilyn Cleanse caps after juice fasting—along with the cleansing diet. Helps pull intestinal mucous and clear mucous congestion from the respiratory system.

**Mucous cleansers:** Use Crystal Star D-Congest as an expectorant to aid mucous release; Herbs Etc. Lung Tonic—A mullein and horehound expectorant to loosen and remove mucous; Herbs Etc. Respiratonic is an all-purpose complex which loosens mucous, clears lung congestion, and dilates the bronchioles.

**Herbs to relieve mucous:** mullein loosens and expels mucous; slippery elm removes excess mucous, soothes and strengthens mucous membranes; sage helps excessive mucous discharge; white pine, an antioxidant expectorant, reduces mucous.

**Better oxygen uptake:** Rhodiola rosea; NutriCology Germanium; Herbs Etc. Chlorenergy.

**Enzyme support:** Crystal Star Dr. Enzyme between meals or Transformation Gastrozyme relieves bouts of mucous congestion. After congestion is relieved, use Enzyme Essentials Digestzyme to assist complete digestion. Improperly digested foods putrefy and cause mucous.

**Electrolyte boosters help digestive efficiency up to 80%:** Alacer Emergen-C; Nature's Path Trace-Lyte Liquid Minerals; Arise & Shine Alkalizer.

**Probiotics help maintain proper mucous levels:** UAS DDS-Plus; Jarrow Formulas Jarro-Dophilus+Fos; Nutricology Symbiotics with FOS. Bodywork Techniques

## Pick bodywork and relaxation therapies to accelerate and round out your cleanse

**Enema:** Take an enema the first, second and last day of your juice fasting to help thoroughly clean out excess mucous. Irrigate: Or, have a colonic for a more thorough colon cleanse.

**Exercise:** Take a brisk, walk on each day of your cleanse. Breathe deep to help the lungs eliminate mucous.

**Massage therapy with percussion:** a rubdown stimulates circulation and loosens mucous. Most people have several congestion-releasing bowel movements and expectoration incidences within 24 hours after a massage therapy treatment.

**Compress:** Apply wet ginger/cayenne chest compresses to increase circulation and loosen mucous.

**Essential oil support:** aromatherapy oils help clear mucous congestion in the lungs:

- Eucalyptus (inhale) - antiviral action works on respiratory tract to loosen mucous - treats asthma, bronchitis and sinusitis.

- Tea tree oil (inhale) - antiviral and antibacterial decongestant.

- Oregano oil (inhale) - antiviral and antibacterial properties help eradicate lung infection.

**Flower remedies:** Nelson Bach Rescue Remedy to calm difficult breathing.

**Visualize your detox:** Close your eyes—inhale and exhale long and slowly. As you exhale, visualize mucous dislodging and leaving your lungs and also from your colon. As you inhale, visualize oxygen and nutrients renewing all your cells.

**Bathe & Sauna:** long warm baths and saunas help loosen mucous congestion. Add to your bath 5 drops of eucalyptus, tea tree oil or oregano oil.

## For your continuing diet

Eliminate junk foods and fried foods. Avoid pasteurized dairy foods, heavy starches and refined foods that are a breeding ground for continued congestion. Drinking eight glasses daily helps flush body toxins and prevent the build up of excess mucous. Eat plenty of enzyme-rich foods like fresh vegetables (salads) and fruits. They form the least amount of mucous and they are the easiest to digest, passing through the body in less transit time.

---

# brown rice cleanse

A brown rice cleanse is a 7-day cleansing diet. I've found it's an effective option to a juice cleanse. It's especially useful for dropping a few quick pounds and a great way to transition from an unhealthy diet into a better diet. It's amazingly easy to fit into your lifestyle. A brown rice cleanse is based on macrobiotic principles for body balance. Brown rice adds a building, warming factor to a cleanse, making your meals more satisfying, and ensuring that you get plenty of fiber and minerals.

A brown rice cleansing diet encourages an approach to eating that provides complex carbohydrates, quality protein, and energy fats by using rice as a nutrient building food, and using vegetables and vegetable juices as concentrated cleansing supplements.

## Is your body showing signs that a brown rice cleanse would do you some good?

- Is your immune response low?
- Do you feel like you need to clear cobwebs from your brain?
- Do you need to lose about 10 pounds? A brown rice diet is a healthy way to lose weight!
- Are you feeling log-y and out-of-sorts?
- Are you looking for a gentle, easy transition to an improved diet? A brown rice diet is cleansing, yet filling. You don't feel like you're on a cleanse at all, yet it does the trick. It's the best cleansing diet for colder times of the year.

## Pointers for best results from your brown rice cleanse

- Drink 8 to 10 glasses of water (or herbal teas) a day to hydrate and flush wastes and toxins from all cells.
- Add 1 tbsp. of a green drink mix or superfood powder to each juice you take during the day.
- Use non-fat seasonings to your own taste. Use only 1 tbsp. of a healthy oil dressing on salads (like flax, olive or perilla oil). Better yet, I like to use only sea greens or herbal seasoning salts on both my salads, soups and rice during this diet.
- Follow this diet for at least seven days. You need one week to set up an ongoing body balance, Then, ease yourself into a good, ongoing diet. Include other wholesome grains like millet, amaranth, quinoa and buckwheat after you complete the brown rice cleanse.

## Benefits that you may notice as your body responds to a brown rice cleanse

- Most people notice an improvement in vitality and energy levels right away.
- Almost everybody loses some weight during this cleanse. Most people experience about a 2 to 5 pound weight drop.

- People who have heart problems regularly notice a more stable heartbeat and better circulation. A fiber-rich cleansing diet with sea vegetables, that eliminates animal (meat and dairy) protein, almost invariably lowers the risk of heart problems, high blood pressure and diabetes risk. The diet is stimulating to the heart and circulatory system.

- A brown rice cleanse is high in potassium, natural iodine, other minerals and trace elements. Most people notice improvement in their hair, skin texture and nail growth.

## Brown rice cleanse nutrition plan

*Start with this 7 day nutrition plan.*

## The night before your brown rice cleanse…

A green leafy salad for dinner sweeps your bowels.

## The next 7 days…

**On rising:** take a glass of 2 fresh squeezed lemons, 1 tbsp. maple syrup and 8 oz. of pure water.

**Breakfast:** have a drink like Pulsating Parsley Juice: 6 carrots, 1 beet, 8 spinach leaves and ¼ cup fresh parsley leaves.

**Mid-morning:** take a cup of Crystal Star Cleansing & Purifying Tea or Daily Detox by M.D.

**Lunch:** have a veggie juice like Super V-7: juice 2 carrots, 2 tomatoes, handful of spinach leaves and a handful of parsley, 2 celery ribs, ½ cucumber, ½ green bell pepper. Add 1 tsp. green superfood: Crystal Star Energy Green; Fit For Life Miracle Greens; Barleans Greens or Aloe Life Daily Greens.

**Mid-afternoon:** have a glass of carrot juice.

**Dinner:** have steamed brown rice and mixed steamed vegetables. Sprinkle with sea vegetables (like dulse or kelp, easily purchased in flakes or granules). Use 1 tbsp. flax or olive oil, if desired, and 1 tbsp. Bragg's Liquid Aminos. Add flavor and nutrition by sprinkling with nutritional yeast.

**Before Bed:** have a cup of herbal tea such as peppermint, spearmint or chamomile.

**The next 6 days:** have 2 to 3 glasses of mixed vegetable juices throughout the day. Any blend of your favorite vegetables is fine. Don't eat any solid food during the day. Have steamed brown rice and mixed vegetables for an early dinner each evening. Either steamed or raw vegetable salads can be used. The enzymes in raw vegetables provide a greater cleansing quality.

## Herbs & supplements

*Choose two to three cleansing boosters.*

**Cleansing boosters:** Crystal Star Herbal Laxa Caps stimulate the body to eliminate wastes rapidly; Nature's Secret Ultimate Cleanse helps detoxify all five channels of elimination and is taken along with a cleansing diet.

**Cleansing teas:** Crystal Star Cleansing & Purifying Tea helps cleanse and detoxify the system while providing strength and nourishment; Daily Detox by M.D. is a mild cleanser, gentle enough to take on a daily basis, yet stimulates all the major elimination organs.

**Enzyme support:** Enzyme Essentials Digestzyme.

**Cleansing support formulas:** Crystal Star Toxin Detox caps; or Pure Essence Antioxidant protect against oxidative damage and environmental assault.

**Electrolyte boosters:** electrolytes play a major role in detoxifying cells, and enhance uptake of essential nutrients, macro minerals and proteins from food sources and other supplements. Trace Mineral Research Concentrace; Arise & Shine Alkalizer.

**Probiotics:** the number one factor in creating and maintaining health and well-being of the intestines. UAS DDS-Plus; Wakunaga KYO-Dophilus; Jarrow Formulas Jarro-Dophilus EPS.

**Essential Fatty Acids:** Evening primrose oil 1000mg.

**Chlorella:** Chlorophyll is the most powerful cleansing agent found in nature. Green algae are the highest sources of chlorophyll in the plant world—Sun Wellness Sun Chlorella or Pure Planet Chlorella.

## Bodywork techniques

*Pick bodywork and relaxation therapies to accelerate your cleanse.*

**Enema:** Take an enema the night before or the morning of your cleanse. Flushing the colon is one of the best ways to jump-start any cleanse. Cleansing the colon allows more expedient release of toxins from all other body cells.

**Exercise:** Take a brisk walk, or workout on an exercise bicycle or a treadmill. Exercise increases oxygen uptake, and boosts blood transport to carry nutrients to cells and waste products and toxins away from the cells.

**Massage therapy:** It's one of my cardinal cleansing points. Get a massage once a week for the month of your cleanse. Health experts agree that a regular massage promotes the movement of body fluids. There's also noticeable improvement in overall health because most of the body's processes rely on movement of fluids, including getting nutrients to cells, oxygenating tissues and removing wastes from all body parts.

**Flower remedies:** Nelson Bach Rescue Remedy or Crab Apple.

**Essential oils:** Aromatherapy supports relaxation, detoxification and healing. Wyndmere Stress Relief or Meditative Mood are good choices for this cleanse.

**Visualize your detox:** Close your eyes and inhale and exhale long and slowly. Visualize a free movement of body fluids. As you exhale, visualize toxins dislodging from cells, being carried by the bodies fluids, and leaving your body. As you inhale, visualize oxygen and nutrients flowing to and renewing all your cells.

## For your continuing diet

Eating whole foods is the first principle to remember as you choose the foods for your continuing diet. Eating from the sea is the second important principle. Include fish or shellfish, or sea vegetables at least three times a week. Work at eliminating (completely if possible) fried and fast foods. Reduce your consumption of meats and dairy foods. Consciously add more grains and vegetables. Eat your fruits and fruit juices in the morning or late at night.

# pollutant/heavy metal cleanse

Chemical pollutants and toxic by-products affect every facet of our lives, from our water and food supply to the workplace and our homes. Heavy metal poisoning and pollutant toxicity are now major health problems of the American culture. We have moved from fetid air to undrinkable water to severe allergy reactions to serious diseases caused by pollution. There seems to be no way to avoid toxic exposure. The main effect of an unhealthy environment is reduced immune response, especially in the way that our filtering organs, the liver and kidneys, are impacted. Periodic detoxification needs to be a part of life to keep our bodies able to defend us… against yet more pollutants. (An astounding 25,000 NEW chemicals enter our society every year.) A hair analysis can help you determine which heavy metals are lodged in your body, and also what nutrient deficiencies you may have that result from toxin overload.

Your immune response will improve quickly as heavy metals and chemicals leave your body. Provide a highly nutritious diet for yourself right away after your cleanse to build up resistance. Your cells and tissues will benefit from nourishing nutrients and more easily release toxins that would otherwise lodge in them.

## Is your body showing signs that it needs a pollutant/heavy metal cleanse?

- Are you far more sensitive to odors like perfumes and strong cleansers than most people? Do you feel worse in certain stores?

- Do you have an unusually small tolerance for alcohol?

- Are there medications you can't take? Even some vitamins and supplements that make you feel worse?

- Do you have small black spots along your gum line? Unusually bad breath or body odor?

- Is your reaction time when driving noticeably poorer in city traffic?

- Do you have unexplained seizures, memory failure or psychotic behavior?
- Have you become infertile or impotent?

## Pointers for best results from your pollutant/heavy metal cleanse

- Drink 8 – 10 glasses of bottled water each day of your cleanse.

- A heavy metal, pollutant detox is one of the most likely cleanses for a "healing crisis" to occur. You may feel head-achy, a slight upset stomach or nausea as toxins are released into the bloodstream for elimination. The feelings should pass quickly, usually within 24 hours. But I don't recommend an all-liquid diet if you're trying to release heavy metals or chemicals. They may enter the bloodstream too fast and heavily for your body to handle safely. Eat solid cleansing foods instead to release the toxins more slowly and safely.

- Chlorophyll is the most powerful cleansing agent found in nature. Green veggie drinks and green superfoods are a must.

- Sea greens are potent environmental toxin, heavy metals and radiation releasers. They can be sprinkled on salads, steamed veggies, baked potatoes, into vegetable juices, etc.

## Nutrition plan for your pollutant/heavy metal cleanse

*Start with this 7 day nutrition plan.*

**On rising:** take 2 – 3 tbsp. cranberry concentrate in 8 oz. water with ½ tsp. ascorbate vitamin C crystals; or Crystal Star Green Tea Cleanser; or blend half a lemon with pit, 1 tsp. honey, 1 cup water and 1 tsp. acidophilus in 8 oz. aloe vera juice.

**Breakfast:** have a glass of fresh carrot juice, with 1 tbsp. of a green superfood like Crystal Star Energy Green or Green Foods Green Magma, and whole grain muffins or rice cakes w/ kefir cheese or yogurt; or a cup of rice milk or plain yogurt blended with a cup of fresh fruit, walnuts, and ½ tsp. Nutricology Symbiotics (or acidophilus powder) in 8 oz. aloe vera juice.

**Mid-morning:** take a cup of green tea, with ½ tsp. ascorbate vitamin C

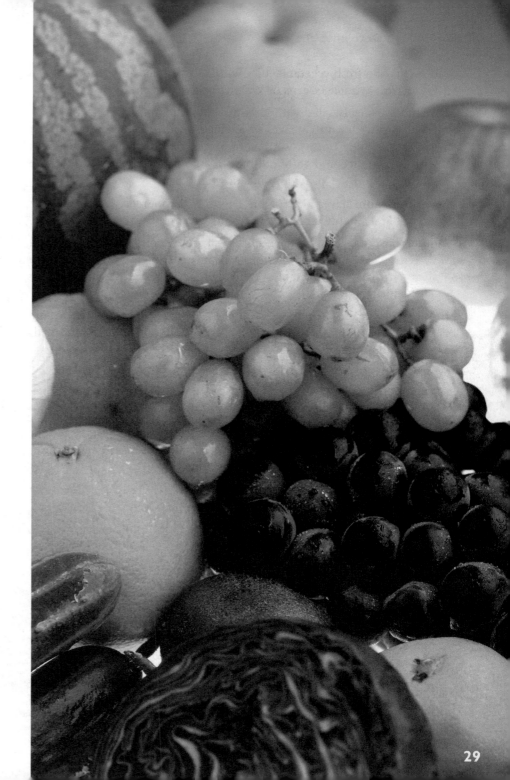

crystals; or a fresh vegetable juice with 1 tbsp. green superfood such as Fit for You Miracle Greens or Wakunaga Kyo-Green.

**Lunch:** have a leafy salad with lemon/flax oil dressing; or have an open-faced sandwich on rice cakes or a chapati, with rice cheese and fresh veggies; or a cup of miso soup with brown rice; or steamed vegetables with brown rice and tofu; and pau d'arco tea with ½ tsp. ascorbate vitamin C and ½ tsp. acidophilus powder.

**Mid-afternoon:** have a carrot juice with 1 tbsp. green superfood like Crystal Star Energy Green; or a shot of wheatgrass juice.

**Dinner:** have a baked potato with Bragg's Liquid Aminos and a fresh salad w/ lemon/flax dressing; or a black bean or lentil soup; or a Chinese steam/stir fry with vegetables, shiitake mushrooms and brown rice; or a tofu and veggie casserole.

**Before Bed:** take a 8 oz. glass of aloe vera juice with ½ tsp. ascorbate vitamin C with bioflavs; and another carrot juice, or papaya juice with 1 tsp. acidophilus powder.

## Herbs & supplements

*Choose two to three cleansing boosters.*

**Deep Cleansing product:** Along with the cleansing diet use a deep cleanser like Arise & Shine Cleanse Thyself Program.

**Pollutant/Heavy Metal cleansers:** Crystal Star Toxin Detox; or Cleansing & Purifying tea; or Nature's Answer Seacentials Gold.

**Herbal immune protection:** astragalus extract; propolis extract; panax ginseng; Siberian ginseng; aloe vera and garlic.

**Liver enhancers:** Crystal Star Liver Renew caps or Liver Cleanse Flushing tea; Milk Thistle Seed extract; dandelion extract.

**Antioxidants defeat pollutants:** Alpha Lipoic Acid is among the most powerful liver detoxifiers ever discovered. Jarrow Formulas Alpha Lipoic Acid or Alpha-Lipoic Acid by MRI; New Chapter Supercritical Antioxidants; Pure Essence Labs Antioxidant tabs.

**Chelation:** Oral chelation cleanses circulatory of heavy metals. Metabolic Response Modifiers Cardiochelate; Golden Pride Formula One, oral chelation with EDTA.

**Enzyme support:** Protease binds to heavy metals, sparing metabolic enzyme destruction: Crystal Star Dr. Enzyme.

**Probiotics help deactivate drugs:** UAS DDS-Plus with FOS; Jarrow JarroDophilus EPS.

**Chlorella supplements:** chlorella's high chlorophyll content and powerful detox ability are available through its unique cell wall. Sun Wellness Sun Chlorella or Pure Planet Chlorella.

**Sea Vegetables:** Seaweeds bind with and neutralize many heavy metals and environmental toxins. Nature's Path Trace-Min-Lyte; Crystal Star Ocean Minerals cap; New Chapter Ocean Herbs caps.

## Bodywork techniques

*Pick bodywork and relaxation therapies to accelerate your cleanse*

**Enema:** Enemas greatly assist removal of toxins and relieving stress on the body. Take an enema the first and second day of your cleansing program. Take additional enemas as you feel the need. See enemas in this book. Better yet—have at least one colonic irrigation during your cleanse.

**Detox Bodywork:** consider VIBE machine therapy with biophotonic light and EB footbath (you can see toxins being released in the water!).

**Exercise:** Exercise only moderately during this cleanse. Allow your body to use its energy for healing and repair. Take a walk every day, breathing deeply. Get plenty of tissue oxygen. Do deep breathing exercises on rising, and in the evening on retiring to clear the lungs and respiratory system.

**Shower:** Take a hot and cold hydrotherapy treatment at the end of your daily shower. Alternating hot for 1 minute, then cool for 1 minute to stimulate circulation. Use a dry skin brush before and after the shower to remove toxins coming out on the skin (quite common in a heavy metal cleanse).

**Bathe:** A detoxifying, relaxing mineral bath: Add 1 cup Dead Sea salts, 1 cup Epsom salts, ½ cup regular sea salt and ¼ baking soda to a tub. If you have access to seaweed (either dried or freshly gathered), add it to the bath to help draw out toxins. If you wish to add essential oils, swish in 4 drops lavender oil, and 4 drops chamomile oil or try my favorite: Crystal Star Hot Seaweed Bath.

**Visualization Exercise:** Close your eyes and inhale and exhale long and slowly. As you exhale, visualize toxins dislodging and leaving your body. As you inhale, visualize pure, nourishing nutrients building health and vibrancy.

## For your continuing diet

Protection against pollutants begins with a healthful whole foods diet. Eat organically grown foods as much as possible to reduce the intake of toxins. Green drinks are a key against all kinds of contaminants. One of the easiest ways to do this is to add 1 – 2 tbsp. of a green superfood mix to juice or water at least once a day.

# fat/cellulite detox

Cellulite is a combination of fat, water and trapped wastes beneath the skin—usually on otherwise thin women. When circulation and elimination processes become impaired, connective tissue loses its strength. Unmetabolized fats and wastes become trapped in pockets just beneath the skin instead of being expelled through normal means. Over time, the waste materials harden and form the puckering skin effect we know as cellulite. Because it is unattached material, dieting and exercise alone can't dislodge cellulite.

Do you have cellulite? It looks like lumpy, rippled skin around thighs, hips and love handles. When regular fat is squeezed, the skin appears smooth—cellulitic skin will ripple like an orange peel, or have the texture of cottage cheese.

Cellulite is also characterized by heaviness in the legs, soreness and tenderness when tissue is massaged. Why do you get it? Sometimes its a family trait, more often it's linked to poor nutrition resulting in liver exhaustion, excess estrogen build up, and poor fat metabolism. Inadequate exercise, poor elimination and insufficient water intake increase trapped wastes and toxins. Other causes? Crash dieting with rapid regain of weight increases cellulite formation. Smoking impedes both circulation and metabolism. Don't get too much sun. UV rays contribute to cellulite.

## An effective program for cellulite release should be in four parts

1. Stimulate elimination functions.
2. Increase circulation and metabolism.
3. Control excess fluid and waste retention.
4. Re-establish connective tissue elasticity.

### Is your body showing signs that it needs a fat/cellulite detox?

- Do you have bulging, dimply cellulitic skin on hips, buttocks, thighs and knees (women); torso and stomach (men)? Cellulite is a combination of fat, water and trapped wastes beneath the skin.
- Are your upper arms flabby or your waistline noticeably thicker?
- Does your face look jowl-y or puffy? Have your wrists and ankles thickened?
- Do you have a thick waist that doesn't go away even with exercise and diet improvements?

### Pointers for best results from your fat/cellulite detox

- Add daily flushers to free trapped toxins: pineapple (bromelain), apples and berries (pectin fiber) and citrus (vitamin C). Carrot/beet/cucumber juice cleans the liver so it can metabolize fats better. Drink 6 to 8 glasses of water, juices and green tea every day. Graze—eat smaller, more frequent meals, instead of 2 to 3 large ones to keep fat burning.
- Fruits and juices each morning. Two fresh or steamed vegetables at every other meal. A fresh salad and brown rice once a day.
- The cellulite blacklist: all fried, fatty dairy foods; high caffeine, carbonated sodas, hard liquor; red meats; extra salty foods (use herbal seasoning instead).
- Balance estrogen: add cruciferous veggies like broccoli to keep excess estrogen flushed. Have omega 3-rich fish and seafood twice a week. Have 2 tbsp. chopped dried sea greens 3 or 4 times a week in a soup, salad or rice; or 6 pcs. sushi daily.
- Drink plenty of water! Eight glasses of bottled water each day of your

cleanse (can include herbal teas).

- Enzymes are a dieters best friend! Enzyme-rich juices and foods help you lose and maintain your ideal weight.

- Include a superfood drink once or twice a day for energy and nutrient content.

- Boost your fiber intake. Fiber is another key to weight and cellulite control.

- Watch your fats like a hawk! Unhealthy fats make you gain weight... healthy fats assist weight loss.

## Nutrition plan for your fat/cellulite detox

*Start with this 3 to 7 day nutrition plan. Begin with a 3 day juice/liquid diet and follow with 1 to 4 days of all fresh cleansing foods.*

**Note:** Drink plenty of water during this cleanse. Water naturally suppresses appetite and helps maintain a high metabolic rate. In fact, water is the most important catalyst for increased fat burning. It enhances the liver's main function of detoxification and metabolism, and allows it to process more fats. Don't be concerned about fluid retention; high water intake actually decreases bloating, because it flushes out sodium and toxins. Expert dieters drink 8 glasses of water a day.

**On rising:** take a glass of lemon juice and water in the morning.

**Breakfast:** have a Fat Melt Down Juice: juice 2 apples, 2 pears, 1 slice of fresh ginger to help reduce fat from places where it is stored in cellulite. The ginger stimulates better blood circulation.

**Mid-morning:** have a carrot/beet/cucumber juice to flush the liver. Add 1 tbsp. green superfood into the juice: Crystal Star Energy Green; Pure Planet Spirulina; or Barleans Greens.

**Lunch:** have a liquid Salad Special: juice 3 broccoli flowerets, 1 garlic clove, 5 carrots or 2 tomatoes, 2 celery stalks, ½ red or green pepper.

**Mid-afternoon:** have a cup of Crystal Star Liver Cleanse Flushing tea or green tea.

**Dinner:** have an electrolyte broth: In 3 cups water, cook 2 cups fresh mixed vegetables (carrots, broccoli, dark leafy greens, celery and parsley), and 2 tsp. miso. Add in mixed sea vegetables. Seaweeds add minerals and improve sluggish metabolism.

**Before Bed:** have licorice or peppermint tea with a dash of honey.

## Herbs & supplements

*Choose two to three cleansing boosters.*

**Deep liver cleanser:** The liver is your body's chemical plant responsible for fat metabolism. Weight gain and energy loss are often the result of a liver which has become enlarged through overwork, alcohol exhaustion or congestion. Try: Crystal Star Cellulite Release caps; Health from the Sun Sunpower CLA; Milk thistle seed extract or Artichoke leaf extract for liver congestion.

**Essential fatty acids:** Without essential fatty acids (EFAs), poor fat metabolism is certain. Unhealthy excess fluid retention is also controlled by EFAs. EFA deficiency increases appetite and promotes obesity.

EFAs to consider:

- Flax Oil - 1 or 2 tbsp. over a salad, or Barleans Total Omega.

- Evening Primrose Oil - 1000mg daily.

- CLA - an Omega-6 fatty acid with fat-burning properties, 1800mg daily.

**Capillary strengthening:** you must tighten capillary walls in order to keep extra fat and cellulite from returning. Bioflavonoids are important: Ethical Nutrients Turmeric Flavonoid Complex; or Jarrow Gentle Fibers.

**Herbal weight loss help:** Crystal Star Will Power with hoodia helps keep you from overeating; Nature's Secret Ultimate Weight Loss; Gaia Herbs Diet Slim; Source Naturals Diet-Phen.

**Enzyme support:** Crystal Star Dr. Enzyme; Bromelain 1500mg daily to break down proteins and help metabolize fats; Enzyme Essentials Balance-Zyme for weight loss.

**Electrolytes dramatically boost energy levels:** Trace Mineral Research Concentrace; Trimedica Alkamax; Nature's Path Trace-Lyte Liquid Minerals.

## Bodywork techniques

*Pick bodywork and relaxation therapies to accelerate your cleanse.*

**10-minute daily cellulite exercises work:** They support a slim subcutaneous fat layer, increase circulation, maintain underlying tissue integrity. Do them all each day for 10 minutes.

1. Standing arm swings 50 count both arms.

2. 100 tummy sucks.

3. 100 torso twists.

4. Wall pushups with each arm and both arms.

5. Standing leg circles, 50 each leg.

6. Weight lifting that focuses on the lower body helps develop the muscles in the hips and thighs.

7. Deep breathing moves out lymph congestion that shows as cellulite (one reason why yoga and pilates are so effective).

**Dry brushing:** Fatty wastes can get trapped beneath the skin's surface easily (especially in women) when the liver or lymphatic systems are sluggish. Use a natural bristle brush—brush vigorously in a rotary motion and massage every part of your body in this order: feet and legs, hands and arms, back and abdomen, chest and neck. Five to fifteen minutes is the average time.

**Rub-on cellulite-fighting essential oils:** Antioxidant oils rosemary and thyme. Peppermint oil increases metabolism. Juniper stimulates circulation.

**Massage:** Have a massage therapy treatment at the beginning and end of your cleanse to move excess fluid wastes and unattached fats into elimination systems, and to stimulate skin circulation.

**Bathe away excess fats:** Crystal Star Hot Seaweed Bath; or a sea salt bath: add 1 cup Dead Sea salts, 1 cup Epsom salts, ½ cup regular sea salt and ¼ baking soda to a tub; swish in 3 drops lavender oil, 2 geranium drops oil, 2 drops sandalwood oil and 1 drop neroli oil.

## For your continuing diet

Drink plenty of water for good weight maintenance. Water can help you move past weight loss plateaus; decreasing water intake causes increased fat deposits. Drink all liquids before eating, to suppress appetite and maintain a high metabolic rate. Make sure at least 50 percent of your diet is composed or fresh foods and juices. Fresh food calories are relatively non-stimulating to glands and tend to stabilize weight.

---

# bladder-kidney cleanse

Your kidneys are largely responsible for the elimination of waste products from protein breakdown. Concentrated protein wastes can cause chronic inflammation of the kidney filtering tissues (nephritis), and can overload the bloodstream with toxins, causing uremia. If the movement of salts, proteins or other bio-chemicals goes awry, health problems from mild water retention to major kidney failure arise.

But your bladder and kidneys do more than just remove water wastes. Channeling pollutants and chemicals out of our systems before they build up and contaminate our cells is obviously crucial to the body's internal hygiene. The bladder and kidneys are primary removal sites for toxic and potentially toxic chemicals in the bloodstream. The urinary system is also part of a complex process that maintains your body's fluid stability. Urinary controls are involved with the brain, hormones, and receptors all over the body. They are smart controls that register your body needs for fluids. Sometimes, they remove very little salt or water; at other times, they remove a lot. By the way… dehydration is the most common stress on the kidneys. Natural medicine emphasizes the importance of high quality water for kidney health.

## Is your body showing signs that it needs a bladder-kidney cleanse?

Do you have chronic lower back pain, irritated urination, frequent unexplained chills, fever, or nausea or unusual fluid retention? If you do, a gentle, natural, three to five day cleansing course might be just the thing to keep you from getting a full-blown, painful bladder infection.

## Pointers for best results from your bladder-kidney cleanse

- Drink 10 glasses of bottled water each day of your cleanse. Body purification systems can operate efficiently only if the volume of water flowing through them is sufficient to carry away wastes.
- Avoid dietary irritants on the kidneys, such as coffee, alcohol, and excessive protein.
- Herbal supplements provide excellent support for a kidney cleanse. Take them as liquids (drinks or teas) for best results.
- Take a liquid green supplement each day of your cleanse, such as Barleans Greens, or Pure Planet Chlorella.
- Apply wet, hot compresses on the lower back to speed cleansing; or take alternating hot and cold sitz baths.

## Improvement signs show that your body is responding to the cleanse

- The flow of urine will be increased.
- Infection of the bladder and/or irritated urination will abate.
- The kidneys will be relieved of any undo stress from their detoxification duties.

*If you have been diagnosed with kidney stones or think you may have them, turn to page 86 for a kidney stone removal cleanse.*

## Bladder-kidney cleanse nutrition plan

*Start with this 3 to 5 day nutrition plan. Water is the key to this cleanse. Drink 8 to 10 glasses of pure water each day.*

## The night before your bladder cleanse...

Take a cup of bladder cleansing herb tea, (see next column). Add ¼ tsp. non-acidic C crystals.

## The next 3 – 5 days...

**On rising:** take 1 lemon squeezed in a glass of water, with 1 tsp. acidophilus liquid; or 3 tsp. cranberry concentrate in a small glass of water, add ¼ tsp. non-acidic vit. C crystals. (Cranberry juice reduces ionized calcium in the urine by over 50% to create an unfavorable environment for urinary tract infections.)

**Breakfast:** have a glass of watermelon juice or cranberry juice with ¼ tsp. non-acidic vit. C crystals or a glass of organic apple juice with ¼ tsp. acidophilus powder.

**Mid-morning:** take 1 cup watermelon seed tea (grind seeds, steep in hot water 30 minutes, add honey); or a potassium broth (page 101) with 2 tsp. Bragg's Liquid Aminos; or a cleansing tea like Crystal Star Bladder Comfort tea.

**Lunch:** have a carrot/beet/cucumber juice, or a chlorophyll-rich superfood drink, or a glass of carrot juice.

**Mid-afternoon:** take a cup of healing herb tea, (parsley/oatstraw, plantain, watermelon seed tea or cornsilk tea); or a cleansing tea.

**Dinner:** have a carrot juice, add 1 tsp. spirulina powder; or another cranberry juice, add ¼ tsp. ascorbate vitamin C crystals.

**Before Bed:** take a glass of papaya or apple juice with ¼ tsp. acidophilus powder.

## Herbs & supplements

*Choose 2 to 3 cleansing boosters. Liquid supplements are best with this cleanse.*

**Bladder/kidney cleansers:** Crystal Star Bladder Comfort tea or extract; cornsilk tea; Jean's Greens P.P.T. tea; Nature's Apothecary Detox Formula.

**Anti-biotic/anti-infective/anti-inflammatory:** Crystal Star Anti-Bio caps or extract; marshmallow tea; vitamin C-1,000mg 3x/day; Solaray Cran-Actin or Nature's Plus AquaActin.

**Enzyme support:** Enzyme Essentials Excell-zyme (kidney antioxidant), and Dr. Enzyme, a protease supplement that helps breaks apart stone sediment.

**Bladder/kidney healing tonics:** Crystal Star Tinkle tea; Herbs Etc. Kidney Tonic; Nature's Apothecary Kidney Support; plantain extract (especially for incontinence); dandelion tea; parsley tea. Tahoma Clinic U-Tract (D-Mannose) for chronic UTI, ½ tsp. 2 times daily.

**Electrolyte mineral support:** Nature's Path Trace-Lyte Liquid Minerals; Trimedica Alkamax.

**Probiotic support:** Jarrow Fem-Dophilus (esp. for chronic UTI and candida); American Health Acidophilus liquid.

**Chlorophyll rich superfoods:** Sun Wellness Chlorella drink or tablets; Crystal Star Energy Green drink or capsules; spirulina powder.

**Fiber supplements reduce risk of stones:** All One Whole Fiber Complex; Nature's Secret Ultimate Fiber.

## Bodywork techniques

*Pick bodywork and relaxation techniques to accelerate and round out your cleanse*

**Exercise:** Take a daily brisk walk to keep kidney function flowing.

**Enemas:** Take a spirulina or catnip enema the first, second and the last day of your kidney cleanse to help release toxins. See enema instructions (page 151) in this book.

**Heat therapy:**

- Take hot saunas to release toxins and excess fluids, and to flush acids out through the skin.

- Apply hot compresses to the kidney area. Combine your choice—ginger and oatstraw, or cayenne and ginger, or mullein and lobelia.

**Massage therapy:** Have at least one massage during your cleanse to stimulate circulation.

**Bladder/Kidney Baths:** Add 8 – 10 drops of essential oils to your bath—a combination of two or three oils, like juniper, cedarwood, sandalwood, lemon, chamomile, eucalyptus or geranium. Stir the water to disperse. (Or use about 15 drops essential oil in 4 oz. of jojoba oil and rub on kidney area).

**Note:** Avoid commercial antacids during healing. Some NSAIDS drugs have been implicated in kidney failure cases.

## For your continuing diet

After your cleanse, add sea foods and sea vegetables, whole grains and vegetable proteins. Continue with a morning green drink or Crystal Star Green Tea Cleanser. Kidney healing foods include garlic and onions, papayas, bananas, watermelon, sprouts, leafy greens and cucumbers. Take these frequently for the rest of the month. Avoid heavy starches, red or prepared meats, dairy foods (except yogurt or kefir), salty, fatty and fast foods. They all inhibit kidney filtering.

# blood purifying cleanse

Your blood is your river of life. Your blood supplies oxygen to your body's sixty trillion cells, transports nutrients, hormones and wastes, warms and cools your skin, wards off invading organisms, seals off wounds and much more. It is the chief neutralizer against bacteria and toxic wastes. Toxins ingested in sublethal amounts can eventually add up to disease-causing amounts. For example, slow viruses that lead to nerve diseases like M.S. can enter the cells and remain dormant for years, mutating and feeding on toxic substances. While your body has its own self-purifying complex for maintaining healthy blood, the best way to protect yourself from disease is to keep those cleansing systems in good working order. A modified blood purifying detox may be followed for 1 to 2 months, or longer if the body is still actively cleansing. A blood detox diet may also be returned to when needed, to purify against relapse or additional symptoms.

Cautionary note: for persons suffering from severe blood toxicity: Most immune deficient diseases are the result of blood toxins and can benefit from a blood purifying diet. However, in serious degenerative conditions like AIDS, Lupus, Chronic Fatigue Syndrome or Fibromyalgia, there may be large amounts of toxins and pollutants in the blood. In these cases, an all-liquid fast is not recommended. It is often too harsh for an already weakened system, and in fact may dump more toxins out into the bloodstream than the body can handle. In these severe cases, an initial diet should be as pure as possible in order to be as cleansing as possible—totally vegetarian—free of all meats, dairy foods, fried, preserved and refined foods and saturated fats.

## Is your body showing signs that it needs a blood cleanse?

- A simple blood-color test monitors blood improvement. Make a small, quick, sterilized razor cut on your finger. If the blood is a dark, bluish-purplish color it is not healthy. A bright red color indicates healthy blood.
- unexplained depression, memory loss, unusual insomnia, schizophrenic behavior, seizures, periodic black-outs
- sexual impotence or dysfunction
- black spots on the gums, bad breath/body odor, unusual, severe reactions to foods and odors; a deep, choking, chronic cough
- loss of hand/eye coordination, especially in driving

## Pointers for best results from your blood cleanse

- Food should be organically grown. Avoid canned, frozen, prepackaged foods or foods with colors, preservatives and flavor enhancers.
- Avoid sodas, artificial drinks, concentrated sugars, fried foods and sweeteners.
- Mild herb teas and bottled mineral water (6 to 8 glasses) are recommended throughout each day, to hydrate, and alkalize.
- For optimum results, add ½ tsp. ascorbate vitamin C crystals with bioflavonoids to any drink.

## Blood purifying cleanse nutrition plan

*Start with this 4 to 7 day nutrition plan. Begin with a 3 day juice/liquid diet; follow with 1 to 4 days of 100% fresh solid and liquid foods.*

## The night before your blood cleanse…

Take your choice of gentle herbal laxatives or Gaia Herbs Supreme Cleanse.

## The next day…

**On rising:** Take 2 to 3 tbsp. cranberry concentrate in 8 oz. water with ½ tsp. ascorbate vitamin C crystals, or use a green tea blood cleansing formula, such as Crystal Star Green Tea Cleanser; or cut up a half lemon with skin and blend in the blender w/ 1 tsp. honey, and 1 cup distilled water; and ½ tsp. Nutricology Symbiotics in 8 oz. aloe vera juice.

**Breakfast:** have a glass of fresh carrot juice, with 1 tbsp. Bragg's Liquid Aminos added; or an 8 oz. aloe vera juice with ½ tsp. Nutricology Symbiotics.

**Mid-morning:** take a potassium broth (page 101) and ½ tsp. ascorbate vitamin C crystals; and another fresh carrot juice, or pau d'arco tea.

**Lunch:** have a glass of fresh Personal Best V-8 juice (page 106) or a carrot or apple juice. Mix in 1 tbsp. of a green superfood such as Crystal Star Systems Strength or Barleans Greens.

**Mid-afternoon:** have a vegetable juice such as Blood Regenerator Juice: handful spinach, 4 romaine leaves, 4 sprigs parsley, 6 carrots, ¼ turnip.

**Dinner:** have a cup of miso soup with 2 tbsp. dried sea vegetables (dulse, nori, wakame, kombu or sea palm) snipped over the top.

**Before Bed:** take a 8 oz. glass of aloe vera juice with ½ tsp. ascorbate vitamin C with bioflavs and ½ tsp. Natren Trinity lactobacillus powder.

## Herbs & supplements

*Choose 2 to 3 cleansing boosters.*

**Herbal blood cleansers:** Crystal Star Blood Detox caps; Herbal Magic Col-Liv Herbal Base; Planetary Formulas Complete Pau D'arco Program.

**Blood cleansing herbs:** red clover, dandelion, burdock, yellow dock, echinacea, Oregon grape root, sarsaparilla, astragalus, pau d' arco, goldenseal root, garlic and cayenne, or Nature's Answer Blood Support.

**Enzyme support:** Crystal Star Dr. Enzyme, removes undigested proteins in the bloodstream that can lead to autoimmune reactions. A potent blood purifier: Rainbow Light Advanced Enzyme System.

**Electrolytes establish healthy blood and strengthen the immune system:** Arise & Shine Alkalizer; Nature's Path Trace-Lyte Liquid Minerals.

**Probiotics provide nutrients for building blood:** UAS DDS-Plus; American Health Acidophilus liquid; Jarrow Jarro-Dophilus.

**Chlorophyll enhances blood cleansing:** Sun Chlorella by Sun Wellness; Pure Planet Chlorella.

**Antioxidants strengthen white blood and T cells:** Solgar Advanced Antioxidant Formula; Jarrow Formulas Coenzyme Q10; Enzymatic Therapy Grape Seed Phytosome 100.

**Antioxidant blood cleansers:** germanium, 100 to 150mg; Vitamin E 1000IU with selenium 200mcg; CoQ10 180mg daily; Vit. C-1,000mg w/ bioflavs. 3x daily; Quercetin and bromelain 500mg 3x daily, for auto-immune reactions; Lane Labs shark cartilage to stimulate interferon, interleukin, lymphocytes.

## Bodywork techniques

Pick bodywork and relaxation techniques to accelerate and round out your cleanse.

**Enema:** Take an enema the first, second and the last day of your blood cleansing program to help release toxins out of the body.

**Irrigate:** Take a colonic irrigation or Nature's Secret Supercleanse once a week to remove infected feces.

**Exercise:** Exercise daily in the morning, if possible. Aerobic oxygen intake alone can be an important nutrient.

**Massage therapy:** Have a massage to stimulate blood circulation.

**Essential oil support:** To assist your blood cleanse use rosemary, cypress & vetiver. You can use one or a combination of all three oils. Put a total of 15 drops essential oil in 1 oz. of a carrier oil (such as jojoba) and rub on the skin.

## Stress & relaxation techniques

**Bathe/Sauna:** Take several saunas or long hot baths if possible during a blood cleanse for faster, easier detoxification. Add a total of 8 – 10 drops of essential oil to your bath. Stir the water briskly to disperse evenly. Use a combination of two or three of the following essential oils: rosemary, cypress & vetiver.

## For your continuing diet

Vegetable and fruit juices stimulate rapid, heavy waste elimination, a process that can generate mild symptoms of a "healing crisis." A slight headache, nausea, bad breath, body odor and dark urine occur as the body accelerates release of accumulated toxins. If you are detoxifying from alcohol or drug overload, 5000 to 10,000mg. of ascorbate Vitamin C is recommended daily during serious cleansing, to help keep the body alkaline and encourage oxygen uptake.

# colon cleanse

A colon elimination cleanse is a cleanse most of us need. As the solid waste management organ for the entire body, mucous and trapped waste can easily adhere to colon walls. The colon is also the easiest breeding ground for putrefactive bacteria, viruses and parasites. (A nationwide survey reveals that one in every six people has parasites living somewhere in the body.)

The latest estimates show that over 90% of disease in America is related in some way to an unhealthy colon. Headaches, skin blemishes, senility, bad breath, fatigue, arthritis and heart disease can be linked to a congested colon. Colon and bowel problems are a big factor in early aging, too. When waste backs up, it becomes toxic, then releases the toxins into the bloodstream. Other elimination organs become overburdened in their detoxification duties, and it's easy to see why health problems begin. Cleansing your colon lightens the toxic load on every other part of your body... even your mind (mental dullness is a sign of colon congestion). In fact, hardly any healing program will work without a colon cleanse as part of it. Real healing takes place at the deepest levels of your body, your cells. All cells are fed by your blood. The nutrients that reach your blood get there by the way of the colon. So a clogged, dirty colon means toxins in your blood.

## Is your colon toxic?

Here are some questions to ask yourself:

**Is your elimination time slow?** Bowel transit time should be approximately twelve hours. Slow bowel transit time allows wastes to become rancid. Blood capillaries lining the colon absorb these poisons into the bloodstream, exposing the rest of your body to the toxins.

**Do you eat too much fast food?** Highly processed, chemical laced food? Synthetic foods? A clean, strong system can metabolize or eliminate many pollutants, but if you are constipated, they are stored as unusable substances. As more and different chemicals enter your body they tend to interact with those that are already there, forming second generation chemicals more harmful than the originals. Colon cancer, now the second leading cancer in the United States (only slightly behind lung cancer in men and breast cancer in women), may be related to accumulated toxic waste. Colitis, irritable bowel syndrome, diverticulosis, ileitis and Crohn's disease, are all signs of poor waste management. They're on the rise, too. Over 100,000 Americans have a colostomy every year! An incredible fact.

**Is your digestion poor?** The most common signal of toxic bowel overload is poor digestion. If you're eating a lot of rich, red meats and cheeses, white bread, sugary, salty foods, or fried foods, they're robbing your body of critical electrolytes and they have almost no fiber for digestion. A high fiber, whole foods diet is both cure and prevention for waste elimination problems. Eating high fiber means you're moving food through the digestive system quickly and easily. A low residue diet causes a gluey state—your intestinal contractions can't work efficiently. You can picture this if you remember the hard paste formed by white flour and water when you were a kid. A lot of the food we eat today is simply crammed into the colon and never fully excreted.

**So much media attention has been focused on high fiber foods, you might think everybody in America has changed their diet for better colon health.** This is simply not the case. Americans target their diets to reduce fats at all costs, often at the expense of a fiber-rich diet. Even a gentle, gradual change from low fiber, low residue foods helps almost immediately. In fact, a gradual change is better than a sudden, drastic about-face change, especially when the colon is inflamed.

## Check your fiber

The protective level of fiber in your diet is easily measured:

- The stool should be light enough to float.
- Bowel movements should be regular, daily and effortless.
- The stool should be almost odorless, signalling decreased bowel transit time.
- There should be no gas or flatulence.

## Is your body showing signs that it needs a colon cleanse?

- Are you constipated most of the time? (a colon cleanse softens, removes clogging colon congestion)
- Do you feel heavy and logy? (a colon cleanse helps you lose colon congestive weight)
- Do you have gas, audible bowel rumbling, bloating or flatulence after you eat? (a colon cleanse helps you remove gluey materials impairing your digestion)
- Do you catch a cold, or flu every few weeks? (a colon cleanse releases excess mucous that harbors hanging-on cold and flu viruses)
- Are you tired most of the time for no real reason? (a colon cleanse boosts immune and liver response to give you more energy)
- Do you have a white-coated tongue, bad breath or body odor frequently? (a colon cleanse removes rancidity that causes smells)
- Do you feel mentally slow and tired? (a colon cleanse lets more blood circulation get to your brain)
- Is your skin unusually sallow and dull? (a colon cleanse removes toxins that come out through your skin)
- Do you have a degenerative disease like cancer, arthritis, M.S. or lupus? (a colon cleanse can remove disease-causing toxic elements.)
- Are your cholesterol numbers too high? (a colon cleanse increases absorption of cholesterol-lowering foods) You can easily combine a colon cleanse with a cholesterol cleanse.

## Pointers for best results from your colon cleanse:

- A colonic irrigation is a good way to start a colon/bowel cleanse. (See how to take a colonic, page 153) Grapefruit seed extract (15 to 20 drops in a gallon of water) is effective, especially if there is colon toxicity along with constipation. Or take a catnip or diluted liquid chlorophyll enema every other night during the cleanse. Note: Enemas may be given to children. Use smaller amounts according to size and age. Allow water to enter very slowly; let them expel when they wish.
- Drink six to eight glasses of water daily during your colon cleanse.
- Take a brisk walk for an hour every day to help keep your colon elimination channels moving.
- Take several long warm baths during your cleanse. A lower back and pelvis massage and dry skin brushing will help release toxins coming out through your skin.

**Note 1:** Drugstore laxatives aren't really body cleansers. They offer only temporary relief, are usually habit-forming and destructive to intestinal membranes and don't even get to the cause of the problem. The laxative so irritates the colon that the bowels expel whatever loose material is around.

**Note 2:** Bowel elimination problems are often chronic, and may require several rounds of cleansing. You can space out more than one colon cleanse by alternating it with periods of eating a healthful diet.

## Colon cleanse nutrition plan

*Start with this 3 to 5 day nutrition plan.*

## The 4 keys:

1. High chlorophyll plants for enzymes.
2. Fruits and vegetables for fiber.
3. Cultured foods for probiotics.
4. Eight glasses of water a day.

## The night before your colon cleanse…

- Take your choice of gentle herbal laxatives.
- Soak dried figs, prunes and raisins in water to cover; add 1 tbsp. molasses, cover, leave over night.

## The next 3 – 5 days…

**On rising:** take a cleansing and flushing booster product, or 1 heaping teaspoon of a fiber drink like All One Totally Fiber in juice or water. Add 1000mg of vitamin C with bioflavonoids 3x a day to raise body glutathione levels, an important detox compound.

**Breakfast:** discard dried fruits from soaking water and take a small glass of the liquid.

**Mid-morning:** take 2 tbsp. aloe juice concentrate in a glass of juice or water.

**Lunch:** take a small glass of potassium broth (page 101); or a glass of fresh carrot juice.

**Mid-afternoon:** take a large glass of fresh apple juice; or an herbal colon cleansing tea.

**About 5pm:** take another small glass of potassium broth, another fresh carrot juice, or a vegetable drink (page 106).

**Supper:** take a glass of apple or papaya juice. (**Note:** Finish your cleanse with a small raw foods salad on the last night.)

**Before Bed:** repeat the herbal cleansers that you took on rising, and take a cup of mint tea.

## Herbs & supplements

*Choose 2 to 3 cleansing boosters .*

**Gentle herbal laxatives:** Zand Cleansing Laxative tabs; Crystal Star Herbal Laxa Caps, M. D. Labs Daily Detox Tea.

**Note:** If you have a sensitive colon or irritable bowel disease (IBS), heal your colon before you cleanse. Avoid products with senna or psyllium. Use a gentle herbal cleansing formula, with peppermint oil, like Crystal Star

BWL-Tone I.B.S. to lessen inflammation and irritation of bowel mucosa which make the bowel more permeable to toxins.

**Cleansing and flushing boosters:** Nature's Secret Supercleanse tabs; Planetary Triphala; una da gato extract drops in water.

**Chlorophyll sources:** Pure Planet Chlorella; Futurebiotics Colon Green; Crystal Star Energy Green drink; Green Foods Green Magma if you have IBS.

**Enzymes:** Crystal Star Dr. Enzyme with Protease & Bromelain; Transformation Digestzyme.

**Electrolyte boosters speed up the cleanse:** Trace Mineral Research Concentrace; Nature's Path Trace-Lyte Liquid Minerals; Arise & Shine Alkalizer.

**Probiotics replenish healthy bacteria:** UAS DDS-Plus with FOS; Jarrow Jarro-Dophilus EPS; Arise & Shine Flora Grow.

**Antioxidants defeat pollutants:** Pure Essence Antioxidant caps; NutriCology Antiox Formula ll.

**Fiber support:** All One Fiber Complex; Jarrow Gentle Fibers drink; AloeLife FiberMate.

## Bodywork techniques

*Pick bodywork and relaxation techniques to accelerate and round out your cleanse.*

**Irrigate:** Take a colonic irrigation 2 to 3 times during your cleanse.

**Exercise:** take a brisk walk for an hour every day to help keep your elimination channels moving.

**Bathe:** take several long warm baths during your cleanse. Dry brush your lower back, abdomen, hips and thighs to help release colon toxins coming out through the skin. Lemon Detox Bath: add into warm bath—5 drops lemon and 2 drops geranium essential oil.

**Massage therapy:** get one good lower back and pelvis massage during your cleanse

**Reduce stress:** Deva Flower Remedies Assistance Remedy.

**Visualize your detox:** Close your eyes and inhale and exhale long and slowly. As you exhale, visualizes toxins dislodging and leaving your colon. As you inhale, visualize pure, nourishing nutrients rebuilding your vibrancy.

## For your continuing diet

After the initial cleanse above, the second part of a colon health system is rebuilding healthy tissue and body energy. This stage takes 1 to 2 months for best results. It emphasizes high fiber from fresh vegetables and fruits, cultured foods to replenish healthy intestinal flora, green foods for enzyme production, and alkalizing foods to prevent irritation while healing. Avoid refined foods, saturated fats, fried foods, red meats, caffeine and pasteurized dairy foods.

# gland cleanse

Your glands work at your body's deepest levels. They are involved with every body function and biochemical reaction, so they're a key to good health, especially as you age. The comment "you are as young as your glands" has merit. There are two types of glands in the body: Exocrine glands, like salivary and mammary glands, regulated by the hypothalamus, secreting fluids through ducts. Endocrine glands, like the pituitary, pineal or ovaries that emit their secretions (primarily hormones) directly into the bloodstream and lymph system.

In their turn, hormones are chemical messengers with wide-ranging effects on both glands and organs. Hormones affect our moods, energy levels, mental alertness, even metabolism. The glands and their secretions like adrenaline, insulin, and thyroid hormones, are extraordinarily affected by nutritional deficiencies, environmental pollutants, chemicalized foods and synthetic hormones. In fact, glands and hormones are affected first by harmful toxins and poor nutrition. A mineral deficiency, for instance, something most Americans have today, undermines the health of almost every gland and organ. The chronic stress loads most Americans live under have a direct effect on hormone levels. We can see this easily in low levels of steroidal hormones produced by our "stressed-out" adrenals.

## Is your body showing signs that it needs a gland cleanse?

Look for unexplained weight gain and sluggish metabolism (impaired thyroid activity), and blood sugar problems (unbalanced insulin levels). Poor digestion may mean low enzyme output from a congested pancreas; chronic fatigue may indicate adrenal exhaustion.

## Body improvement signs you can look for to see if your cleanse is working

- Your energy level should noticeably rise indicating less stressed and inflamed adrenal glands.
- Your mood should improve and be more stable, indicating better blood sugar balance from the pancreas.
- Bloating, unexplained weight gain and metabolism should improve, indicating a more active thyroid.
- Your sleep and rest should improve, indicating pineal balance and adrenal health.
- Your digestion should improve, indicating more pancreas, gallbladder and liver vitality.
- You should have noticeably less colds and flu. Glands are always affected by chronic respiratory infections.

## Pointers for best results from your gland cleanse

- The glands are affected first by dehydration. Drink 8 glasses of water a day.
- Trace minerals and protein are important for gland function. Add green superfoods to your diet.
- Long periods of stress deplete your whole gland system. Herbal adaptogens noticeably improve the way your body handles stress. Add herbs from the ginseng family: panax and Siberian ginsengs, suma, gotu kola, dong quai and ashwagandha to your healing program.

## Gland cleanse nutrition plan

*Start with this 4 to 7 day nutrition plan. Begin with a 3 day juice-liquid diet and follow with 1 to 4 days of a diet of all fresh foods.*

## The night before your gland cleanse…

Take your choice of gentle herbal laxatives, like Crystal Star Herbal Laxa caps; or M. D. Labs Daily Detox Tea. (See Product Resources, page 218)

## The next day…

If possible, depending on the season, for the first day of your juice cleanse, go on a watermelon juice only cleanse. Drink throughout the day to rapidly flush and alkalize. If watermelon is not available, start with the following:

**On rising:** take lemon juice in water with 1 tsp. honey. Add 2 tsp. nutritional yeast flakes.

**Breakfast:** have a carrot juice with 1 tbsp. green superfood, like Aloe Life Daily Greens or Pure Planet Chlorella.

**Mid-morning:** take a carrot or mixed vegetable drink. Add 1 tsp. sea veggie flakes (dulse or kelp).

**Lunch:** have a bowl of miso soup. Sprinkle with dulse flakes and 1 tsp. nutritional yeast.

**Mid-afternoon:** have a mixed vegetable juice like Personal Best V-8 (page 106), a high vitamin/mineral drink for body balance.

**Dinner:** have a Mineral Rich Broth: Simmer 30 minutes: 3 carrots, 1 cup parsley, 1 onion, 2 potatoes, & 2 stalks celery. Strain and add 1 tbsp. Bragg's Liquid Aminos.

**Before Bed:** have an apple or pineapple/ papaya juice. If desired, blend in 1 fresh fig.

## Herbs & supplements

*Choose 2 to 3 cleansing boosters.*

**Deep gland cleanser:** Gaia Herbs Supreme Cleanse.

**Herbal gland support:** Use herbal compounds that contain phytohormone-rich herbs, like ginseng, licorice root, sarsaparilla, dong quai, and black cohosh. Bioflavonoid-rich complexes like Jarrow Gentle Fibers drink have gland balancing properties. For gland homeostasis, Crystal Star Great Ginseng! or Adrenal Energy, or Planetary Formulas Schizandra Adrenal Support; mineral compounds for the glands, Crystal Star Ocean Minerals; Crystal Star Toxin Detox caps, or sea vegetables 2 tbsp. daily if you are regularly exposed to toxic pollutants.

**Essential Fatty Acids:** Barlean's Total Omega, Health from the Sun Total EFA; Crystal Star Evening Primrose Pearls.

**Enzyme support:** Crystal Star Dr. Enzyme rejuvenates glands and immune response; or Transformation PureZyme.

**Electrolytes expedite the cleanse:** Nature's Path Trace-Lyte Liquid Minerals; Arise & Shine Alkalizer.

**Probiotics assist detoxification & protection from toxins:** UAS DDS-Plus; American Health Acidophilus liquid; Jarrow Fem-Dophilus (if you also have yeast infections).

**Chlorophyll rich superfoods for glands:** Aloe Life Daily Greens; Wakunaga KyoGreens; Futurebiotics Vital K Liquid.

## Bodywork techniques

*Pick bodywork and relaxation techniques to accelerate and round out your cleanse.*

**Enema:** Take an enema the first, second and the last day of your gland cleansing program to help release toxins out of the body. Or have a colonic irrigation to deep cleanse the glands.

**Exercise:** Take a regular 20 minute "gland health" walk every day.

**Environmental concerns:** Avoid air and environmental pollutants as much as possible. Your glands are the first to feel their damaging effects.

**Acupressure points:** Stroke the top of the foot on both feet for 5 minutes each to stimulate endocrine and hormone secretions.

**Massage therapy:** Have a massage therapy treatment to stimulate circulation and re-establish clear meridian pathways in the body.

**Essential oil support:** To assist your gland cleanse use bergamot, chamomile, eucalyptus and lavender. You can use one or more of the oils in a combination. Put a total of 15 drops essential oil in 1 oz. of a carrier oil (such as jojoba) and rub on the skin.

**Bathe/Sauna:** Try a relaxing mineral bath. Add 1 cup Dead Sea salts, 1 cup Epsom salts, ½ cup regular sea salt and ¼ baking soda to a tub; swish in 3 drops lavender oil, 2 drops chamomile oil, 2 drops marjoram oil and 1 drop ylang-ylang oil.

## For your continuing diet

**Good gland foods:** sea foods and sea veggies, fresh figs and raisins, pumpkin and sesame seeds, green leafy veggies, broccoli, avocados, yams and dark fruits. Trace minerals, essential fatty acids and protein are important for glandular function. Herbal digestive tonics (especially with ginger), mineralizers (especially from dark leafy greens like spinach) and herbal adaptogens (like ginseng) are helpful when you feel your glandular system is weak.

# liver cleanse

Your liver is your most important organ of detoxification. Your life depends on your liver. To a large extent, the health of your liver determines the health of your entire body. The liver is really a wonderful chemical plant that converts everything we eat, breathe and absorb through the skin into life-sustaining substances. The liver is a major blood reservoir, forming and storing red blood cells, and filtering toxins at a rate of a quart of blood per minute. It also manufactures natural antihistamines to keep immune response high. Without the liver, digestion would be impossible and the conversion of food into living cells and energy nonexistent. It is the primary metabolic organ for proteins, fats and carbohydrates. It synthesizes and secretes bile, a substance that not only insures good food assimilation but is critical to the excretion of toxic material from the gastrointestinal tract. Blood flows directly from the gastrointestinal tract to the liver, so it can neutralize or alter toxic substances from our food before they are distributed to the rest of the body. Blood also keeps returning to the liver, processing toxins again and again through the lymph system until they are excreted by the bile or kidneys.

Liver congestion and exhaustion interfere with all of these vital functions. Unfortunately, since the common American diet is high in calories, fats, sugars and alcohol, with unknown amounts of toxins from preservatives, pesticides and nitrates, almost everybody has liver malfunction to some extent. Still, a healthy liver can deal with a wide range of toxic chemicals, drugs, solvents, pesticides and food additives. Your liver also has amazing rejuvenative powers, continuing to function when as many as 80% of its cells are damaged. Even more remarkable, the liver can regenerate its own damaged tissue.

Even in life-threatening situations, like cirrhosis, hepatitis, acute gallstone attacks, mononucleosis or pernicious anemia, the liver can be rejuvenated, and major surgery or even death averted. Health problems occur after many years of abuse, when the liver is so exhausted it loses the ability to detoxify itself. We can help the liver take a "deep cleansing breath"… something I've found you can almost feel as its miraculous powers of recovery begin to flow. A liver detox is often the first vital step for the body to begin to heal itself.

## Look at all the health problems you can improve or prevent with a liver cleanse

Liver health normalizes other gland and organ functions, especially adrenal, pituitary, kidney, gall bladder, and spleen problems. In fact, gland function and digestion often improve right away. You will notice this in terms of fewer instances of swollen glands during cold and flu season, and less lower back fatigue (adrenal swelling). Weight and cellulite control difficulties may be solved, especially if you notice unusual stomach distension, a clear sign of a swollen liver. Both gallstone and kidney stone accretions lessen. Drug and alcohol cravings reduce. Most women notice that PMS and other menstrual difficulties like endometriosis are far less

severe. Seemingly unrelated problems like breast and uterine fibroids or infertility, even osteoporosis may be corrected. Male impotence is normally improved. Inflammatory conditions like shingles flare-ups, neuritis pain, herpes outbreaks are helped. Brown skin spots and spots before the eyes (signs that the liver is congested and eliminating poisons by other body avenues) begin to fade.

## Is your body showing signs that it needs a liver cleanse?

As the world becomes more prosperous, more people are suffering from liver disorders, mostly due to too many rich foods and alcoholic beverages, but also environmental, air and water pollutants. We lose energy and our sense of well-being when the liver is congested.

**Body signals that your liver needs some TLC include:**

- Unexplained fatigue, listlessness, depression or lethargy, lack of energy; numerous allergy reactions
- Unexplained weight gain and the appearance of cellulite even if you are thin
- A distended stomach even if the rest of the body is thin
- Mental confusion, spaciness
- Sluggish elimination, general constipation alternating to diarrhea
- Food and chemical sensitivities, usually accompanied by poor digestion, and sometimes unexplained nausea
- PMS, headaches and other menstrual difficulties; bags under the eyes
- A yellowish tint to the skin and/or liver spots on the skin; poor hair texture and slow hair growth; skin itching and irritation.
- Anemia and large bruise patches indicate severe liver exhaustion.

## Pointers for best results from your liver cleanse

- Relieve your liver of toxic build-up and strain by eliminating red meats, partially hydrogenated fats and oils (except for essential fatty acids), refined sugars, food preservatives and food dyes.
- Drink 8 glasses of bottled water each day of your cleanse to encourage maximum flushing of liver tissues.

- Liver regeneration needs optimum nutrition for three to four months. Have a dark green leafy vegetable salad every day.

- Get adequate rest and sleep during a liver cleanse. The liver does some of its most important work while you sleep!

I recommend a short liver detox twice a year in the spring and fall, using the extra vitamin D from the sun to help. Your liver is probably the most stressed in the spring and early summer (one of the reasons that people with skin problems get more flare-ups in the spring). A movement of energy in the spring as plant sap rises and nature springs to life is mirrored in the human body with ascending, outgoing energy that can quite readily get rid of waste products accumulated during the fall and winter.

## Improvement signs show that your body is responding to the cleanse

- Many skin conditions can be traced back to digestive and liver problems, so skin conditions will show signs of clearing. If there are no skin problems, the skin will become more radiant.

- Stiff and aching muscles will receive relief as the liver is replenished.

- Warmth may come to cold hands and feet.

## Liver cleanse nutrition plan

*Start with this 3 to 5 day nutrition plan. Follow with a diet of 100% fresh foods for the rest of the week. Add ¼ tsp. vitamin C crystals to each drink you take. It's a natural chelator of heavy metal toxins that deteriorate liver function.*

**Don't forget: 8 glasses of water through the day.**

## The night before your liver cleanse…

Take a cup of miso soup with sea veggies.

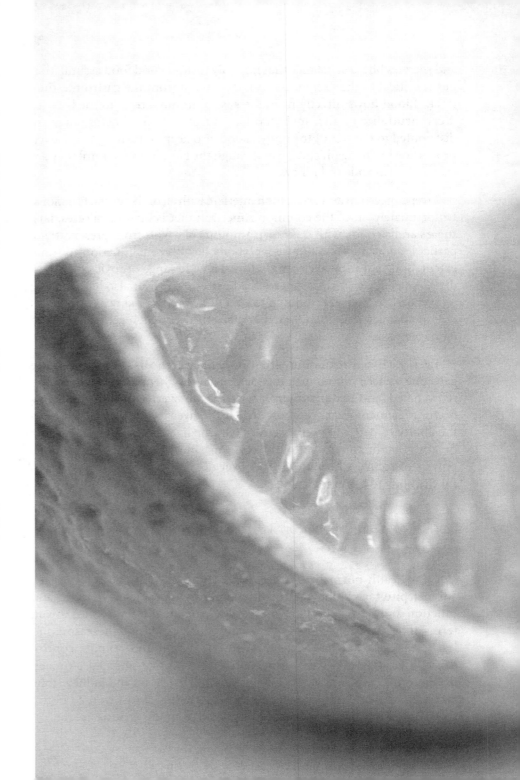

## The next day…

**On rising:** take 1 lemon squeezed in a glass of water; or 2 tbsp. lemon juice in water; or 2 tbsp. cider vinegar in water with 1 tsp. honey.

**Breakfast:** take a glass of potassium broth, (page 101) or carrot/beet/cucumber juice, or organic apple juice or Crystal Star Systems Strength drink. Add 1 tsp. spirulina to any drink for protein and chlorophyll support.

**Mid-morning:** take a green veggie drink (See the Green Cuisine for juicing recipes); or take a green superfood powder mixed into water or vegetable juice (Some superfood choices: Green Foods Green Magma, Crystal Star Energy Green or Barleans Greens).

**Lunch:** have a glass of fresh carrot juice or a glass of organic apple juice.

**Mid-afternoon:** have a cup of peppermint tea, pau d' arco tea, or Crystal Star Liver Cleanse Flushing Tea; or another green drink.

**Dinner:** have another carrot juice or a mixed vegetable juice; or have a hot vegetable broth (See the Green Cuisine for recipes).

**Before Bed:** take another glass of lemon juice or cider vinegar in water. Add 1 tsp. honey or royal jelly; or a pineapple/papaya juice with 1 tsp. royal jelly.

## Herbs & supplements

*Choose 2 to 3 cleansing boosters.*

**Bitters herbs stimulate the liver and bile flow:** Crystal Star Bitters & Lemon extract; Floradix Herbal Bitters; Solaray turmeric caps; roasted dandelion root and leaf tea.

**Liver cleansers:** Crystal Star Liver Renew caps, or Green Tea Cleanser tea; Nature's Apothecary Liver Cleanse; Gaia Herbs Supreme Cleanse; Planetary Bupleurum Liver Cleanse.

**Liver tonics and vitality support:** Milk thistle seed extract (accelerates liver regeneration by a factor of four); Nature's Way Super Thisilyn; Enzymatic Therapy Super Milk Thistle Complex with Artichoke; Herbs Etc. Liver Tonic.

**A liver tonic tea:** 4 oz. hawthorn berries, 2 oz. red sage (salvia miltiorrhiza: use burdock root if salvia is not available), and 1 oz. cardamom seeds. Steep 24 hours in 2 qts. water. Add honey. Take 2 cups daily.

**Enzyme support:** Enzyme Essentials Digestzyme; Herbal Products and Development Power Plus Enzymes.

**Lipotropics prevent fatty accumulation:** Phos. Choline or choline 600mg, or Solaray Lipotropic Plus; sea vegetables (any kind) every day; dandelion tea; gotu kola or fennel seed tea.

**Chlorophyll rich superfoods:** Green Foods Green Essence or Sun Wellness Chlorella.

**Antioxidants for the liver:** Alpha-Lipoic Acid by MRI. (Lipoic acid is one of the most powerful liver detoxifiers ever discovered) 300 – 600mg daily; Carnitine 1000mg; Solaray Centella Asiatica or Solaray Alfa-Juice caps; Enzyme Essentials Excellzyme; vitamin E 400IU with selenium 100mcg.

## Bodywork techniques

*Pick bodywork and relaxation techniques to accelerate and round out your cleanse.*

**Enema:** Take a coffee enema (1 cup coffee to 1 qt. water) the first and last day of your liver cleansing program to help release toxins out of the body. See enemas in this book for instructions. Or, apply castor oil packs to the liver area three times a week to aid liver detoxification.

**Exercise:** Take a brisk, daily walk on each day of your cleanse. Breathe deep to help the liver eliminate toxins. The liver is dependent on the amount and quality of oxygen coming into the lungs. Exercise, an air filter, or time spent walking in the forest and at the ocean can be of great benefit.

**Massage therapy:** Have a massage to stimulate circulation.

**Heat therapy:** a sauna every day possible to induce sweating and faster elimination.

**Early morning sunlight** will boost your cleanse with natural vitamin D.

## Stress & relaxation techniques

**Flower remedies:** Deva Flowers Crab Apple.

**Essential oil support:** To assist your liver cleanse use the essential oils of fennel, lemon & rosemary. You can use one or a combination of all three oils. Put a total of 15 drops essential oil in 1 oz. of a carrier oil (such as jojoba) and rub on the skin.

**Bathe:** Take several long hot baths if possible during a liver cleanse for faster, easier detoxification. Add to your bath 5 drops fennel, 5 drops lemon and 5 drops of rosemary essential oils.

## For your continuing diet

Keep fat low in your nutrition plan. It's crucial to liver regeneration and vitality. Beets, artichokes, radishes and dandelions are good liver foods because they promote the flow of bile, the major pathway for chemical release from the liver. A permanent diet for liver health should be lacto-vegetarian, low in fats, rich in vegetable proteins, with plenty of vitamin C foods for good iron absorption. A complete liver renewal program can take from 3 to 6 months.

# lung and respiratory cleanse

In any two week period during high risk seasons, almost one-third of the U.S. suffers from a cold. Air, water and environmental pollutants may have finally reached an overload point on the general population. Cold symptoms are usually your body's attempt to cleanse itself of wastes and toxins that have built up to the point where natural immunity cannot handle or overcome them. Your glands are always affected, (since the endocrine system is on a 6 day cycle, a cold usually runs for about a week) as the body works through all of its detoxification processes.

Your lungs are on the front line of toxic intake from viruses, allergies,

pollutants, and mucous-forming congestants. If you are highly sensitive to chemicals and pollutants, you're probably already having a variety of respiratory problems. An occasional lung cleanse is a wise way to help your respiratory system release pollutant-caused infections.

Any program to overcome any chronic respiratory problems is usually more successful when begun with a short mucous elimination plan like a lung cleansing diet. This allows the body to rid itself first of toxic accumulations that cause congestion before an attempt is made to change eating habits that support better health.

## Is your body showing signs that it needs a lung and respiratory cleanse?

- Do you have a chronic phlegm producing cough?
- Do you wheeze with asthma?
- Is your head stuffy with congestive allergies?
- Do you have bronchitis or severe sinusitis?
- Do you have a runny nose in any weather?
- Are you a cigarette smoker?

These are signs that you might need a lung cleanse.

## Pointers for best results from your lung and respiratory cleanse

- Drink plenty of non-dairy fluids, like water, juices, herb teas or broth, to hydrate and flush the body. Milk congests and constipates.
- Stimulate the immune system. Maintaining a healthy immune system is a primary way to support lung/respiratory health.
- Alkalize your body during a lung cleanse. Acid-forming foods tend to aggravate or prolong colds, flus and other respiratory problems. Alkalizing foods like fresh fruits, high chlorophyll vegetables, sea veggies and non-gluten grains like brown rice or millet should be used in a ratio of about 4:1 over acid-forming foods during a lung and pulmonary detox.

- Chlorophyll-rich super green foods like chlorella, spirulina and barley grass speed up lung cleansing, increase oxygen in the body and help treat respiratory tract infection.
- Get plenty of quality sleep, fresh air and sunshine.
- Consciously steer clear of air pollution to the best of your ability. Environmental and heavy metal pollutants, like chlorofluorocarbons, tobacco smoke (even secondary smoke) contribute greatly to respiratory problems and can undo all your hard cleansing work.

## Lung and respiratory cleanse nutrition plan

*Start with this 4 to 7 day nutrition plan.*

Begin with a 3 day juice/liquid diet and follow with 1 to 4 days of a diet of 100% fresh foods.

## The night before your lung cleanse…

Take your choice of gentle herbal laxatives.

## The next day…

**On rising:** take 2 squeezed lemons in water with 1 tbsp. maple syrup.

**Breakfast:** have a water-diluted grapefruit juice with 1 tbsp. of a green superfood, such as Fit for You Miracle Greens or Crystal Star Energy Green or water-diluted pineapple juice as a natural expectorant—add in 1 tbsp. of a green superfood for additional detox support.

**Mid-morning:** take a carrot juice or mixed fresh vegetable juice such as Personal Best V-8 (page 106).

**Lunch:** have a Potassium Juice (page 101). This juice is cleansing, neutralizes acids and rebuilds the body. It provides rapid energy and system balance.

**Mid-afternoon:** have a cup of mucous cleansing tea with mullein, marshmallow, comfrey, pleurisy root, rose hips, calendula, boneset, and ginger; or add Crystal Star D-Congest spray in hot water.

**Dinner:** have a Potassium Essence broth (page 101), for energy and mineral electrolytes. Or try this broth, soothing to gastric mucosa, rich in zinc, vitamin A, C, potassium and magnesium electrolytes: In 2 ½ cups water, cook 1 ½ cups fresh mixed vegetables (carrots, broccoli, dark leafy greens, celery and parsley) with 1 tbsp. miso. Strain and take broth. Blender blend veggies, broth and 4 tbsp. sunflower seeds for a hearty version.

## Herbs & supplements

*Choose 2 to 3 cleansing boosters.*

**Deep Cleansing:** Nature's Secret Ultimate Cleanse.

**Lung cleansers:** Yogi Breathe Deep; or Zand Decongest caps.

**Herbal lung support:** Now Oregano Oil soft gels for lung conditions like cough, asthma, colds, flu, bronchitis and pneumonia; Crystal Star D-Congest spray to aid mucous release; Herbs Etc. Lung Tonic supports lung cleansing.

**Immune support:** Immunity herbs: panax ginseng, echinacea, ashwagandha, astragalus, Siberian eleuthero, goldenseal, licorice, ligustrum, suma, codonopsis, pau d' arco, chaparral, dumontiaceae (red marine algae), garlic and immune-enhancing mushrooms, like reishi & shiitake. Chlorophyll rich superfoods: Pure Planet Chlorella or Spirulina.

**Enzyme support:** Enzyme Essentials Gastrozyme (clears mucous congestion); Crystal Star Dr. Enzyme (strengthens immune system).

**Electrolyte increase oxygen uptake:** Nature's Path Trace-Lyte Liquid Minerals; Trimedica Alkamax; Trace Mineral Research Concentrace.

**Probiotics inhibit growth of harmful organisms:** UAS DDS-Plus; Jarrow Jarro-Dophilus; Nature's Path, Flora-Lyte.

**Anti-infective agents:** NutriCology Prolive With Antioxidants (olive leaf extract); Now Oregano Oil soft gels.

**Antioxidants are linked to improved lung function:** Vit. C 1,000mg 3x day raises body's glutathione levels to protect the lungs; Country Life Carotenoid Complex; Source Naturals Proanthodyn.

## Bodywork techniques

*Pick bodywork and relaxation techniques to accelerate and round out your cleanse.*

**Enema:** Take an enema the first, second and the last day of your lung cleansing program to thoroughly clean out excess mucous.

**Detox foot bath:** Energy Balancing (EB) foot bath technology helps clear toxins and bacteria-laden mucous. See pg. 161 for more.

**Exercise:** If you are cleansing your lungs and not ill with a cold, flu, or other respiratory infection, take a brisk, daily walk on each day of your cleanse. Breathe deep to help the lungs eliminate mucous.

**Compress:** Apply wet ginger/cayenne compresses to chest to increase circulation and loosen mucous.

**Essential oil support:** To assist your lung cleanse use oregano, tea tree, and eucalyptus oils (singly or in combination). Put a total of 15 drops essential oils in 1 oz. of a carrier oil (such as jojoba) and rub on the chest.

**Inhalant:** 6 drops of the essential oils can be added to one quart hot water—inhale the steam:

• Eucalyptus has antiviral action to loosen mucous, and treat asthma, bronchitis and sinusitis.

• Tea Tree has decongestant, antiviral and antibacterial properties.

• Oregano oil has antiviral and antibacterial properties help eradicate lung infection. Also thins mucous and stops excessive mucous secretion.

**Bathe/Sauna:** Take a hot 20 minute bath or sauna at the onset of a cold, flu or beginning of a respiratory cleanse to stimulate your body's defenses and increase toxin elimination.

## For your continuing diet

After your initial juice cleanse, your diet for lung health should be high in vegetable proteins and whole grains, low in sugars and starches. Include cultured foods like raw sauerkraut, yogurt, and kefir for probiotics to assist friendly G.I. flora. Include lung-specific pitted fruits such as apricots, peaches and plums. Include nutritional yeast 2 tsp. daily. Take a green superfood drink at least three mornings a week for a month after your cleanse to "set" the cleanse benefits.

---

# lymph cleanse

The lymphatic system includes lymph vessels and nodes, thymus gland, tonsils and spleen. It's really a network of tubing that drains waste products from tissues, produces disease-fighting white blood cells (lymphocytes) and antibodies, and carries the bulk of the body's waste from the cells to the final elimination organs. Experts call the lymphatic system a secondary circulatory system, because it assists the bloodstream with millions of tiny ducts that collect tissue fluid not needed by the capillaries or skin and returns it to the heart for recirculation, because special filtering lymph nodes remove infective organisms, so your lymph system is also a key to your body's immune defenses.

Liver health is a key to lymphatic health. The liver produces the majority of lymph, and lymph a major route for nutrients from the liver. The integrity of the lymph system is dependent on immune cells in the liver that filter out harmful bacteria and destructive yeasts.

The spleen is the largest mass of lymphatic tissue. It destroys worn-out red blood cells, and serves as a healthy blood reservoir for fresh red blood. During times of high demand, such as hemorrhage, the spleen can release its stored blood and prevent shock from occurring.

## Here's an amazing fact

The valves of the lymph system move the waste-filled fluids to be flushed and filtered. But since there is no pump as there is with the heart, lymph circulation depends solely upon your breathing and muscle movement. Physical exercise and diaphragmatic deep breathing are critical to lymph cleansing and to healthy immune response.

## Is your body showing signs that it needs a lymph cleanse?

If you are under chronic stress; if you are constantly tired (indicating liver exhaustion); if your skin is very pale; if you are extremely thin; if your memory is noticeably failing; if you have low immune response with frequent colds, a revitalizing lymph cleanse can make a difference. If your body looks uncharacteristically soft and pudgy or has newly noticeable cellulite (indicating too many saturated fats and sugary foods), you probably need a lymph-draining cleanse.

## Pointers for best results from your lymph cleanse

- Drink 8 glasses of bottled water each day of your cleanse. Add potassium-rich foods—sea greens, broccoli, bananas and seafood.
- Avoid caffeine, sugar, dairy foods and alcoholic drinks for the duration of your cleanse. They contribute to lymphatic stagnation.
- Spicy foods like natural salsas, cayenne pepper, horseradish and ginger boost a sluggish lymph system and cut mucous congestion.

## Improvement signs show that your body is responding to the cleanse

- Most people notice an energy increase in their daily activity, with far fewer stress reactions as body chemistry normalizes.
- Most people notice they no longer catch every cold that comes their way, and the illnesses they do get don't last as long.
- Most people notice better weight control (especially if they were overweight) and less cellulite formation as congestion lessens.

## Lymph cleanse nutrition plan

*Start with this 4 to 7 day nutrition plan. Begin with a 3 day juice-liquid diet and follow with 1 to 4 days of a diet of 100% fresh foods.*

**Note:** Nutrient deficiency is the most frequent cause of a sluggish lymph system. Immune-boosting vegetables for juicing: cabbage, kale, carrot, bell pepper, collards and garlic. Lymph-enhancing juice fruits: apple, pineapple, blueberry and grape.

**On rising:** take a glass of lemon juice and water regularly in the morning for lymph revitalization.

**Breakfast:** have a fresh mixed vegetable lymph juice builder: handful parsley, 1 garlic clove, 5 carrots, and 3 celery stalks. Add 2 tbsp. of a green superfood like Crystal Star Energy Green drink mix or Green Kamut.

**Mid-morning:** have two cups of Crystal Star Liver Cleanse Flushing tea tea for liver and lymph cleansing, or a lymph tea blend of white sage, astragalus, echinacea root, Oregon grape root and dandelion root.

**Lunch:** have a vitamin A/carotene/vitamin C rich drink: 3 broccoli flowerets, 5 carrots, 1 garlic clove, 2 celery stalks and ½ green pepper. Add 2 tbsp. of a green superfood like Crystal Star Energy Green drink mix or Green Kamut.

**Mid-afternoon:** a glass of apple or grape juice.

**Dinner:** have a Potassium Essence Broth (page 101), for mineral electrolytes. Or try a broth rich in zinc, vitamin A and C, potassium and magnesium electrolytes: In 2 ½ cups water, cook 1 ½ cups fresh veggies (carrots, broccoli, dark leafy greens, celery and parsley) and 1 tsp. miso. Strain and use broth. Hearty version: blend warm broth and vegetables. Add 4 tbsp. sunflower seeds.

**Before Bed:** have a glass of papaya juice.

## Herbs & supplements

*Choose 2 to 3 cleansing boosters.*

**Deep lymph cleanser:** Gaia Herbs Supreme Cleanse; echinacea extract and astragalus extract are highly successful deep lymph cleansing single herbs.

**Lymphatic cleansers:** Crystal Star Anti-Bio caps for white blood cell formation, a lymph purifier with immune-stimulant properties. Herbs Etc. Lymphatonic, with echinacea, (reduces lymphatic swelling and congestion), red root (powerful lymphatic cleanser, synergistic with echinacea), and ocotillo (flushes lymph congestion); Nature's Apothecary Lymph Cleanse; Gaia Herbs Echinacea Red Root Supreme, a lymphatic and liver cleanser.

**Immune Support:** Silica decisively affects the functions of the lymphatic nodes and system, increasing the phagocytes to strengthen the immune response. Eidon Silica Mineral Supplement; Flora Vege-Sil.

**Supporting lymph nutrients:** Vitamins A, C, E, B-complex, carotenes, iron, zinc and selenium.

**Herbal lymph immune support:** Maitake Products Mushroom Emperors or Reishi caps.

**Enzyme support:** Protease is a powerful lymph immune booster. Crystal Star Dr. Enzyme.

**Electrolyte boosters:** Mineral electrolytes play a major role in detoxifying the lymph glands, helping to remove acid crystals. Nature's Path Trace-Lyte Liquid Minerals; Trace Mineral Research Concentrace.

**Deficiencies to watch for:** Protein and B12 deficiency also affect efficiency of the lymphatic system.

## Bodywork techniques

*Pick bodywork and relaxation techniques to accelerate and round out your cleanse.*

**Colonic irrigation:** take a colonic irrigation or a Sonné Bentonite Clay Cleanse once a week to remove lymph congestion and infected feces from the intestinal tract.

**Exercise:** exercise is critical to lymphatic flow. To stimulate lymph flow activate muscles with regular exercise and stretching. Start every exercise period with deep, diaphragmatic breathing. Mini-trampoline exercise clears clogged lymph nodes.

**Massage therapy:** elevate feet and legs for 5 minutes every day, massaging lymph node areas.

**Lymph supporting therapies:** acupuncture and acupressure have both been successful.

**Essential oil support:** to assist your lymph cleanse use geranium, juniper and black pepper. Use one or a combination of all three oils. Put a total of 15 drops essential oil in 1 oz. of a carrier oil (such as jojoba) and rub on the skin.

**Shower:** Take an alternating hot and cold hydrotherapy treatment at the end of your daily shower to stimulate lymph circulation.

## Stress relaxation techniques

The mind and emotions have a great affect on immune response. The following techniques are important.

**Bathe:** A relaxing mineral bath. Add 1 cup Dead Sea salts, 1 cup Epsom salts, ½ cup regular sea salt and ¼ baking soda to a tub; swish in 3 drops lavender oil, 2 drops chamomile oil, 2 drops marjoram oil and 1 drop ylang ylang oil. Or, try a Crystal Star Hot Seaweed Bath (great for cellulite, too).

**Lymph support essential oil bath mixture.** Add a total of 8 – 10 drops of essential oils (see above) to your bath. Stir the water briskly to disperse evenly.

**Eliminate aluminum:** cookware, food additives and alum-containing foods and deodorants.

## For your continuing diet

Poor nutrition profoundly impairs the immune system. Excessive dietary sugars and alcohol over consumption especially inhibit white blood cell activity. Be sure to eliminate or limit their use. Adequate protein intake is critical to immune health and the ability to heal. The best sources for immune response are those with plenty of EFAs: salmon and fresh tuna, sea vegetables, green superfoods like spirulina and barley grass and sprouts.

# skin cleanse

Your skin is the surest mirror of your lifestyle. Almost everything that's going on inside you shows on your skin. Your skin is the essence of renewable nature… it sloughs off old, dying cells every day, and gives the body a clean, new start.

Your skin is your body's largest organ of elimination and detoxification.

The skin is a backup for the other elimination organs. If your colon becomes overloaded and stagnant with toxins, or your liver can't efficiently filter impurities coming from the digestive tract, your skin tries to compensate by releasing toxins from your body. It sweats them out, or throws them off through rashes or abscesses.

Your skin is also your body's largest organ of absorption and ingestion— both for nutrients and toxins. A good diet shows quickly. By the same token, chemicalized foods and nutritional deficiencies from a poor diet show up first on your skin. Toxins eliminated through the oil glands in the skin, for example, show up as acne and boils. Your skin mirrors your emotional state and hormone balance, too. Stress reactions and hormone disruption show up as poor skin texture, or spots and blemishes.

## Is your body showing signs that it needs a skin cleanse?

**Do you have sallow skin?** Poor skin coloring may indicate waste build-up from liver malfunction or drug residues. Do you have age spots? Brown mottled spots on the hands, neck or face may reflect waste accumulation in the liver.

**Do you have adult acne, or uneven skin texture?** Waste build-up from environmental pollutants, poor diet, liver exhaustion and stress allow increased free radical formation which attack skin cell membranes.

**Do you have wrinkles, or sagging skin contours?** Free radical activity also affects skin collagen and elastin proteins, resulting in wrinkling and dry skin.

**Do you have puffy or swollen eyes, dark circles under your eyes, or crusty, mucous formations in your eyes?** If your breath is also bad, it's a pretty solid sign your body has an overload of fluid wastes.

**Do you have a skin disorder?** Psoriasis, dermatitis and seborrhea all indicate its time for a skin cleanse.

**Do you have skin sores or rashes that aren't healing?** or hard bumps on the skin? Your body may be overloaded with wastes that you're not eliminating.

**Do you have unusually oily skin?** or scaly, itchy skin? or chronically chapped and red skin? A skin cleanse will probably help.

**Note:** Poor circulation (cold hands and feet, swollen ankles), poor digestion and chronic constipation are also signs that your body lacks tissue oxygen uptake. Poor skin tone is a sign of antioxidant deficiency.

## Pointers for best results from your skin cleanse

Your diet is the fastest way to change your looks. You can make improvements easily. Skin tissues need a rich, high oxygen blood supply, and plenty of mineral building blocks. Silica, sulphur, calcium and magnesium are specific minerals for your skin. Plants are the most absorbable way for your body to get them.

Soft smooth skin depends on a diet rich in fresh fruits and vegetables. Beautiful skin tone needs vitamin A, vitamin C, mineral-rich foods, and high vegetable protein foods, for collagen and interstitial tissue health. Eliminate or limit sugary foods, fried foods and trans-fats, like those in milk and dairy products, margarine, shortening and hydrogenated oils. Avoid red meats and refined foods of all kinds.

- Include a green superfood drink daily during your skin cleanse. Superfood powders can be mixed into any juice or water.

- Don't forget good bodywork for your skin:

1. The healthiest skin needs some fresh air and sunlight every day. Early morning sunlight on the body for natural vitamin D is a key.

2. Daily mild exercise keeps your skin's circulation free and flowing.

3. Dry brush your skin once a week to increase circulation and slough dead cells.

- Drink 8 glasses of bottled water each day of your cleanse (herbal "skin" teas are fine, too). Water keeps you flushed, so waste and toxins won't be dumped out through the skin as blemishes or rashes. Bottled water is best. Fluoridated water may leach Vitamin E out of your body.

## Benefits you may notice as your body responds to skin cleansing

Most people experience noticeable appearance improvement in about 3 weeks.

- Your face will look rested, rejuvenated and revitalized.

- Your skin's natural glow will return as capillary circulation and lymphatic drainage improve.
- Skin blemishes, blotches and spots diminish or disappear.
- The whites of your eyes will become whiter; dark circles will disappear.
- Your skin texture will appear smoother and softer; fine lines will appear less noticeable.

## Skin cleanse nutrition plan

*Start with this nutrition plan. Begin with a 3-day liquid elimination diet and follow with 1 to 4 days of a diet of fresh foods.*

**On rising:** take a glass of lemon juice and water; add New Chapter Ginger Wonder syrup if desired.

**Breakfast:** make a Complexion Booster: juice 2 slices of pineapple and 2 apples. Add 1 tsp. nutritional yeast and 1 tsp. wheat germ oil. Or try Beautiful Skin caps or tea.

**Mid-morning:** have watermelon juice when available (rich in natural silica), or a skin tonic drink: juice 1 cucumber, 1 handful fresh parsley, 1 4 oz. tub fresh sprouts and sprigs of fresh mint. Or have a superfood green drink, such as Crystal Star Energy Green or Barleans Greens.

**Lunch:** have a fresh carrot juice; or a Skin Nutrient drink: juice 5 carrots, 2 apples and add 15 drops Ginger Extract.

**Mid-afternoon:** have a carrot/beet/cucumber juice (once a week for the next month) to keep the liver clean and support the skin's health.

**Dinner:** have a warm potassium essence broth for mineral electrolytes. Or make this high luster skin broth: In 2 ½ cups water cook 2 cups chopped fresh mixed vegetables, add 1 tsp. miso and 2 tbsp. chopped dried sea vegetables (you can snip some wakame into pieces). Hearty version: Blend luster skin broth above; then add 4 tbsp. sunflower seeds for a protein boost. Vegetable protein aids faster healing for damaged skin.

**Before Bed:** have Crystal Star Beautiful Skin Tea or Japanese green tea for skin support; or a pineapple/papaya, papaya or apple juice; or Red Star yeast broth for high B complex vitamins.

## Herbs & supplements

*Choose 2 to 3 cleansing boosters.*

**Deep skin blood cleansing:** Planetary Yellow Dock Skin Cleanse; Crystal Star Red Skin Relief; sage or burdock root tea. White tea daily: I regard white tea as an outstanding choice for detoxification programs of all kinds. It produces an especially noticeable difference in a skin detox, offering a lovely clear texture to the skin. I use white tea for this effect in my skin formulas.

**Smoothing/hydrating herbs for skin:** Crystal Star Beautiful Skin Caps and tea for blemishes and skin maintenance; Immudyne Rejuvenating Serum with beta glucan. Source Naturals Skin Eternal caps and serum.

**Skin vitamins and minerals:** Diamond Herpanacine superior skin support; Futurebiotics Hair, Skin & Nails—results in just 2 weeks; Crystal Star Ocean Minerals caps.

**Skin herbal support:** Crystal Star Beautiful Skin Caps, for blemishes and skin maintenance; Nature's Apothecary Skin Support, blood purifiers and mineralizers; Herbs Etc. Dermatonic, stimulates waste elimination; burdock root normalizes production of the skin's beneficial oils.

**Antioxidants are important for skin health:** Beta carotene protects against the effects of the sun's free radicals; Vitamin E protects against the lipid peroxidation caused by UV rays; Bioflavonoids improve vascularization of the skin.

**Essential fatty acids:** deficiency reflected by skin dehydration and wrinkling: Crystal Star Evening Primrose Pearls; Spectrum Organic Essential Max Efa Oil.

**Enzyme support:** Protease heals skin disorders; Crystal Star Dr. Enzyme.

**Electrolyte boosters:** Nature's Path Trace-Lyte.

**Silica, a mineral for collagen support,** reduces dry, wrinkled skin. Eidon Silica Mineral Supplement; Flora Vegesil; Crystal Star Iodine Source extract with horsetail (for silica).

**MSM (Methyl Sulfonyl Methante):** MSM enhances tissue pliability and helps repair damaged or scarred skin: Nature's Path Msm-Lyte.

## Bodywork techniques

*Pick bodywork and relaxation techniques to accelerate and round out your cleanse.*

**Enema:** Take an enema the first, second and the last day of your skin cleansing program to help release toxins out of the body and help clear the skin. Or have a colonic for a more thorough cleanse.

**Dry brushing:** Use a natural bristle brush. Start with the soles of your feet, brush vigorously making rotary motions and massage every part of your body, starting at the feet and work up to the neck.

**Massage:** Skin circulation for better tone.

## Healing, beautifying skin application treatments

**Crystal Star Healthy Skin Gel:** a cleansing, restorative phytotherapy gel; or AloeLife Skin Gel.

**Skin Beauty Face tea:** steep chamomile, calendula, rosehips, juice of 1 lemon and 2 tsp. rose water. Strain; apply with cotton balls to the face.

**Herbal Answers Herbal Aloe Force Gel:** boosts circulation and stimulates new cell growth.

**Fruit acid treatment:** Rub face with the insides of papaya and cucumber skins. They alkalize wastes that come out on the skin.

**Essential oil support:** Essential oils assist a skin cleanse: lavender, geranium, sandalwood and neroli. Use one or a combination of all three oils. Put a total of 15 drops essential oil in 2 oz. of a carrier oil (such as jojoba) and rub on the skin.

**Skin Mineral Bath:** Add 1 cup Dead Sea Salts, 1 cup Epsom salts, ½ cup regular sea salt and 4 tbsp. baking soda to a tub: swish in 3 drops lavender, 2 drops geranium, 2 drops sandalwood and 1 drop neroli oil. Or, try a high iodine-potassium Crystal Star Hot Seaweed Bath for soft, silky, glowing skin all over.

**Flower remedies:** Natural Labs Stress/Tension; Nelson Bach Rescue Remedy.

## For your continuing diet

Follow a whole foods diet. Eat mineral-rich foods such as leafy greens, bell peppers, broccoli, sesame and sunflower seeds, fish and sea vegetables. Include 4 to 5 servings of vegetables day—if possible eat half raw—as salads. Eat fruits 1 to 3 times per day. Increase fiber to help keep your colon clean. Besides the fiber of vegetables and fruits include: flax seed meal, whole grains (like oats and rice), and beans (pinto and black beans).

- Use essential fatty acids. People with skin problems may be deficient in these nutrients. Use cold-pressed flaxseed oil as an excellent source of omega-3 fatty acids. Evening primrose oil helps the skin.

- Drink 8 glasses of water a day (can include herbal teas).

- Eliminate sugars, trans-fatty acids, fried foods and junk food.

# addiction detox

## Do you need a cleanse from drug or alcohol dependency?

Americans take $19 billion worth of prescription drugs each year. Ten million Americans are officially classified as addicted to alcohol, at a cost to taxpayers of $276 billion dollars a year. The use of "hard" or "pleasure" drugs in today's society is also prevalent. Still, experts believe the most serious addictions are those to pharmaceutical drugs. More than one million people a year, 3 to 5 percent of admissions, end up in hospitals as a result of reactions to prescription drugs.

Clearly, modern drugs play lifesaving roles in emergency situations and they can help numerous health problems, especially short term, but most people begin taking drugs to alleviate boredom and fatigue, or to relieve physical or psychological pain. A detox program helps release drugs and alcohol from your system, but withdrawing after long time use can produce harsh effects (see following page). I highly recommend the supervision of a qualified health professional for an addictions cleanse, especially if dependency has been long term. Sometimes, the best way is to wean yourself gradually off the addictive substance while you're doing a detox.

The symptoms that drugs or excessive alcohol address are merely the warning signs of deeper problems. Alcohol abuse especially is marked by stress and depression. Drugs and alcohol may aggravate an original health problem by adding to poisons in your body. Drug detoxification is a process of releasing the stored substances while changing lifestyle habits so that you are no longer dependent on them. It is critical to fortify your body enough to give it the power to resist returning to the addictive substance. Only a well-nourished body can offer both your body and mind enough of a sense of well being and strength to melt the relapse urges and desires.

## Is your body showing signs that it needs an addiction cleanse?

- Do you only feel happy and relaxed after having a drink or taking a mood elevating drug?
- Do you find that you can't relieve stress, or escape daily problems without alcohol or drugs?
- Do you have liver problems? Does your stomach protrude but you are thin everywhere else? It could be a sign of liver enlargement and inflammation.
- Do you have esophagus impairment, high blood pressure, or pancreatitis? Are your stools pale?
- Are the whites of your eyes dingy? Is the eye lower lid yellow? Is your skin slightly jaundiced? Do you sweat a lot?
- Have you lost your appetite? Have you gotten noticeably, or unusually thin? Do you have a marked intolerance for fatty foods?
- Is your digestion always bad? Do you have a metallic taste in your mouth? Are you drowsy after meals? In the overwhelming number of cases, habitual drug and alcohol users suffer from chronic subclinical malnutrition, and from multiple depletions of critical nutrients. Vitamins, minerals, amino acids, fatty acids and enzymes are all depleted, some by 50 to 60 percent.
- Are you often foggy mentally? Do you have a lot of food allergies or chemical sensitivities? Do you crave sweets? Is your blood sugar usually low? These signs indicate rampant hypoglycemia from alcohol or drug overload.

- Do you feel shaky and sweaty? Do you often get a "wired," nervous feeling, sometimes with heart palpitations? Central nervous system overload is a sign of addiction.
- Do you have frequent memory loss? Short term memory loss is one of the first signs of alcohol abuse; brain damage is another.
- Are you unusually anxious, even paranoid? Do you lose your temper or get in a bad mood easily? Do you feel depressed and cry a lot? Do you ever get dizzy or black out? These are typically late symptoms of alcohol abuse.
- Is your immune response low? Do you seem to have a cold or flu all the time? All drugs weaken the immune system over time.
- Do you avoid spending time with friends and family? Withdrawal from normal social and family contacts is often a clear sign of dependency.
- Are you missing more and more work or school days? Late stage addicts focus on only one goal, getting more of the addictive substance and using it.
- Do you blame others or circumstances for your drug use? Do you deny that you have a problem? Denial and blame run deep in addictions. An addict feels he is victim of life's injustices, rather than chemically dependant

## Pointers for best results from your addiction cleanse

- Drink 8 glasses of water each day of your cleanse (can include herb teas). Water flushes alcohol and drugs from every corner of your body.
- Natural mood enhancers that our bodies are equipped to handle, like the herbs St. John's Wort and Kava Kava, help in the weaning process from addictive substances.
- Use green superfoods. They are rich in chlorophyll, antioxidants, vitamins, minerals, enzymes, and more. Superfoods nourish your body quickly, rebuild immunity and help stave off cravings.

## What does it feel like to withdraw from drugs or alcohol?

Breaking destructive habits is hard. Your body reacts when a substance it thinks it depends on is removed. The initial withdrawal phase is usually the most difficult part of the detox and can last from a day or two to a week or more. Withdrawal symptoms are the same as addiction symptoms, only worse and more frequent. You'll start getting chronic headaches, usually with diarrhea as your body tries to release toxins faster, and a lot of irritability. Some people experience hallucinations, disorientation or irrational thinking. Some go into depression. You'll probably sleep poorly, and your sleep will be interrupted during the night. Most people in withdrawal are sensitive to light and noise, experience hot and cold flashes, and sweating.

I encourage people to look at each episode of discomfort as a little victory on the road to recovery. Every day gets easier. One of the laws of the universe is that we don't have to fight the same battle twice. As your body dislodges and removes more toxins day by day, you have the satisfaction of knowing they are gone for good.

## Benefits you'll notice as your body responds to an addiction cleanse

- Your mood will lift as your nerves heal.
- Memory and thinking improve. Take ginkgo biloba extract for a month to help speed up brain processes.
- Your skin will become clearer—less muddy; your eyes will become brighter.

## Addiction cleanse nutrition plan

*Start with this 3 to 7 day nutrition plan.*

The overwhelming majority of habitual drug and alcohol users suffer from malnutrition, metabolic upset and nutritional imbalances. The following drug detox diet not only helps remove alcohol and drug residues, but also helps rebuild a depleted system.

**On rising:** a superfood/aloe drink gives energy and controls morning blood sugar drop: add 1 tsp. each to aloe vera juice: spirulina, bee pollen granules (for GLA), nutritional yeast; or use 1 tbsp. of a superfood mix: Crystal Star Energy Green Drink; Arise & Shine Power Up; Green Foods Green Magma.

**Breakfast:** make a mineral mix—1 tsp. each: sesame seeds, wheat germ, bee pollen granules, nutritional yeast. Add to fresh fruit with yogurt; oatmeal or rice pilaf with maple syrup; whole grain cereal or granola with apple juice.

**Mid-morning:** have fresh carrot juice or Super V-7 veggie juice: 2 carrots, 2 tomatoes, handful each spinach and parsley, 2 celery ribs, ½ cucumber, ½ bell pepper. Add 1 tbsp. green superfood—Crystal Star Energy Green Drink; Barleans Greens.

**Lunch:** have a fresh veggie salad topped with almonds or sunflower seeds. Sprinkle on chopped sea vegetables, 1 tsp. nutritional yeast, 1 tsp. flax or olive oil 1 tsp. lemon juice and Bragg's Liquid Aminos.

**Mid-afternoon:** have a glass of carrot juice with 1 tbsp. green superfood (see above); or Crystal Star Systems Strength broth mix, or a ginseng restorative tea.

**Dinner:** have brown rice and steamed vegetables with chopped onions, nutritional yeast, chopped shiitake mushrooms.

## Herbs & supplements

*Choose 2 to 3 cleansing boosters*

**Herbal support:** Crystal Star Addiction Withdrawal caps and Depress-ex extract help overcome drug-related depression. Ginseng is a key: Y.S. Royal Jelly/Ginseng vials; Superior Renshenwangjiang.

**Cleansing support:** Crystal Star Toxin Detox or Blood Detox caps 4 daily; Sun Chlorella Tabs; Yogi Detox Tea; Herbal Clean Quick Tabs (results temporary). Pacific BioLogic Recovery America, morning and evening formulas show excellent results in treatment facilities.

**Liver support:** It's the key to recovery from alcohol and drug abuse. Alpha Lipoic Acid—among the most powerful liver detoxifiers ever discovered. Milk thistle seed, licorice and kudzu root are key herbs: Planetary Formulas Kudzu caps; Gaia Milk Thistle Seed extract; Crystal Star Liver Cleanse Flushing Tea.

**Lessen withdrawal discomfort:** Crystal Star Relax caps (fast acting), Valerian-wild lettuce extract for sleepless anxiety; Natural Balance HTP. Calm; gotu kola caps; glutamine 1000mg; DLPA 750mg for cravings and depression. Try Chamomile for stress, scullcap for nerves, ginkgo biloba for memory loss, chromium to rebalance sugar levels.

**Replenish neurotransmitters:** Enzymatic Therapy Thyroid/Tyrosine caps (fast results), NADH 10 mg daily; Country Life Relaxer (GABA with taurine). Vitamin C crystals, up to 10,000mg daily, with niacin 1000mgdaily.

**Enzyme support:** cleans up cellular debris from drug abuse. Enzyme Essentials Purezyme; Crystal Star Dr. Enzyme.

**Green superfoods:** Crystal Star Energy Green Drink Mix; Sun Wellness Sun Chlorella; All One Multiple Vitamins & Minerals green phytobase; Enzyme Essentials Super Cellzyme caps; Nature's Secret Ultimate Green tabs.

## Bodywork techniques

Pick bodywork and relaxation techniques to accelerate and round out your cleanse.

**Enema:** especially important when detoxing from alcohol and drugs—take an enema the first and second day of your cleansing program.

**Irrigate:** Or have a colonic for a more thorough colon cleanse.

**Exercise:** every day if possible. Exercise helps the movement of toxins out of the body—it also brings oxygen to the cells. Exercise also helps reduce the stress of detoxing from addictions. Take a walk every day of your cleanse, breathing deeply.

**Guided imagery:** give your body some active encouragement. Guided imagery is a relaxation technique to use frequently during an addictions detox. Actively imagine each gram of the addictive substance dislodging itself from your tissues, floating into your bloodstream and into your bladder or bowel for elimination. Make sure you visualize it leaving your body.

**Deep breathing exercise:** Do deep breathing exercises on rising, and in the evening on retiring to clear the lungs and respiratory system, and to bring oxygen into the cells.

**Hot and cold hydrotherapy:** alternating hot and cold showers are effective. Spasmodic pain and cramping, circulation, muscle tone, bowel and bladder problems, system balance, relaxation, and energy all show improvement with hydrotherapy.

Begin with a comfortably hot shower for three minutes. Follow with a sudden change to cold water for 2 minutes. Repeat this cycle three times, ending with cold. Follow with a full or partial massage, or a brisk towel rub and mild stretching exercises for best results.

## For your continuing diet

- Eat magnesium-rich foods: green leafy and yellow vegetables, citrus fruits, whole grain cereals, fish, legumes.

- Eat potassium-rich foods: oranges, broccoli, green peppers, seafoods, sea vegetables, bananas, tomatoes.

- Eat chromium-rich foods: nutritional yeast, mushrooms, whole grains, seafoods and peas. Increase alkalinity with fresh foods.

- Cravings and withdrawal symptoms intensify in an acid body, from foods like meats, milk products, refined flours and sugars.

# allergy/asthma detox

Allergies have become an epidemic of the 21st century. Once merely a nuisance, today more than 60 million Americans suffer from allergies—over 20% of our population! Environmental chemicals, acid rain, chemically treated and genetically altered foods, radiation levels, air and soil pollutants all add to the allergen load our bodies are faced with. Irresponsible use of antibiotics and steroid drugs taken over a long period of time for allergy symptoms can reduce immune response, and our ability to deal with allergens permanently. Allergy reactions are often an unrecognized cause of other illnesses, too—with problems like chronic sinusitis, cyclical headaches, epilepsy seizures, hypoglycemia, candida albicans infections and emotional over-reactions.

Asthma, inflammation of the bronchial tubes, is a severe respiratory allergy reaction. Since 1980, asthma has increased by 75% in America, with a 50% rise in the last decade, mainly due to more environmental pollutants. It now affects 4 percent of the U.S. population, about 18 million people, 2.5 million of whom have needed emergency treatment. More alarming, a new study by The Pew Environmental Health Commission concludes that 29 million people will have asthma by 2020! Drug-free natural therapies can help reduce the need for medication. Still, emergency medical measures may be necessary to arrest severe asthma attacks which can be life threatening.

## Do you have seasonal allergies?

Respiratory allergies to environmental allergens like air pollutants, and seasonal allergens to dust, pollen, spores and mold, are called Type 1 allergies. This type of allergy develops more easily if your body has excess mucous accumulation to harbor the allergen irritants.

Spore and pollen allergens produce congestion, making you feel symptoms of sinus clog, stuffiness, headaches and puffy eyes. Sometimes your body throws this excess off through the skin, and you get skin irritations or a sore throat. An allergic response to spores and pollen may cause a histamine release that swells nasal passages and membranes, producing symptoms like runny, itchy nose and eyes, sneezing, coughing attacks, bronchial and sinus infections, skin rashes, asthma, insomnia, menstrual disorders and hypoglycemia.

## Allergies to chemicals and contaminants

Repeated chemical exposures set off rampant free radical reactions, as well as allergic responses. (Histamine reactions like itching, sneezing and runny nose are related to free radical damage to liver function from chemicals and pollutants.) Research shows 60% of people with chemical sensitivity have a vitamin B6 deficiency; 30% have a vitamin C deficiency; and 30% are deficient in vitamins B1, B2, B3, and B5. While many physicians do not recognize MCS as an official disorder, natural health practitioners regularly treat it with encouraging results.

Allergies to chemicals and contaminant allergens are called Type 2 allergies. Reactions to chemicals are frequently a defense mechanism, the body's attempt to isolate an offending substance by storing it in fatty tissue.

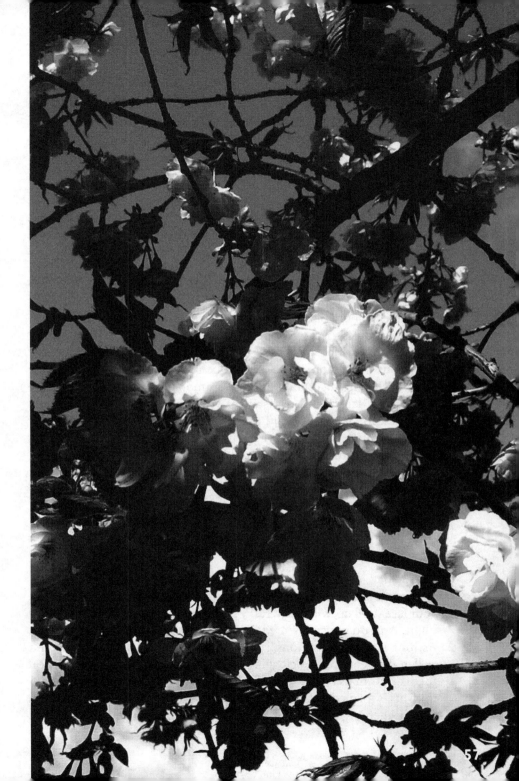

An allergic reaction of this type only occurs after the second exposure to the irritant when your body's histamine response is alerted. Repeated exposures set off massive free radical reactions as the body's contaminant toleration levels are reached; toxic overload results and a severe allergic reaction sets in.

## Allergies, intolerances to foods or food additives are also called Type 2 allergies

They're the fastest growing form of allergic reactions in the U.S. today, as more people are more exposed to chemically altered foods. Food intolerances are often confused with food allergies. A food allergy is an antibody reaction, involving an immune system response to a food it views as a pathogen or parasite. Food allergies may be hereditary, with a child being twice as likely to develop allergies if one parent has them, or four times as likely if both parents have them. A food intolerance is an enzyme deficiency to digest a certain food. For example, people with a lactose intolerance experience the bloating, cramping and diarrhea of an allergy reaction. But the symptoms are really due to a deficiency of the enzyme lactase, which helps digest milk sugar. Common food intolerances include those to wheat, dairy foods, fruits, sugar, yeast, mushrooms, eggs, corn and greens. These foods may be healthy in themselves, but they are often heavily sprayed or treated; in the case of many animal products, also affected by antibiotics and hormones. Food sensitivities are similar to allergy reactions, but differ in that no antigen-specific antibodies are present. In general, they are not a permanent condition.

## Is your body showing signs that it needs an allergy/asthma cleanse?

- Do you have chronic sinus congestion with itchy, watery nose and eyes? Do you get headaches with sneezing, coughing and scratchy throat? Does your face swell up, with itchy, rashy skin? Do you have trouble sleeping at night? Are you unusually tired? You may have a Type 1 seasonal allergy. Asthma is the most serious Type 1 allergy reaction. (**Note:** Spore and pollen allergens produce clogging and congestion as the body tries to seal them off from its regular processes, or tries to work around them. Extra mucous is formed as a shield around the offending substances, and we get the allergy symptoms of sinus clog, stuffiness, hayfever, headaches and watery, puffy eyes. Sometimes the body tries to throw this excess off through the skin, and we get skin irritation symptoms or scratchy sore throat.)

- Do you have difficulty breathing with lots of mucous congestion ( a sign of asthma)?

- Do you get unexplained migraine headaches? Are you frequently moody and depressed for no reason? Do friends and family tell you that your personality changes, that you are often space-y or that your memory is getting unusually bad? Do you have a child that's chronically hyperactive? You may have a Type 2 allergy to chemicals and contaminants.

- Do you get headaches and mental fuzziness after eating? Do you get heart palpitations, sweating, rashes or puffiness around the eyes after eating? Does your abdomen become swollen after eating with heartburn or cramps? Have you gained significant weight even though your diet hasn't changed? Do you have a child that's irritable, flushed and hyperactive after eating? You may have an allergy or intolerance to certain foods or food additives, another kind of Type 2 allergy.

**Note:** Regardless of the food, most food allergy symptoms are similar. Inflammation is generated by a release of histamines into tissue mast cells, walling off the affected body area until immune response agents can restore health. But this process takes time. If the body is re-exposed before health is renewed, inflammation and symptoms, especially mucous congestion become chronic.

## Pointers for best results from your allergy/asthma cleanse

An ample supply of water will expedite a mucous cleansing program. Drink 8 – 10 glasses of bottled water each day of your cleanse to lubricate and flush out allergens (can include herbal teas).

Empowering your immune response is the key to overcoming allergies. I regularly recommend green superfoods because they are so rich in allergen neutralizers like chlorophyll, antioxidants, minerals and enzymes, and such powerful immune builders.

## Benefits you may notice as your body responds to an allergy/asthma cleanse

- Congestion will noticeably begin to clear in the body. Mucous from the lungs and throat will break up and be eliminated.
- Respiratory inflammation will give way to relief as the cleanse progresses.
- Mucous from the colon is also often noticeably expelled.

## Allergy/asthma cleanse nutrition plan

*Start with this 3 to 7 day nutrition plan.*

## The night before your allergy cleanse…

Have a green leafy salad for dinner to give your bowels a good sweeping.

## The next day…

**On rising:** take 2 squeezed lemons in water with 1 tbsp. maple syrup; or take a glass of cranberry, apple, pineapple or grapefruit juice.

**Breakfast:** have a vitamin E-rich drink (vitamin E has antihistamine activity): one handful spinach, 5 carrots, 4 asparagus spears (or mix Crystal Star Systems Strength Broth Mix into hot water for an instant broth and add 1 tsp. nutritional yeast and a pinch of cayenne pepper).

**Mid-morning:** have a glass of fresh carrot juice with 1 tsp. Bragg's Liquid Aminos added. Try a congestion clearing extract, like Crystal Star D-Congest to aid mucous release.

**Lunch:** have a mixed vegetable juice, like V-8, or a potassium broth (page 101); or make this Mucous Cleansing Tonic by juicing: 4 carrots, 2 celery stalks, 2 – 3 sprigs watercress or parsley, 1 radish and 1 garlic clove.

**Mid-afternoon:** have a veggie drink (page 106), or Pure Planet Chlorella; or a greens and sea vegetable mix, such as Crystal Star Energy Green Drink.

**Dinner:** have a hot vegetable broth (page 120) with 1 tbsp. nutritional yeast; or miso soup with sea veggies snipped on top; or a mixed fresh vegetable juice or fresh carrot juice with 1 tbsp. of a green superfood mixed in.

**Before Bed:** have a glass of apple juice or papaya/pineapple juice.

## Herbs & supplements

*Choose 2 to 3 cleansing boosters.*

**Herbal allergy aids:** Try Crystal Star Anti-HST caps (very fast acting, usually within 25 minutes); Dandelion-nettles tea; or Pure Essence Aller Free; or Baywood Dr. Harris Original Allergy Formula.

**For mucous congestion:** Crystal Star Anti-Bio 4 caps at a time, or XLEAR nasal wash with xylitol flushes out allergens, take Crystal Star D-Congest spray for clearer breathing at night; Zand Decongest Herbal; Apply cayenne-ginger chest compresses. Apply Breathe Right post nasal strips.

**Antioxidants are a key:** Pure Essence Antioxidants tabs; Country Life Super 10 Antioxidant; American Health Ester C up to 5000mg daily with bioflavonoids, and CoQ10 30mg 3x daily helps the liver produce antihistamines; Vitamin E 400IU with selenium 200mcg; Quercetin up to 2000mg daily with bromelain; Nutricology Germanium 150mg with B12 SL 2500mcg; Golden Pride Formula One oral chelation w/ EDTA, 2 pkts daily.

**Enzyme support:** Bowel toxicity leads to a constant assault on the immune system. Use Enzyme Essentials Digestzyme with meals—especially helpful for food allergies. Other digestive formulas: Herbal Products and Development Power-Plus Enzymes; Rainbow Light Advanced Enzyme System.

**Immune system herbal support:** panax ginseng, echinacea, ashwagandha, Siberian ginseng (eleuthero), goldenseal, licorice, ginger, astragalus, ligustrum, suma, yellow dock, dandelion and cayenne. Immune formulas: Allergy Research Thiodox (lipoic glutathione complex); Silica for immune enhancement—Flora Vegesil; Eidon Silica Mineral Supplement; Body Essentials Silica gel.

**Green superfoods are potent immune builders:** Crystal Star Energy Green Drink Mix; NutriCology Pro-Greens; Barleans Greens; Fit For You, Intl. Miracle Greens.

**Adrenal support:** Crystal Star Adrenal Energy caps or extract; Planetary Schizandra Adrenal Support; Herbs, Etc. Adrenotonic.

**Probiotics help maintain proper mucous levels, and boost the immune system:** UAS DDS-Plus; Jarrow Prod. Jarro-Dophilus + FOS; American Health Acidophilus liquid.

## Bodywork techniques

*Pick bodywork and relaxation techniques to accelerate and round out your cleanse.*

**Enema:** Take an enema the night before or the morning of your cleanse. Flushing the colon is one of the best ways to jump start a cleanse and allows a more expedient release of toxins. Irrigate: a colonic offers a more thorough colon cleanse.

**Exercise:** Exercise increases oxygen uptake. Take a daily walk with deep breathing exercises.

**Body work:** Acupuncture and chiropractic have both proven effective for allergies.

**Release mucous:** Sessions with an EB (Energy Balancing) foot bath technology can release excess mucous. (Look for results in your bath water.)

**Acupressure points:** During an attack, press tip of nose hard or hollow above the center of upper lip as needed for relief. Press underneath cheekbones beside nose, angling pressure upwards.

## Stress & relaxation techniques

Mental stress depresses immunity and aggravates allergies. Try this following calming technique:

If your mind is racing and you're feeling anxious, shift your focus. Make a sincere effort to turn your attention to your breathing. It's the simplest form of concentrative meditation, the connection between the breath and one's state of mind, a basic principle of yoga relaxation.

Consciously take slow, deep regular breaths, for at least one minute.

To enhance the calming effect, recall a positive or pleasant past experience. Try to feel appreciation or love about the good things and people you have in your life. The effort to shift focus to this positive feeling helps to neutralize stress.

**Avoid allergens:** Invest in an air filter. Stop smoking and avoid secondary smoke. It magnifies all allergy reactions.

## For your continuing diet

Make sure your diet has plenty of organically grown fresh foods. Eat a fresh salad every day. I believe it's your best diet defense against allergy reactions. Cultured food, like yogurt, cottage cheese, miso and tofu help your body keep a good supply of friendly digestive flora. Green superfoods can be a key for extra rich concentrated nutrients to keep the immune system strong.

# alzheimer's/parkinson's detox

### Does someone you know need an Alzheimer's/Parkinson's detox?

The number one fear of older Americans (and their families) isn't heart disease or cancer… it's Alzheimer's. As more people live into their '80s, '90s, and beyond, cases of Alzheimer's and dementia are rising fast. Alzheimer's disease now affects 4 million Americans at a cost of over $100 billion in nursing care and lost wages of family members. As many as 10% of all seniors over 65 have Alzheimer's; 50% of those over 85 are affected. By 2050, as many as 14 million Americans are expected to fall victim to the disease! Alzheimer's disease progresses slowly, but inexorably, with increasing rapidity to the final devastating stages where communication is almost non-existent, feeding and elimination functions uncontrolled.

Alzheimer's disease is a progressive, degenerative condition that attacks the brain, forming neurofiber tangles and plaques believed to result in dementia symptoms. Memory loss and disorientation are the first symptoms as the brain shrinks and nerves degenerate, but eventually there is almost complete loss of physical function, the body breaks down and reverts to childhood in terms of care. It's a devastating, relentless assault that's rising at a rapid rate in industrialized countries worldwide. A substantial number of those diagnosed with Alzheimer's appear to really be victims of too many drugs, or have nutritional deficiencies that can be reversed. Although orthodox medicine has been unable to make a difference in this relentless disease, natural therapies have been successful in slowing brain deterioration. Ask a holistic physician about chelation therapy to reduce heavy metal toxicity.

Parkinson's disease, often a risk factor for Alzheimer's, is the progressive deterioration of specific nerve centers in the brain. The disease process changes the balance of acetylcholine and dopamine, two brain chemicals essential for transmission of nerve signals. The altered balance of these two neurotransmitters results in a lack of control of physical movements. Although the direct cause of Parkinson's is unknown, it is believed that a neurotoxin causes oxidative damage to the basal ganglia that control muscle tone.

## What body signs indicate the need for an Alzheimer's/ Parkinson's detox?

- Is there a noticeable loss of ability to think clearly or remember familiar names, places or events?

- Is there loss of touch with reality, impaired judgement, confusion, difficulty in completing thoughts or following directions?

- Are there clear, unexplained personality or behavior changes?

- Is there a slight tremor in the hands with numbness and tingling in the hands and feet?

- If you noticed a hand tremor, has it become more evident with shaking of the head as well?

- Is there slight dragging of the feet, pronounced with stress or fatigue? Has movement become increasingly difficult?

- If movement is lethargic, has speech also become slow and difficult to follow?

- Has the face lost expression (because of muscle rigidity)? Is there slight drooling? Is vision noticeably impaired?

- Is there unexplained depression? (certain supplements like SAMe may offer dramatic improvement)

## Benefits you may notice as your body responds to the Alzheimer's/Parkinson's detox

- A cleanse helps remove some of the scar-like deposits of proteins and cellular debris that compose Alzheimer's plaques. This toxin release brings a feeling of ease and sense of well being.

- Energy levels increase and circulation improves.

- Mental clarity increases and awareness heightens.

## Pointers for best results from your Alzheimer's/ Parkinson's detox

- Boost your B-complex nutrients. Important food sources are soy foods, seafoods and sea vegetables, nutritional yeast, brown rice, nuts, poultry and leafy greens. Supplementing the diet with B12 (about 2500mcg daily and folic acid (400 to 800mg daily) have shown almost complete reversal in some Alzheimer's patients. I especially like food sources of these vitamins as they appear in bee pollen, royal jelly and sea vegetables. Prolonged B12 deficiency may lead to irreversible changes that will not respond to supplementation.

- Oxidative damage is significant in the progression of both Alzheimer's and Parkinson's. An antioxidant-rich diet with plenty of organic fresh fruits and vegetables offers significant protection and may slow the progression of both conditions.

- Considerably higher aluminum levels are found in the brains of those with Alzheimer's than in people with other types of dementia or in normal people. Do you regularly use aluminum pots and pans or aluminum foil in your cooking? Check on your water supply (aluminum may occur naturally in water, but it's added as alum). Foods like relishes or condiments, antacids that are regularly taken, deodorants or baking powder are other aluminum culprits. Calcium citrate supplements may increase aluminum absorption.

## Continuing diet watchwords after the Alzheimer's/Parkinson's detox

Mental function is directly related to nutrition—especially in the elderly. Good nutrition has a noticeable (sometimes rapid) effect.

**Besides your focus on nutrient-rich foods, avoid foods that create toxic build-up—preserved meats like lunch meats, foods with coloring added, and pesticide-sprayed fruits and vegetables.** Pesticides are full of environmental estrogens which disrupt the delicate hormone balance of the brain, and are thought to be implicated in Alzheimer's symptoms. Wash fruits and vegetables with a food wash (available in health food stores), or better yet, eat organically grown foods. Especially avoid fatty, fried foods. Both too much fat and too many total calories are associated with Alzheimer's and Parkinson's.

**A diet rich in magnesium is important in protecting against aluminum absorption.** Good magnesium sources are dark green vegetables, seafoods and sea vegetables, whole grains, nuts, beans and seeds, tangy spices and cocoa.

**Antioxidant-rich foods are critical.** More than any other nutrient group, they slow the progression of Alzheimer's and Parkinson's. Focus on vitamin E and selenium-rich foods for antioxidant activity—wheat germ and wheat germ oil, sunflower seeds and oil, almonds, pecans, hazelnuts, whole grain cereals, legumes like soy foods, peas and beans, seafoods and sea greens, broccoli, cabbage, garlic and onions. Note: Protease is a potent antioxidant enzyme nutrient. It may even help prevent the formation of neurofibrillary tangles and amyloid plaques. Keep an enzyme like Crystal Star Dr. Enzyme with Protease & Bromelain in your supplement program.

**Add zinc-rich foods.** They show noticeable results in Alzheimer's patients, with positive progression in memory, understanding and communication. Good zinc food sources include nutritional yeast, beans, nuts, seeds, wheat germ and seafood.

**Try to limit prescription and over-the-counter drugs.** A John Hopkins study reveals many Alzheimer's patients are really victims of too many drugs—most taking more than 6 different drugs simultaneously. One-quarter of the medications were either unsafe or ineffective, and the side effects from both the drug interactions or the inappropriate medication affected brain neurotransmission. Most harmful were pain killers and sleeping pills that tended to leach acetylcholine from brain tissues, and diuretics which leached potassium needed by the brain.

While it is sometimes necessary to take medication, drugs are so powerful that I feel it is critical for older people (indeed everyone) to be well informed about the drugs they are taking—dosage, side effects and interaction with other drugs.

**Dehydration contributes to Alzheimer's and Parkinson's.** Drink plenty of water, ideally, eight 8 oz. glasses daily.

## Alzheimer's/Parkinson's detox nutrition plan

*Start with this 2 to 4 day nutrition plan.*

**Note:** Eliminating or at least reducing toxicity from food, water and the environment is critical.

**On Rising:** take an antioxidant rich fruit juice—grape, grapefruit, lemon and cherry—sources of bioflavonoids; or orange, a source of selenium.

**Breakfast:** have cranberry, grape or papaya juice, mix in 1 tbsp. Jarrow Gentle Fibers Drink for antioxidants; or have fresh cherries, bananas, oranges or strawberries with yogurt, and sprinkle on 2 tsp. daily of the following mix: Two tbsp. each: sunflower seeds, lecithin granules, nutritional yeast and wheat germ.

**Mid-morning:** have an antioxidant-rich vegetable juice: Carrot, kale, parsley and spinach, sources of beta-carotene. Kale, garlic, parsley, green pepper and spinach, sources of vitamin C, vitamin E and selenium (slows the progression of Alzheimer's and Parkinson's).

**Lunch:** have a large dark green leafy salad with lemon/oil dressing; and/or a hot veggie broth or hearty veggie soup; with marinated tofu or tempeh in tamari sauce.

**Mid-afternoon:** have a glass of fresh carrot juice or fresh apple juice. Add 1 tbsp. of a green superfood such as Crystal Star Energy Green Drink, Pure Planet Green Kamut; or Aloe Life Daily Greens.

**Dinner:** have steamed brown rice and mixed steamed vegetables. Sprinkle with sea vegetables, 1 to 2 tbsp. flax or olive oil, 1 tsp. liquid lecithin, 1 tbsp. Bragg's Liquid Aminos and 1 tbsp. nutritional yeast, sources of choline (a direct precursor of acetylcholine, the key neurotransmitter for memory) and B-complex (low levels linked to Alzheimer's).

**Before Bed:** have a cup of green tea or Crystal Star Green Tea Cleanser, rich in antioxidants.

## Herbs & supplements

*Choose 2 to 3 cleansing boosters.*

**Slow brain deterioration:** Alpha Lipoic Acid 600mg daily (good results in halting Alzheimer's progression in one study); NADH, 10mg in the morning before eating (highly recommended). Phosphatidyl serine 100mg 3x daily for 3 months, or GPC (glyceryl-phoshorylcholine) or DHA for 3 months (Nature's calcium channel blocker, good results). Maitake products Lion's mane mushroom; Lysine 1000mg daily; Acetyl-Carnitine 2000mg; CoQ-10, 200mg. Vitamin E 2000 IU daily (use under a doctor's supervision).

**Antioxidants:** Free radicals destroy brain cells—antioxidants destroy free radicals—critical in overcoming oxidative damage to the brain to slow progression of Alzheimer's and Parkinson's. Biotec Cell Guard, NutriCology Quercetin 300, CoQ10 60mg 2x daily, L-acetyl-carnitine 500mg daily delays progression of Alzheimer's; phosphatidylserine for impaired mental function.

**Antioxidant herbs:** Ginkgo biloba extract treats Alzheimer's by normalizing acetylcholine receptors and increasing cholinergic transmission.

**For Parkinson's:** Increase body's dopamine biosynthesis: Sabinsa Mucuna Pruriens, a natural source of L-Dopa (goods results against PD); NADH, 5 – 10mg in the morning; Tyrosine 1000mg daily or Enzymatic Therapy Thyroid-tyrosine daily;

**Enzymes:** Oxidative damage and formation of amyloid plaques are the two main causes of Alzheimer's. Protease is a powerful antioxidant enzyme and prevents the formation of amyloid tangles. Crystal Star Dr. Enzyme. Note: Zinc links the tissues to antioxidant enzymes. Zinc deficiency can allow amyloid plaques.

**Aloe vera support:** Herbal Answers Herbal Aloe Force enhances immune response for Parkinson's and Alzheimer's, and helps regenerate tissue needed to correct damage to connective tissue.

**Critical essential fatty acids for nerves and brain:** 1 tbsp. flaxseed oil per day or Barleans Total Omega (highly recommended); Evening Primrose Oil 4 – 6 daily; or Nature's Secret Ultimate Oil.

**Green superfoods are restoratives:** Chlorella has the highest amounts of nucleic acids (RNA/DNA) of any food on earth. Crystal Star Energy Green; NutriCology Pro-Greens; Pure Planet Chlorella.

**Magnesium** helps block aluminum absorption. Eidon Magnesium liquid.

**Silica** prevents aluminum absorption. Eidon Silica liquid.

**Oral chelation:** cleanses heavy metals—Metabolic Response Modifiers CardioChelate; Golden Pride Formula One.

## Bodywork techniques

*Pick bodywork and relaxation techniques to accelerate and round out your cleanse.*

**Restore energy, release metals:** consider VIBE machine therapy with biophotonic light and EB footbath (good results).

**Enema:** Take an enema at least once during your Alzheimer's or Parkinson's cleansing program to help release toxins out of the body.

**Exercise:** A steady moderate exercise regime lowers the risk of developing Alzheimer's. Daily mild exercise is also important for Parkinson's therapy. A brisk daily walk is highly recommended.

**Exercise for brain cells:** Keep your brain active and challenged with mentally creative activities. Use hot and cold hydrotherapy showers for brain and circulation stimulation.

**Flower remedies:** Nelson Bach Rescue Remedy for stress; Deva Flowers Studies & Tests for better concentration.

**Effective body work/therapies:** Relaxation techniques like chiropractic treatment, massage therapy, acupuncture and acupressure have had notable success in reversing early Parkinson's and are helpful for Alzheimer's.

**Special tip:** Decrease prescription diuretics if possible. They leach potassium and nutrients needed by the brain.

## For your continuing diet

Excess meat protein and fat facilitate amyloid neurofiber tangle build-up. Reduce them in your diet to help both Alzheimer's and Parkinson's. Alzheimer's is linked to synthetic estrogens, like those injected into red meats and chickens. Eat organically grown foods when possible to avoid environmental estrogens from pesticides. Eat foods rich in antioxidants to feed the brain: include fresh vegetables, sea vegetables, whole grains, seeds, soy foods, and seafood.

# arthritis detox

Do you need an arthritis cleanse for joints, connective tissue and immune system? Arthritis is the country's number one crippling disease, affecting over 40 million Americans—80% of people over 50. Add to that number the people who suffer from arthritis-like diseases—gout, bursitis, tendonitis and lupus—and the figure becomes staggering.

Arthritis is inflammation of the joints, usually accompanied by changes in joint structure. The focus of medical diagnosis is currently on mineral depletion (especially calcium) as the main cause of arthritis. But that's only part of the story. It isn't a simple disease in any form, affecting not only the bones and joints, but also the blood vessels (Raynaud's disease), kidneys, skin (psoriasis), eyes and brain. Its causes are rooted in immune response as well as wear-and-tear. Conventional medicine has not been able to address arthritis with much success. Unfortunately, NSAIDs (non-steroidal anti-inflammatory drugs), commonly used to relieve arthritis pain, send 76,000 people to the hospital and kill 7,600 people each year! Merck has pulled its COX 2 inhibiting drug from the market because of link to blood clots,

heart attacks and stroke. Celebrex and Naproxen have documented links to cardiovascular risks, too.

Some, like glucosamine, actually help rebuild joints and prevent further destruction. Natural treatment relies on improved nutrition to create an environment for the body to support its own healing functions. Even in advanced inflammation and joint degeneration, diet change can affect improvement. I have personally seen notable reduction of swelling and deformity in long-standing cases. Further, COX-2-inhibiting herbs like ginger, turmeric and rosemary can effectively reduce arthritis inflammation without causing intestinal damage or cardiovascular risks.

Even though the medical focus of diagnosis has been on age and joint damage as a cause of arthritis, I find that hormone imbalance and adrenal exhaustion are the keys to repair. Vigorous diet therapy is the most beneficial thing you can do to control the causes and improve the symptoms of arthritis. Arthritic conditions are degenerative processes that take years to develop. Small or subtle changes are not successful in reversing them. Additional actions you can take for noticeable benefits are seaweed baths, an arthritis sweat bath (pg. 65), and morning sunbaths for Vitamin D and better calcium use.

Arthritis has close ties to emotional health. Emotional stress frequently brings onset of the disease. Long held emotional resentments and obsessive-compulsive actions aggravate arthritis. Most arthritis sufferers have a marked inability to relax (relaxation techniques are essential to arthritis healing). Many have a negative attitude toward life that locks up the body's healing ability. Relaxation therapies like yoga, meditation, and massage therapy are beneficial for recovery. Writing about stressful or traumatic life experiences has been shown to help rheumatoid arthritis sufferers.

### Is your body showing signs that it needs an arthritis cleanse?

- Do you notice marked stiffness and swelling in your fingers, shoulders or neck when the weather turns cold and damp?

- Are you unusually stiff when you get up in the morning, especially when the weather is damp?

- Have you started to notice bony bumps on your index fingers? Or bony spurs on any other joints?

- Are your joints starting to crack and pop?

- Are you anemic? Is your complexion unusually pale? Have you recently lost weight but weren't on a diet?

- Is your digestion poor? Do you have food allergies or intolerances?

- If you experience back or joint pain when you move, does it get worse with prolonged activity?

- Are you more than 20 pounds overweight and starting to feel the effects of the extra weight in your knees and hips?

- Do you have a lot of long-standing lung and bronchial congestion?

- Are you usually constipated? Do you suffer from ulcerative colitis?

- Do you take more than 6 aspirin a day on a regular basis? Are you on a long-term prescription of corticosteroid drugs? Either of these may eventually impair the body's own healing powers.

## Pointers for best results from your arthritis cleanse

**Food allergies contribute to osteoarthritis symptoms.** Avoid these foods during and after your detox: fatty meat and dairy foods, wheat pastries high in sugar and fat; highly salted or spiced foods; caffeine, chocolate, colas and soda pop. Avoid nightshade foods like peppers, eggplant, tomatoes and potatoes if you have rheumatoid arthritis. Include plenty of fresh vegetables for enzyme therapy.

**Standard drug therapy with aspirin or NSAIDS drugs suppress pain and inflammation, but may actually promote the progression of arthritis by damaging cartilage and inhibiting the body's ability to repair its collagen structures.** A compound of glucosamine and chondroitin sulfate, body substances that stimulate the production of cartilage components. A Glucosamine-Chondroitin Complex work better than NSAIDS drugs without the side effects. Shark cartilage is natural, easily available chondroitan.

**For bumps on your knuckles, cherries and cherry juice are a specific remedy.** Take a mild herbal diuretic such as Crystal Star Tinkle-eze caps to flush out released material. Accelerate your cleanse with a daily green drink and add enzyme therapy, like Crystal Star Dr. Enzyme.

## Benefits that you may notice as your body responds to the arthritis cleanse

- Reduction in inflammation and swelling is fairly rapid. Using natural supplements along with the diet, offers some people relief within 24 hours. Instead of dulling pain with drugs, you are repairing the damage that causes the pain. Regenerating flexibility takes longer—usually several months as cartilage and connective tissue rebuild, but some stiffness should subside within 2 to 3 weeks.

- As mucous membrane health improves, you should see better skin tone, digestive and bowel health (regularity) and eye moisture.

## An arthritis elimination sweat

An arthritis sweat is an effective, ancient technique to help eliminate offending crystalline deposits in connective tissue and relieve stiffness. A surprising amount of arthritis-aggravating material can be eliminated via the skin. A sweat is also a good way to start an arthritis cleanse. Results increase when diaphoretic herbs like elder flowers, peppermint or yarrow are taken in a hot tea along with the bath.

## Here's how to take the bath

If you have a weak heart or hypertension, consult a health professional before trying an arthritis sweat bath.

Use about 3 pounds of Epsom salts (or as directed for Dead Sea salts). Run hot bath water, add the salts, let cool enough to get in; Stay in the bath for 15 to 20 minutes. Rub affected joints with a stiff brush in the water for 5 minutes. On emerging, do not dry yourself. Instead, wrap up immediately in a clean sheet and go straight to bed, covering yourself with several blankets. The osmotic pressure of the Epsom salt solution absorbed by the sheet will draw off heavy perspiration, (protect your mattress with a sheet of plastic). The following morning the sheet will be stained with yellowish brown material excreted through the skin. Continue treatment once every two weeks until the sheet is no longer stained, a sign that the body is cleansed. Drink plenty of water throughout the procedure to prevent dehydration and loss of body salts. Improvement after the Epsom salt bath experience is notable.

## Lack of water is linked to arthritis pain and stiffness

Chondroitin sulfate, a remedy for arthritis, is the molecule in cartilage that attracts and holds water. Healthy joints are up to 90% water, but since cartilage doesn't have its own blood supply, chondroitin aids the "molecular sponge" that provides joint nourishment, waste removal and lubrication. Include eight 8 oz. glasses of water daily in your arthritis healing diet. Limit use of alcoholic beverages since they are especially dehydrating.

## Arthritis cleanse nutrition plan

*Start with this 3 to 7 day nutrition plan.*

**On rising:** take a glass of lemon juice and water; or a glass of fresh grapefruit juice (Citrus fruits help enzymes alkalize the body); or Crystal Star Green Tea Cleanser.

**Breakfast:** take a Potassium broth (pg. 101); or a glass of carrot/beet/cucumber juice.

**Mid-morning:** have black cherry juice; Green Foods Barley Essence; or Crystal Star Energy Green.

**Lunch:** have miso soup with snipped sea greens, and a glass of carrot juice with Bragg's Liquid Aminos.

**Mid-afternoon:** have a green drink, or alfalfa/mint tea, or Crystal Star Cleansing & Purifying Tea.

**Dinner:** have a glass of cranberry/apple, or papaya juice, or another glass of black cherry juice.

**Before Bed:** take a glass of celery juice, or a cup of miso soup with 1 tbsp. of nutritional yeast.

**Note:** Follow your detox with a fresh foods diet for 1 month.

1. Fresh fruits and vegetables, with lots of green leafy greens are rich in enzymes.

2. There is a link between a sulfur deficiency and arthritis. Eat sulfur-containing foods like broccoli, onions, cabbage and garlic.

3. Fiber keeps crystalline wastes flushed. Eat whole grains like rice and oats.

4. Bioflavonoids strengthen connective tissue. Eat (and drink) cranberries, grapes, papayas and citrus fruits, or arrow Gentle Fibers drink.

5. Have cold water fish like salmon for high Omega-3 oils twice a week.

## Herbs & supplements

*Choose 2 to 3 cleansing boosters.*

**Repair joints, protect cartilage:** Glucosamine-Chondroitin 4 daily (not if you have prostate cancer); Shark cartilage (natural chondroitin sulfates). Use with CMO (cetyl-myristoleate) 500mg, like Jarrow True CMO for EFAs; Lane Labs Advacal Ultra for calcium balance; Omega-3 flax or fish oil 3x daily—expect less pain in about 3 months.

**Effective COX-2 inhibitors and anti-inflammatories:** DLPA 1000mg; New Chapter Zyflamend AM & PM; Source Naturals Minor Pain Comfort; Quercetin 1000mg w/ Bromelain 1500mg daily; MSM 1000 mg.; Herbal anti-inflammatories: Crystal Star Anti-Flam caps; cat's claw caps.

**Antioxidants help regenerate cartilage:** SAMe protects cushioning sinovial fluid and blocks enzymes that degrade cartilage (can be as efective as ibuprofen); CoQ10 300mg daily; Carnitine 2000mg daily for 3 months; Lane Labs Nature's Lining to strengthen the stomach wall (highly recommended for damage caused by Non-Steroidal Anti-Inflammatory Drugs (NSAIDs)).

**Chlorophyll sources stimulate cortisone:** Alfalfa tabs 10 daily; Solaray Alfa Juice caps; Crystal Star Energy Green Drink Mix; NutriCology Pro-Greens; Wakunaga Kyo-Green; Barleans Greens.

**Enzymes help normalize body chemistry:** Crystal Star Dr. Enzyme; Transformation Repairzyme; Crystal Star Bitters & Lemon extract.

**Nettles therapy:** nettles extract suppresses pro inflammatory proteins—their sting on affected joints can dramatically reduce symptoms. Use with guidance from an herbalist or holistic professional.

**Stimulate natural cortisone production:** Crystal Star Adrenal Energy daily with Evening Primrose Oil 3000mg daily; Prince of Peace Royal Jelly/Ginseng vials, one daily; Nutricology Adrenal Cortex caps.

## Bodywork techniques

*Pick bodywork and relaxation techniques to accelerate and round out your cleanse.*

**Enema:** take an enema the first, second and the last day of your arthritis cleanse to release toxins.

**Exercise:** A lack of exercise weakens muscles putting more stress on joints. A daily stretching program and yoga are my favorites for keeping skeletal muscles strong.

**Bodywork therapies:** Massage therapy relieves pain, improves the circulation and hastens elimination of harmful deposits. Another choice? Crystal Star Hot Seaweed Bath normalizes body pH almost immediately.

**To relieve pain:** Press the highest spot of the muscle between thumb and index finger. Press in the webbing between the two fingers, closer toward the bone that attaches to the index finger. Press for 10 seconds at a time into the web muscle, angling the pressure toward the bone of the index finger.

**Exercise:** Lack of exercise weakens muscles putting more stress on joints. A daily stretching program and yoga are my favorites for keeping skeletal muscles strong.

## Healing applications

Home Health Celadrin cream for stiffness; BHI Traumeel healing gel; Arnica gel for soreness; Boswellin creme; Biochemics Pain Relief lotion. Capsaicin creme, cayenne-ginger compresses; Boericke & Tafel Triflora Arthritis Gel.

## For your continuing diet

Mix 2 tbsp. each: sunflower seeds, lecithin granules, nutritional yeast, wheat germ. Mix into yogurt, or sprinkle on fresh fruit or greens. Take 2 tsp. daily. Soy foods, like tofu, tempeh and miso can be a key diet factor for women. They are hormone balancing and immune stimulating with non-meat protein. Fiber foods with protein, like rice, oats, lentils and beans are a key factor for men. Use only olive or canola oil in cooking. Never fry your foods.

# detoxification & blood sugar imbalances: diabetes and hypoglycemia

It's the bittersweet truth: Even after decades of warnings about their dangers we are a nation addicted to sugar and artificial sweeteners like aspartame. Over 60% of the U.S. population suffers from some degree of the "blood sugar blues." Twenty million Americans suffer from diabetes (high blood sugar) or hypoglycemia (low blood sugar).

Sugar has become an entire food group, counting for an astounding 20% of total daily calories for adult Americans. U.S. kids eat enough sugar to account for half of their daily calories! Sugar has so infiltrated our food supply that most of us hardly notice it's there. In August 1999, the Center For Science in the Public Interest filed a petition to the FDA to require more explicit labeling of added sugar in foods. Almost all snack foods and pre-prepared foods have added sugar in their ingredients to enhance their flavor. As a society, we're clearly paying the price in terms of our pocketbooks and our health.

## The diabetes epidemic

Type 2 diabetes has reached epidemic levels in America. The rates of diabetes have doubled in the last three decades! Today, 17 million people suffer from diabetes. Many more have the disease and don't know it. Type 2 diabetes cases are even rising among young adults and children. In type 2 diabetes, the most common type, the pancreas is unable to use insulin properly or has too little insulin, the hormone that allows sugar to be stored or used for energy. It's a vicious cycle where poor fat and sugar metabolism lead to obesity… which then leads to diabetes. The cycle keeps going. Diabetes makes you more hungry, so symptoms are aggravated as well as brought on by eating too much fat and too many sugary foods.

Complications from diabetes are the fourth leading cause of death by disease in the world today. Heart disease, high blood pressure, retinopathy (loss of vision), nerve damage, kidney problems, arteriosclerosis, and circulatory problems are all major problems that face diabetics. But there is a lot of hope. While some cases need to be managed medically, many type 2 diabetics can balance their blood sugar simply by following a low glycemic, low fat diet and getting regular exercise.

An important note on type 1 diabetes: Type 1 diabetes is a juvenile, autoimmune condition where the body destroys its own insulin-producing cells. Today scientists are working with Islet-cell transplants as a possible cure with some success. However, at this point, type 1 diabetes is a chronic problem that is almost entirely dependent on insulin to sustain life.

## Do you have high blood sugar warning signs?

- constant thirst with frequent urination
- slow healing cuts and wounds; chronic infections
- recent weight loss or weight gain without diet changes
- severe, unexplained fatigue
- blurry vision

## Diabetes control diet

Both types of diabetes benefit from diet improvement, exercise and natural supplements. Diet improvement is absolutely necessary to overcoming diabetes. High blood sugar is also an indication of high triglycerides, a risk factor for heart disease. The following diet, in addition to reducing insulin requirements and balancing blood sugar, has the nice "side effects" of healthy weight loss and better heart protection.

This diet supplies slow-burning, complex carbohydrate fuels that do not need much insulin for metabolism. Meals are small, largely vegetarian, and low in fats of all kinds. Proteins come from soy foods and whole grains that are rich in lecithin and chromium. Fifty percent of the diet is based in fresh or simply cooked vegetables for low calories and high digestibility. Avoid caffeine and caffeine foods, hard liquor, food coloring and sodas. Even diet

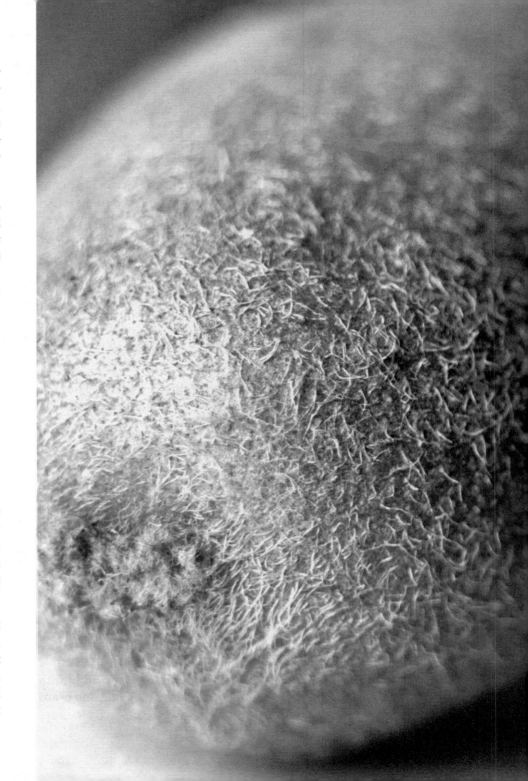

sodas have phenylalanine that can affect blood sugar levels. Check your blood sugar regularly to monitor high and low swings that may require medical attention!

**Note:** Diabetics do poorly on long juice fasts or extended detox diets. The following diabetes detox diet focuses on reducing excess sugar, and including high quality protein and fiber sources for balance and regularity. People with diabetes should not skip meals. Most diabetics should eat 6 mini meals a days, especially if they're on insulin therapy.

**On rising:** take the juice of two lemons in a glass of water with 2 tsp. Sun Wellness Chlorella granules.

**Breakfast:** have aloe vera juice; or All One Vitamin-Mineral drink in apple juice or water to balance sugar curve. Make a mix of 2 tbsp. each: nutritional yeast, toasted wheat germ, lecithin granules and rice or oat bran. Sprinkle into yogurt with fresh fruit and grated almonds on top; or have a poached egg on whole grain toast; or low sugar granola with almond milk; or buckwheat pancakes with a little butter and juice.

**Mid-morning:** have a green drink like Crystal Star Energy Green or Fit for You, Intl. Miracle Greens; or green tea. Recent USDA research shows green tea's catechins enhance insulin activity.

**Lunch:** have a green salad, with celery and sprouts, marinated tofu and mushroom soup; a tofu burger; turkey with steamed veggies and rice or cornbread; or a baked potato with yogurt or kefir cheese, and miso soup with sea greens; or a whole grain sandwich, with avocado, rice cheese, a low fat spread and watercress.

**Mid-afternoon:** have a glass of mixed vegetable juice or a sugar balancing herb tea, such as licorice, dandelion, or pau d'arco tea. If you're still hungry, have a hard boiled egg with sesame salt, or whole grain crackers with veggie dip.

**Dinner:** Keep it light—have baked or broiled seafood with brown rice and peas; or a Chinese stir-fry with rice, veggies and miso soup; or a light Italian polenta with a hearty vegetable soup, or whole grain or veggie pasta salad; or a mushroom quiche with whole grain crust and yogurt sauce, and a green salad. Beware! Consuming any alcohol can cause blood sugar to soar.

**Before bed:** take a cup of miso soup, or mix 1 tsp. Red Star nutritional yeast in 1 tsp. warm water.

## These supplements can help normalize your high blood sugar

*Choose 2 – 3 cleansing boosters.*

- **Stabilize blood sugar:** Crystal Star Sugar Control High capsules help insulin balance; Bitter Melon capsules help both high and low blood sugar attacks. Adapters like GTF Chromium or chromium picolinate 200mcg daily and Vanadium 25 mcg. daily (diabetics usually make enough insulin, chromium and vanadium help them use it). Siberian eleuthero extract or Grifron Maitake SX Fraction caps to enhance insulin sensitivity.

- **Lower blood sugar levels:** Alpha Lipoic acid 600mg daily lowers glucose levels up to 30%; Crystal Star Great Ginseng! caps (ginseng is a proven aid to blood sugar control), or Olive Leaf extract; high dose biotin—3000mcg daily; Vitamin C 3000mg daily with magnesium 400mg daily combats insulin resistance; Herbcare Charantia tea.

- **Normalize pancreas activity and insulin function:** Take gymnema sylvestre extract before meals to help repair damage; Ester C 3000mg daily increases insulin tolerance, normalizes pancreatic activity. Glutamine 1000mg with carnitine 1000mg; Nutricology ProLive olive leaf extract as directed; DHEA 25mg daily increases cell sensitivity to insulin. Burdock, Pau d'arco or Astragalus tea, 2 cups daily for 3 months; raw pancreas glandular or Premier Vanadium 25mcg daily.

- **Prevent nerve damage with EFAs:** Evening Primrose Oil capsules 1000 – 2000mg daily, Omega-3 flax or fish oil (for DHA) 3000mg daily.

- **Raise antioxidants:** Pycnogenol or grape seed PCOs 200mg daily.

- **Boost energy:** Crystal Star Adrenal Energy caps for cortex support with Energy Green Renewal caps for stable energy. Spirulina tablets 6 daily to elevate mood.

## Bodywork and lifestyle techniques are critical to success in overcoming blood sugar irregularities

- **Don't smoke.** Nicotine increases the desire for sugar and sugary foods.

- **Hot tub therapy:** A study reported in the New England Journal of Medicine shows soaking in a hot tub for 30 minutes a day for three weeks lowers blood sugar levels 13%!

- **Walking** is good exercise for diabetics to increase metabolic processes and reduce need for insulin. Insulin resistance drops by nearly 2% for every 200 calories burned through exercise.
- **Lose excess weight.** A fiber weight loss drink, like AloeLife Fiber-mate or All One Totally Fiber complex is effective.
- **A regular deep therapy massage** is effective in regulating sugar use through the body.
- **Strive for eight hours of sleep a night.** Sleep deprivation increases diabetes risk and complications.

## Hypoglycemia control plan

Hypoglycemia and diabetes stem from the same causes. Like diabetes, hypoglycemia is caused by sugar overload, but a hypoglycemic body reacts to the sugar in the opposite way. The pancreas produces too much insulin rather than too little. The blood sugar swings are just as wild, though. The excess insulin lowers blood sugar too much as the body struggles to achieve the proper glucose/insulin balance. The brain bears the brunt of the damage, as it requires 50% of all blood glucose as an energy source to think clearly. If your adrenals are exhausted (they sit atop your kidneys and they hurt when pressed if they're exhausted), if you diet excessively, or if you abuse drugs or alcohol, you're on a road to hypoglycemia. Hypoglycemia can also result from prolonged, strenuous exercise, fasting, and in early pregnancy. Be aware that regular hypoglycemic episodes can be a sign that your body is on the pathway to diabetes.

## There are two types of hypoglycemia

1. Endogenous hypoglycemia, related to a serious medical condition like liver disease, is the most severe and needs immediate medical supervision.

2. Reactive hypoglycemia, which happens a few hours after a meal, is the type we're talking about in this section. Reactive hypoglycemia occurs when the excess insulin secreted by the pancreas lowers blood sugar to the point of body disruption. This form of hypoglycemia is an internal body condition, not a disease. It is less severe than endogenous hypoglycemia, but symptoms become apparent swiftly. Your decision making and thinking abilities are affected first.

## Do you have hypoglycemia?

A blood test is a quick way to determine whether you are suffering from hypoglycemia. Home blood glucose monitoring kits are also available from your pharmacist. And, watch for these low blood sugar body signs:

- memory lapses and mental dullness
- mood swings and aggressive behavior
- depression and anxiety
- insomnia, blurry vision
- frequent headaches or migraines
- ravenous hunger and cravings for sweets
- shakiness, racing heartbeat, temporary incoordination
- PMS

## Detox diet for hypoglycemia control

The key factors in hypoglycemia are stress and poor diet… both a result of too much sugar and refined carbohydrates, like pastries and desserts. These foods quickly raise glucose levels, causing the pancreas to over-compensate and produce too much insulin, which then lowers body glucose levels too far and too fast. This diet supplies your body with fiber, complex carbohydrates and protein—slow even-burning fuel that prevents sudden sugar swings. I recommend a diet like this for 2 – 3 months until blood sugar levels are regularly stable. Note: Like diabetics, hypoglycemics do poorly on long juice fasts or extended detox diets. The following detox diet cleans the "junk" out of the diet and focuses on high nutrition foods to stabilize the system.

## Diet watchwords

- **Eat potassium-rich foods:** oranges, broccoli, bananas, and tomatoes.

- **Eat chromium-rich foods:** nutritional yeast, mushrooms, seafood and sea greens, beans and peas.

- **Eat high quality vegetable protein at every meal.**

**On rising:** take a "hypoglycemia cocktail:" 1 tsp. each in diluted apple or orange juice to control morning sugar drop: glycine powder, powdered milk, protein powder, and nutritional yeast; or a protein/amino drink, like Wakunaga Harvest Blend, or Crystal Star Systems Strength.

**Breakfast:** the most important meal of the day for hypoglycemia. Include ⅓ of daily nutrients; have oatmeal with yogurt and fresh fruit; or poached or baked eggs on whole grain toast with butter or kefir cheese; or whole grain cereal or pancakes with apple juice, soy milk, fruit or yogurt, nuts; or tofu scrambled "eggs" with bran muffins, whole grain toast and a little butter; or my favorite: brown rice with tofu and tamari sauce and steamed veggies for breakfast.

**Mid-morning:** have a Stress Cleanse juice (page 110), Green Foods Green Magma with 1 tsp. Bragg's Liquid Aminos, or Crystal Star Energy Green Renewal drink; or a sugar balancing herb tea, such as licorice, dandelion, or a green and white tea blend; and some crisp, crunchy vegetables with kefir or yogurt cheese.

**Lunch:** have a fresh salad, with cottage cheese or soy cheese, nuts, noodle or seed toppings, and lemon oil dressing; or a seafood or chicken sandwich on whole grain bread, with avocados and low-fat cheese; or a bean or lentil soup with tofu or shrimp salad or sandwich; or a seafood and whole grain pasta salad; or a vegetarian pizza on a chapati crust with low fat cheese.

**Mid-afternoon:** have a a licorice herb or dandelion root tea, or another green drink; and yogurt with fruit, nuts and seeds.

**Dinner:** have some steamed veggies with tofu, or baked or broiled fish and brown rice; or an Asian stir fry with seafood, rice and vegetables; or a vegetable pasta dish with verde sauce and hearty soup (add green beans for pancreatic support); or a Spanish beans and rice dish, or paella with seafood and rice.

**Before bed:** have a cup of Red Star nutritional yeast or miso broth; or papaya juice with a little yogurt.

## These supplements can help normalize your low blood sugar

*Choose 2 – 3 cleansing boosters.*

- **Normalize blood sugar swings** with herbs and nutrients. Crystal Star Sugar Control Low is designed to balance blood sugar levels, support stressed adrenals and encourage a feeling of well-being; or Source Naturals Gluco Science (highly effective nutrient support); Crystal Star Great Ginseng! helps remove excess sugar from the blood; All One Totally Fiber Complex helps insure a low-glycemic diet to balance sugar curve.

- **Supercharge adrenals for long-term recovery:** When blood glucose is low, the adrenals compensate by secreting extra adrenaline which brings sugar levels back up. Eventually, the adrenals become exhausted by repeated attempts to normalize blood sugar. Consider vitamin C with bioflavonoids 1x3000mg or Pure Planet Amla C Plus tabs with spirulina to revitalize the adrenal glands. (Take vitamin C immediately during an attack). Crystal Star Adrenal Energy also provides adrenal support and helps stabilize blood sugar levels. Nutricology Adrenal Cortex extract and Planetary Schizandra Adrenal Complex nourish exhausted adrenals. Gentle whole herbs like kava kava, passionflowers, scullcap and gotu kola caps fight stress linked to hypoglycemia; Evening Primrose Oil caps 2000 mg.; B Complex 100 mg. 2x daily with extra PABA 100 mg., and pantothenic acid 500 mg.

- **Boost energy:** Glutamine 500 mg. daily; 1 tsp. each: spirulina granules and bee pollen granules in apple juice, or Rainbow Light Hawaiian Spirulina between meals. Beehive Botanicals Royal Jelly caps or Prince of Peace Red Ginseng-Royal Jelly vials for a noticeable energy boost. Take aloe vera juice concentrate before meals (add pinches of cinnamon, ginger and nutmeg to help control cravings—good results).

- **Enzyme therapy for glucose homeostasis:** CoQ-10 60 mg. 3x daily for 3 – 6 weeks; Pancreatin 1200 mg. with meals; Crystal Star Dr. Enzyme with protease and bromelain; Transformation BalanceZyme with MasterZyme; Pure Essence Labs Candex before meals, especially if candida yeast is also a problem.

- **Chromium may be critical:** GTF Chromium 200 mcg.; Solaray Chromiacin; Chromium picolinate 200 mcg.

## Bodywork and lifestyle changes for hypoglycemia pay off for total health, too

- Eat 6 – 8 mini-meals throughout the day to keep blood sugar levels up. Large meals throw sugar balance way off, especially at night.

- Eat relaxed, never under stress. Regular massage therapy treatments can do wonders.

- Get some exercise everyday to work off unmetabolized acid wastes.

- Some oral contraceptives can cause glucose intolerance and poor sugar metabolism. Ask your doctor.

# candida detox

Candida albicans yeast normally lives harmlessly in the gastrointestinal tract and genito-urinary areas of the body. Candida may infect virtually any part of the body. The most commonly involved sites include the nail beds, skin folds, feet, mouth, sinuses, ear canal, belly button, esophagus, intestine, vaginal tract and urethra. Candida also infects deep internal organs, which sometimes results in serious disease. Likely sites of infection include the thyroid and adrenal glands, kidneys, bladder, bowel, esophagus, uterus, lungs and bone marrow. In the past, candida infection was regarded as a women's problem because of its connection to a vaginal yeast infection. Today, we know that both men and women are equally likely to develop candida. Candidiasis is really a state of inner imbalance, not a germ or bug. When immunity and resistance are low, the body loses its intestinal balance and candida yeasts multiply too rapidly, voraciously feeding on sugars and carbohydrates in the digestive tract. It's an immune-compromised condition. Unless the body's weakened defenses are given assistance, candida colonies will flourish throughout the body and keep releasing toxins into the bloodstream.

## Lifestyle factors that promote candida infection

1. Poor diet—especially excessive intake of sugar, starchy foods, yeasted breads and chemicalized foods.

2. Repeated use of antibiotics—long term use of antibiotics kill protective bacteria (that keep candida under control).

3. Hormone medications like corticosteroid drugs and birth control pills.

4. A high stress life, too much alcohol, too little rest.

## Is your body showing signs that it needs a candida cleanse?

- Do you have recurrent digestive problems, gas, bloating or flatulence?

- Do you have rectal itching, or chronic constipation alternating to diarrhea?

- Do you have a white coating on your tongue (thrush)?

- Have you been unusually irritable or depressed? Are you bothered by unexplained frequent headaches, muscle aches and joint pain?

- Do you feel sick all over, yet the cause cannot be found? Are the symptoms worse on muggy days?

- Has your memory been noticeably poor? Are you finding it hard to concentrate or focus your thoughts?

- Do you have chronic vaginal yeast infections or frequent bladder infections?

- If you are a woman, do you have serious PMS or other menstrual problems? Do you have endometriosis?

- If you are a man, do you have abdominal pains, prostatitis, or loss of sexual interest?

- Do you have chronic fungal infections like ringworm, jock itch, nail fungus or athlete's foot?

- Do you have psoriasis, eczema or chronic dermatitis? Are you bothered by erratic vision or spots before the eyes?

- Do you catch frequent colds that take many weeks to go away?

- Are you oversensitive to chemicals, tobacco, perfume or insecticides? Do you crave sugar, bread, or alcoholic beverages?

- Have you recently taken repeated rounds for 1 month or longer, of antibiotics or corticosteroid drugs, like Symycin, Panmycin, Decadron or Prednisone, or acne drugs?

Getting rid of a candida yeast infection is not easy. The longer you wait to begin a detox and healing program, the harder the job becomes. Consider a candida test before starting a healing program. Call Immunosciences Lab (1-800-950-4686), for a blood test for candida immune complexes and candida antibodies. For information on electrodermal candida screening, call Harmony Health Systems (770-345-6614).

## Here's what you'll be doing on a candida cleanse

**Killing the candida yeasts:** The diet and supplement program will kill the yeasts. Avoid antibiotics, corticosteroid drugs and birth control pills, unless there is absolute medical need, so you don't get re-infected.

**Eliminating the dead yeasts from your body:** The cleansing diet and cleansing products will release the dead yeasts and their waste from the body. Enemas or colonics will expedite their removal.

**Rebuilding your normal systemic environment and immune defenses:** The program will strengthen your digestive system by enhancing its ability to assimilate nutrients. Afflicted organs, especially the liver, and glands will be strengthened. Metabolism will normalize and probiotic supplementation will promote friendly bacteria in the gastrointestinal tract.

## Pointers for best results from your candida cleanse

- Drug therapy for candidiasis uses Nystatin, Ketaconazole and other antifungal products to try and kill the yeast invader. But this method only relieves the ill effects of candidiasis while the drug is being taken. Drugs do nothing to prevent recurrence, and some of them produce unpleasant side effects. Many of the drugs further suppress the immune system. An effective program must not only kill the yeasts but also strengthen the body's own immune defense mechanisms to keep candida under control. Empowering your immune response is the real key to overcoming candida.

- Early clinical findings show that a program with plant enzyme therapy, probiotics, certain herbal extracts and organic minerals is clinically effective in treating and preventing candida.

- Drink 8 – 10 glasses of bottled water each day of your cleanse (can include herbal teas). Water lubricates and flushes wastes, toxins and dead yeast cells from the body. An ample supply of water will expedite a candida cleansing program.

## Benefits you'll notice as your body responds to a candida cleanse

- Unpleasant symptoms like aversion to odors and allergy reactions will subside.

- You will be reestablishing the vitality of your colon, so alternating constipation and diarrhea will normalize.

- You'll start to regain your energy and stamina.

- Sleep and the ability to rest will improve

- Mental clarity will improve. You won't be feeling so "spaced-out."

- Sugar cravings will begin to subside, but be careful… these cravings have a yo-yo reaction.

- The time line for feeling better varies widely. Some people feel better with one to two weeks; others take one to two months.

## Then what? How do you keep candida yeast under control?

The whole healing-rebuilding process usually takes from three to six months for the yeasts to be eliminated and friendly bacteria re-established. A strong immune system, a vital liver and robust colonies of friendly bacteria are critical to lasting control and prevention. The changes you'll need to make in diet, habits and lifestyle are often radical. Enzyme therapy in conjunction with diet therapy and anti fungal herbs speeds up recovery time for candida. (See supplement recommendations on pg. 75 for more.) Some people feel better within 2 days; others go through a rough "healing crisis." (Yeasts are living organisms—part of your body. Killing them off is traumatic.) But most people with candidiasis infection are feeling so bad anyway, that the treatment and the knowledge that they are getting better, pulls them through the hard times. Be as gentle with your body as you can. Give yourself all the time you need. You want to get better quickly, but multiple therapies all at once can be quite stressful. Just stick to it and go at your own pace.

After your candida cleanse, keep your program going. Here are some watchwords:

**Eat plenty of beta-carotene-rich foods, and iodine and potassium-rich foods.** They are the most effective food nutrients against candida. My favorite food for these nutrients is sea vegetables—all kinds, in soups, on rice or a healthy pizza, or in a salad.

**Use raw sauerkraut in your diet.** It is a superfood for conquering candida. Dr. Elson M. Haas, M.D., director of the Preventive Medical Center of Marin, CA; Gary Ross, M.D. of Health & Medical Clinic of San Francisco, CA; Dr. Paul Yanick, Director of Bio-Health Center, New Hope, PA, and Jack Tips, N.D., C.N.C. author of Conquer Candida, are just four of many candida experts who report that raw cultured vegetables (sauerkraut) are very helpful in controlling and conquering candida. Nutritional authors Patricia Bragg, Donna Gates and Klaus Kaufmann attest to amazing accounts of candida sufferers who report substantial improvement in their condition after eating raw sauerkraut. Use Rejuvenative Foods Raw Sauerkraut or Vegi-delite, or make the cultured vegetables yourself. For a good raw sauerkraut recipe check out www.bodyecology.com.

**Eat three to four small, healthy meals a day.** Provide your body with healing foods during periods of cleansing. But be careful not to overeat or you will divert your body's energy from cleansing to digestion.

**Eat alkalizing foods.** A good rule of thumb is 80% alkaline-forming foods and 20% acid-forming foods. Alkalizing foods are: fresh, steamed, baked or grilled vegetables, sea veggies, brown rice, millet, quinoa and amaranth grains, herbs and herb teas, sprouts and seeds (except sesame seeds), lemons, limes and unsweetened cranberries, cultured foods (like raw cultured vegetables, yogurt, kefir, organic apple cider vinegar), and soaked almonds. Acid-forming foods are: animal foods like beef, poultry, eggs, fish, and shellfish, buckwheat, and organic, unrefined oils,

**Limit or avoid these foods on a continuing basis to keep candida from coming back:** Fruits (except those listed above). Acid-formers like sugary foods or sweeteners such as Saccharin or NutraSweet, soft drinks, wheat flour foods, beans, tofu, nuts and nut butters, wine or other alcoholic beverages, commercial vinegars or condiments. If you crave sweets, use the herb Stevia in your tea.

**Watch your food-combinations.** Overgrowth of yeast will not disappear if you are combining foods that aren't compatible in the stomach. Instead, you'll get fermentation that produces sugars and alcohol, and continue to feed the yeast. People with candidiasis are normally in a weak digestive state so good food combining becomes even more important.

Here are four general food-combining rules to follow:

1. Eat your fruits alone.

2. Eat protein foods like meats and grains with non-starchy vegetables or sea vegetables.

3. Eat starchy vegetables like potatoes with non-starchy vegetables or sea vegetables.

4. Don't combine a large amount of fat with protein foods like meat or grains. Large amounts of fat, especially refined oils, delay the secretion of hydrochloric acid needed to digest the protein. An example is mixing mayonnaise with tuna or chicken. If you make this combination into a sandwich with bread, you'll be making it even more difficult to digest. Use an oil-free or miso dressing to make tuna, egg or chicken salad. Eat it with a vegetable salad instead of with bread.

## Candida cleanse nutrition plan

*Start with this 3 to 7 day nutrition plan. To overcome a candida yeast infection, your diet must simultaneously nourish your body while starving candida of the foods that support its growth.*

**On rising:** take 2 tsp. cranberry concentrate, with 1 tsp. cider vinegar and 1 tsp. maple syrup in water; or a fiber cleanser like AloeLife Fibermate or Crystal Star Herbal Laxa caps; or a cup of Crystal Star Green Tea Cleanser.

**Breakfast:** have a vegetable omelette with broccoli; or scrambled eggs with onion, shiitake mushrooms and red pepper; or brown rice with onions and carrots; or oatmeal with 1 tbsp. Bragg's Liquid Aminos; or cream of buckwheat sweetened with stevia and sautéed veggies.

**Mid-morning:** have a vegetable drink (page 106) with Pure Planet Chlorella or Fit for You, Intl. Miracle Greens; or Crystal Star Systems Strength; or a cup of miso soup with sea veggies; and a cup of pau d' arco, echinacea or chamomile tea.

**Lunch:** have a fresh green salad with lemon/coconut, olive or flax oil dressing and seafood, chicken or turkey; or a vegetable or miso soup with sea veggies; or steamed veggies with brown rice.

**Mid-afternoon:** have potato corn chowder with crackers; or some raw veggies dipped in lemon/coconut, olive, or flax oil dressing; or mineral water and hard boiled egg with sea vegetable seasoning.

**Dinner:** have broiled fish or chicken with raw sauerkraut or green beans; or steamed vegetables or baked potato sprinkled with sea vegetables and Bragg's Liquid Aminos; or a vegetable stir fry with brown rice, sea veggies and miso soup;.

**Before Bed:** chamomile tea, ginger extract drops in water, or miso soup.

## Herbs & supplements

*Choose 2 or 3 cleansing boosters.*

**Cleansing support formula:** Gaia Herbs 2 week Candida Supreme Vital Cleanse.

**Candida cleansing formulas:** Crystal Star Candida Detox; Nature's Secret Candistroy; Gaia Candida Supreme Vital Cleanse; Nutricology Perm A Vite if you also have leaky gut syndrome.

**Probiotics are critical to restore a healthy internal environment: (Choose one and add to your diet either sprinkled on food or taken with water throughout the day):** Garden of Life Fungal Defense; American Health Acidophilus liquid; UAS DDS-PLUS; Percoba Colostrum tabs for extra immune support.

**Enzyme therapy is critical to recovery:** Enzyme therapy along with diet therapy and anti fungal herbs speeds up recovery time. Some people feel better within 2 days!: Pure Essence Candex; Crystal Star Dr. Enzyme; Enzyme Purezyme, high protease formula.

**Oregano oil:** essential oil with amazing antimicrobial powers, strongly inhibits growth of candida albicans. Now Oregano Oil soft gels. Use only as directed.

**Olive leaf extract:** stimulates phagocytosis of all types of pathogenic microfungi and bacteria. NutriCology Prolive; Planetary Full Spectrum Olive Oil extract.

**Coconut oil:** rich source of caprylic acid, a potent anti-fungal. Has 50% lauric acid—a disease-fighting fatty acid. Spectrum Organic Coconut Oil.

**Reishi mushrooms support immunity, discourage infection:** Maitake products Reishi tabs; New Chapter Reishi; Country Life Shiitake/Reishi Complex With Chlorella.

**Green superfoods—potent immune builders:** Crystal Star Energy Green; Kyolic Green Harvest Blend; Fit for You, Itl. Miracle Greens; Barleans Greens.

## Bodywork techniques

*Pick bodywork and relaxation techniques to accelerate your cleanse.*

**Enema:** Take an enema the night before or the morning of your cleanse. Flushing the colon is one of the best ways to jump start a cleanse; it allows a more expedient release of dead yeast cells and toxins from the body. Irrigate: Have at least colonic once during your cleanse for best results.

**Exercise:** Take a brisk walk for more body oxygen, and a positive mind and outlook. They are essential to overcome candida body stress. Try a good hearty laugh every day.

**Rest:** Candida infection often means interrupted sleep patterns.

**Flower remedies:** Deva Flower Assistance; Nelson Bach Rescue Remedy (for stress).

**Effective vaginal treatment:** use one or more.

• Stop candida transmission: Use a cleansing vaginal douche and penis soak, or pau d'arco, or 1 tsp. tea tree oil in 2 cups as a douche or soak.

• Nutribiotic Grapefruit Seed Extract as a vaginal douche or enema.

• Garlic douche or vaginal insertion.

• Acidophilus capsule insertions, or sprinkle powder on a tampon and insert.

• Make up a garlic, echinacea, myrrh solution in a squirt bottle and wash perineum after defecating to keep from reinfecting.

**Nail fungus soak:** Pau d' Arco tea.

**For thrush (yeast infection of the mouth):** use tea tree oil-based mouth washes, homeopathic thuja, and Black Walnut extract. Disinfect toothbrush with 3% hydrogen peroxide frequently.

**Note:** Nutritional yeast does not cause or aggravate candida albicans yeast overgrowth. It is one of the best immune-enhancing foods available. While it is well known that candida yeasts feed on dietary sugars, it is not well known that the yeasts also need minerals, and they deplete the minerals from our bodies. Restricting sugar in your permanent diet is essential. Supplement minerals to shore up mineral defiencies caused by the yeast… try Trace Mineral Research Concentrace; Arise & Shine Alkalizer.

# detox for female/male fertility problems

In America, 20% of married couples of child-bearing age have trouble conceiving and completing a successful pregnancy. The latest statistics show that around one in five U.S. couples is "infertile," which means that they have tried unsuccessfully to become pregnant for at least one year. The fertility industry is big business, grossing $2 billion a year. Fertility problems are complex and usually correctable without invasive procedures or fertility drugs.

Nutritionally, our diets are still lackluster, with an abundance of fats, sugars and processed foods forming the foundation for the meals many of us eat on a daily basis. Nature tries to avoid conception under conditions of inadequate nutrition or obesity. Environmentally, we're exposed to more toxic chemicals than any other generation, and many of these chemicals are known hormone disrupters that can affect ovulation and lower sperm count. And, both men and women are facing an epidemic of Sexually Transmitted Diseases, some of which can lead to sterility and increased risks during childbirth.

## Women's imbalances: overcoming fibroids and endometriosis

Reproductive blockages like fibroids, adhesions and endometriosis can impede conception efforts. An astounding 40% of American women 35 and older have fibroids. Uterine fibroids are actually more common than blue eyes! A hysterectomy is the common medical solution, but most women tell me they would rather deal with the fibroids! Uterine fibroids are benign growths between the size of a walnut and orange that appear on uterine walls. Their symptoms can be mild to severe with excessive menstrual bleeding, abdominal pain, bladder infections, painful intercourse and infertility topping the list.

Most uterine fibroids are not cancerous, and have less than ½ of 1% chance of becoming cancerous before menopause. Most fibroids go away on their own after menopause. Breast fibroids are also common, although they do not impact fertility. They feel like moveable, rubbery nodules near the breast surface. In a small number of cases, breast fibroids can be fast-growing and may require medical diagnosis. Even then, false cancer positives are reported in 30% of cases.

## How is endometriosis different?

Endometriosis is specifically caused by excess growth of endometrial tissue that is not shed during menstruation. The tissue escapes the uterus and spreads, attaching to other areas of the body—ovaries, lymph nodes, fallopian tubes, bladder, rectum, even kidneys and lungs. It grows abnormally, bleeding severely during the menstrual cycle, from the vagina or rectum, or bladder or back through the fallopian tubes, instead of normally through the vagina.

Endometriosis means heavy periods and pain all month long, and it increases risk for benign uterine and breast fibroids, and infertility. In fact, endometriosis is credited with up to 50% of infertility cases in American women. Still, even in advanced cases, fibroids and endometriosis can be reduced, even eliminated entirely by making simple diet changes and following specific herb and supplement protocols.

## Do you have warning signs of fibroids or endometriosis?

A visit to your holistic physician will give you a definitive diagnosis, but two or more yes answers to the symptoms below should alert you to a potential problem.

- severe abdominal cramping and shooting pain; and abdominal-rectal pain
- excessive, painful menstruation; passing large clots; prolonged abnormal menstrual cycles
- chronic fluid retention, bloating
- irregular bowel movements or diarrhea during menses

## What causes endometriosis and fibroids?

Scientists are still not entirely certain why endometriosis and fibroids develop, but here are major risk factors:

**Excess estrogen levels / Low progesterone levels:** Excess estrogen fuels abnormal tissue growth and is a direct cause of both fibroids and endometriosis for the majority of women. And, as I mentioned, when estrogen production declines during menopause, fibroids normally go away on their own. However, quite understandably, this isn't nearly soon enough for women who are suffering from the problem.

**X-Ray consequences:** Even low dose radiation may mean increased risk for fibroids. Breast tissue is so sensitive that the time between a mammogram and fibroid growth is sometimes as little as three months.

**High fat diet with too much caffeine and commercial meat:** This is especially a problem for breast fibroids. Eliminating caffeine and hormone-injected meats dramatically reduces fibrocystic breasts for many women.

**Oral contraceptives may play a role:** Your physician will tell you that newer pills are much better, and they are. Still, feedback I've had from birth control users has me convinced that even the newest low dose oral contraceptives can cause breast swelling, and aggravate fibroid problems and endometriosis for susceptible women.

## Get the best results from your fresh foods detox

- Trace minerals and protein are important. Add green superfoods to your diet for the most rapid results.
- Herbal adaptogens like ginseng noticeably improve the way your body handles stress. Add herbs like panax ginseng, suma, jiaogulan, Siberian eleuthero, gotu kola, dong quai and ashwagandha to your program.
- Eat smaller meals. Overeating can suppress hormone production.
- Limit dairy foods and meats (especially beef), notoriously high in hormone-disrupting chemicals. Look for natural poultry at health food stores—Petaluma Poultry Rosie the Organic Chicken, Diestel and Coleman Natural Products.
- Wash produce to reduce hormone disrupting pollutant residues; Healthy Harvest Fruit/Vegetable Rinse.
- Add fermented soy foods (tofu, tempeh, miso, etc.) to your diet for hormone normalizing isoflavones.
- Drink green tea to flush out fats that harbor estrogen-disrupting chemicals.
- Eat cruciferous veggies like steamed broccoli and cauliflower to help flush excess estrogens out.

## A 3 – 5 day fresh foods detox diet for female fertility

A fresh foods cleansing diet is recommended to clear your body of toxins and allow it a brief rest before trying to conceive. Hormone imbalance disorders like PMS, fibroids and endometriosis can be overcome or reduced as congestive wastes leave the body. Eliminate caffeine during your cleansing diet for the best improvement of female problems. Avoid red meats, excess dairy, hard alcohol (too much sugar), sodas and tobacco. Note: Avoid all liquid diets, long cleanses (more than 24 hours) or strong laxatives if you're already pregnant.

The night before your cleanse… have a green leafy salad to give your bowels a good sweep. Take an herbal laxative. Drink 8 to 10 glasses of water a day to hydrate, and flush wastes and toxins from all cells.

**On rising:** take lemon juice in water with 1 tsp. maple syrup; or a glass of aloe vera juice with herbs and 1 tsp. Red Star nutritional yeast flakes; or green tea, or Crystal Star Conceptions tea to support female fertility.

**Breakfast:** take 2 tsp. of cranberry concentrate in water with 1 tsp. honey for bladder kidney support; or Jarrow Fermented Soy Essence drink for estrogen balancing; and fresh fruit with yogurt and toasted wheat germ.

**Mid-morning:** have a mixed vegetable juice with carrot, dandelion greens, beet, cucumber and parsley for a liver detox; or Knudsen's Very Veggie Juice with 1 tsp. Bragg's Liquid Aminos.

**Lunch:** have a Potassium broth (pg. 101) or a bowl of miso soup with 1 tsp. nutritional yeast for B vitamins; or have a green salad with sprouts, carrots and lemon/oil dressing and sea vegetables sprinkled on top.

**Mid-afternoon:** have a green drink like Crystal Star Energy Green for balance; and some raw crunchy veggies (especially broccoli and cauliflower) with a vegetable dip.

**Dinner:** have brown rice and steamed vegetables and a balancing herb tea, like Crystal Star Conceptions tea to support female fertility; or a high fiber fruit smoothie with bananas, peaches, pears, berries and a handful of flax seeds.

**Before Bed:** have an apple-alfalfa sprout juice; or 1 tsp. cranberry concentrate in chamomile tea; or a cup of Crystal Star Stress Arrest tea for easier sleep.

## Supplement choices for women's fertility

**For women with abnormal periods:** Crystal Star Female Harmony caps or tea, Fertility aids: Crystal Star Conceptions tea (highly recommended) with Vitex extract or Rainbow Light Vitex-Black Cohosh Complex; For longterm balance, Moon Maid Botanicals Pro-meno wild yam cream, or Crystal Star Pro-Est Balance gel roll-on; Note: New Research shows taking standardized St. John's wort with oral contraceptives can increase intracyclic bleeding (J. Clin Pharmacol 2003; 56:683-90).

**For uterine fibroids and endometriosis:** Crystal Star Women's Best Friend 6 daily for 3 months, then Breast & Uterine Fibro Defense 4 daily for 3 months (highly recommended); or Pacific Biologic GynoEase. Protease enzyme therapy shows excellent results. Consider Crystal Star Dr. Enzyme with Protease & Bromelain to help dissolve abnormal growths.

Note: Protease may thin the blood. Ask your natural health practitioner if protease enzyme therapy is right for you.

**For breast fibroids:** Crystal Star Fibro Defense caps for 3 months, then Vitex extract 2x daily with Burdock tea 2 cups daily for one month. Also: Evening Primrose Oil 3000 mg. daily, vitamin E 800IU with folic acid 800 mcg. daily; and Nature's Way Dim-Plus.

**Hormone tonics for more energy:** Crystal Star Great Ginseng! and Adrenal Energy; Planetary Schizandra Adrenal Support; Crystal Star Toxin Detox if you are regularly exposed to pollutants.

**Essential fatty acids normalize hormone production:** Evening primrose oil, 3000 – 4000 mg. daily; Barleans Essential Woman; Nature's Secret Ultimate Oil; Udo's Perfected Oil Blend.

**Hormone support nutrients:** Calcium-magnesium 2000 mg. daily, iron 20 mg.; B-complex 100 mg.; Iodine, potassium and silica from sea veggies are key to endocrine health: Crystal Star Ocean Minerals or Iodine Source extract (highly recommended).

## Bodywork techniques

**Exercise:** Exercise is a cleansing nutrient in itself because it changes body chemistry.

1. Take a regular 20 minute "gland health" walk every day (especially good to help overcome fibroids and endometriosis).

2. Do yoga stretches every morning.

3. Get morning sunlight on the body every day possible, on the arms for women.

4. Do deep breathing.

**Castor oil packs:** Castor oil has been used medicinally since the times of ancient Egypt. Used in a pack, castor oil is part of a traditional naturopathic protocol for reduction and relief of endometriosis, ovarian cysts, fibroids, mild pain and digestive complaints. A castor oil pack applied to the skin enhances circulation, detoxifies and supports healing of tissues, and digestive and reproductive organs.

**How to make a castor oil pack:** First, soak a piece of flannel in castor oil and place it on the area you want to treat (low abdomen for menstrual problems, ovarian cysts, endometriosis or fibroids,). Cover with a plastic sheet, and a hot water bottle to keep it warm. (Watch out because castor oil can stain clothing.) Relax with the pack on for 1 hour. Use 5 days a week for best results.

- **Bathe/Sauna:** Hot ginger baths increase circulation to the pelvic region for relief; just add 2 strongly brewed cups of ginger tea to the bath water; or try Crystal Star Hot Seaweed Bath for pH balance.

## Men's imbalances: low sperm count

Today twenty million U.S. men are characterized as semen infertile. Millions more are described as semen sub-fertile. Poor sperm motility (rather than low sperm count) affects about 10% of infertile men. Further, while age does not impact male fertility to the extent that it does female, a gradual lessening of semen quality does occur for men each decade after age 40. Testosterone levels start to decline around age 40, falling up to 10% each decade. This phenomenon, called "andropause" is now recognized by almost eight in ten family physicians as a real condition that affects quality of life for men.

Apart from the more common problems of low sperm count and motility, men's infertility can also be caused by sickle cell anemia, metabolic disorders, testicular cancer or trauma, undescended testes, anatomical obstructions, and varicocele (abnormally dilated testicular veins which affect sperm production). 19 to 41% of infertile men have a varicocele which may require medical treatment for reversal. Note: Some herbs can decrease varicocele. The Chinese combination Guizhi-Fuling-Wan (Cinnamon and Poria Formula) and the herb tribulus terrestris have been shown clinically to reduce infertility caused by varicocele.

## The chemical link to male infertility

A healthy human male produces about 1500 sperm with every heartbeat. However, worldwide studies show sperm counts have dropped on average by more than half over the last 50 years (one report from Britain shows a drop of 160 per milliliter to 66 million per milliliter). Sperm are rich in lipids, highly sensitive to free radical damage from toxic chemicals and pollutants. In one study, high free radical levels in the male reproductive tract was linked to infertility in 40% of men. In another study, a significant decline of sperm quality was seen in men with high exposure to three pesticides: alachlor, diazinon and atrazine, all commonly found in today's water supplies.

Long term exposure to solvents like paint, printing presses, and dry cleaning chemicals is also linked to male infertility. Over 1,000 workplace chemicals have been linked to reproductive problems. Exogenous estrogens from pesticides can lower sperm count, affect sperm viability and reduce the amount of seminal fluid produced by men. The highest risk jobs are: livestock and dairy farmers, fruit and flower growers, and gardeners. Men who work in plastic production, welding or who work with lead or other heavy metals face reproductive hazards, too.

## What other nutritional and lifestyle factors reduce male fertility?

A fast food diet high in trans fat and low in protective antioxidants decreases male fertility. Deficiencies of vitamin C and E are linked to male fertility problems. Too much workplace stress is a fertility blocker for men. Research from the University of Calgary shows men with the most daily work stress produce ⅓ less sperm than men under low stress. Heavy drinking and recreational drug use are other factors in low sperm count, sperm abnormalities and decreased sexual performance. Smoking is a major infertility factor that reduces the ability of sperm to bind to an egg. As with women, being overweight or underweight can also lead to fertility problems in men.

## A 3 – 5 day fresh foods detox diet for male fertility

A healthy detox for men's fertility is full of antioxidant-rich foods to fight free radical damage, and high quality protein for foundation body strength. Further, the mineral zinc is crucial for male reproductive health. Zinc is involved in sperm formation and motility, and testosterone metabolism, too. Low zinc levels reduce testosterone levels and seminal volume. Low prostate zinc levels have especially been connected to prostate cancer. Your long term diet should include more zinc-rich foods like fish and seafood (especially shellfish like oysters), seeds (sunflower, pumpkin and caraway), nutritional yeast, eggs, mushroom and wheat germ. For reproductive health, avoid or reduce consumption of tobacco, caffeine, and alcohol. Note: Pesticide residues on commercially grown foods can disrupt male fertility by lowering sperm count. Buy organic!

**On rising:** Have a protein drink like Metabolic Response Modifiers Whey Pumped or Pure Form Whey Protein drink. Add 1 – 2 tsp. of Herbs America Maca Magic powder for extra fertility help.

**Breakfast:** Have a glass of fresh squeezed orange, tangerine or pomegranate juice for antioxidants; or a "Prostate Sediment Cleanser" juice on pg. 108 if you also have BPH. Or, have a high fiber fruit bowl with apple, pear, pineapple or papaya.

**Midmorning:** Make a mix of nutritional yeast, bee pollen granules, wheat germ and oat bran: blend 2 tsp. into a superfood drink like Green Foods Green Magma, Barleans Greens or Aloe Life Daily Greens.

**Lunch:** Have a green leafy salad with a lemon oil or Italian dressing. Include celery, avocados and some grilled fresh fish like wild salmon if available.

**Mid-Afternoon:** Have a cup of ginseng or licorice root tea (avoid licorice if you have high blood pressure) and a handful of pumpkin seeds for zinc.

**Dinner:** Have a bowl of vegetarian minestrone soup or lentil soup. Have another protein drink like Metabolic Response Modifiers Whey Pumped or Pure Form Whey Protein drink. Add 1 – 2 tsp. of Herbs America Maca Magic powder for extra fertility help.

**Before bed:** Have a nutritional yeast broth or small bottle of mineral water.

The male system responds quickly to nutritional changes. In addition, supplementation can produce dramatic renewed fertility results for men. Consider the following supplements for a man's fertility and virility program.

## Supplement Choices for Men's Fertility

*Choose 2 or 3 supplement recommendations.*

**Natural vitamin E,** 400IU daily. New studies show vitamin E fights free radical damage and significantly improves sperm motility and fertility in men. A selenium supplement can improve sperm function. Try Vitamin E 400IU with selenium 200mcg daily (tests show pregnancies rise 21%).

**Folic acid,** 800mcg daily (a key fertility nutrient for men, too) with **Zinc** 50 – 75mg daily or Ethical Nutrients Zinc Status (tests for deficiency, too). A 2002 study published in Fertility and Sterility showed men who took folic acid and zinc together had a 74% increase in total sperm count.

**B12** helps about half of men with low sperm count.

Tests show the amino acid **L-carnitine,** 500 – 3000mg daily, boosts sperm quality in subfertile men.

**L-arginine,** 2000 – 4000mg can raise sperm count and motility (contraindicated if you have herpes).

**Pycnogenol** shows good results for sperm quality. In a clinical test with subfertile men, 200mg daily of pycnogenol improved sperm quality and motility by 38%.

**Vitamin C,** 3000mg daily and **niacin** 500mg (good results for low sperm count or sperm clumping).

To remove heavy metals, especially lead from pesticides, consider Crystal Star Toxin Detox caps, 6 daily. Add extra glutathione for antioxidant defense. I like Carlson Glutathione Booster.

## Bodywork for men

**Exercise is a key fertility nutrient for men.** Exercise stimulates circulation to the genitals and increases body oxygen. In one study, 78 healthy, but sedentary men were studied during nine months of regular exercise. The men exercised for 60 minutes a day, three days a week. Every man in the study reported significantly enhanced sexuality, including increased frequency, performance and satisfaction. The rise in sexuality was even correlated with how much each man's fitness improved!

**Consider acupuncture:** There are many reports of acupuncture improving sperm count, motility and morphology (shape) for infertile or subfertile men. In one 1987 study reported in the Journal of Chinese Acupuncture, of 248 men who received acupuncture to treat infertility, 89 were cured, 77 made significant improvements and 85 experienced no change.

**Avoid electric blankets, hot tubs and hot water beds.**

**Sun bathe in the morning, nude if possible for 15 minutes.**

# gallstone cleanse

In America, high bile cholesterol levels are the main cause of gallstones, with most stones (80 – 90%) composed of cholesterol, bile salts, bile pigments and inorganic calcium salts. About 20 million Americans have gallstones, and gallbladder cholecystitis (acute gallbladder inflammation); three fourths of them are women. Gallstones are far easier to prevent than to reverse. New research shows eating just one large orange a day may reduce gallstone risk. When bile in the gallbladder becomes supersaturated with cholesterol (bile cholesterol does not necessarily correlate with blood cholesterol), it combines with other particulate matter and begins to form a stone. A stone may grow for 6 to 8 years before symptoms occur. Since continuing formation of the gallstone is dependent on either more cholesterol accumulation or less bile acid or lecithin levels, it's easy to see that anywhere along the way, diet improvement will deter, even arrest, stone development. What else causes gallstones? High risk factors for gallbladder disease include a poor diet with high cholesterol and low bile acids, chronic indigestion and gas from too much dairy and refined sugars, obesity, certain drugs (notably HRT (hormone replacement therapy) drugs), age, and Crohn's disease. Yo-yo dieting increases risk of gallstones. (I personally knew a 64-year-old woman who died from her gallstones that became severe through twenty-five years of yo-yo dieting.) Gastrointestinal diseases, like Crohn's disease and diverticulitis may be involved along with dietary factors like high blood sugar, high calorie and saturated fat intake. Oral contraceptives and some estrogen replacement drugs have been implicated.

## Is your body showing signs that it needs a gallstone cleanse?

Gallstones are present in 95% of people suffering from cholecystitis (gallbladder inflammation). There may be no identifiable symptoms, except for periods of nausea and intense abdominal pain that radiates to the upper back. Ultrasound provides a definitive diagnosis.

**Important note:** Have a sonogram before embarking on a flush to determine the size of the stones.

Traditional naturopathic medicine has relied on natural gallbladder cleansing flushes as an effective method for passing and dissolving gallstones. Depending on the size of the stones and the length of time they have been forming, the flushing programs may last from 3 days to a month. If your sonogram shows that your gallstones are too large to pass through the bile and urethral ducts (less than 1% of cases), they must be dissolved first. Try using the Crystal Star Stone-ex herbal program for 1 month (2 caps 3x daily with 3 to 5 cups of Chamomile tea). If pain and symptoms do not improve, you should consult a health professional. Surgical methods may be necessary. **Note:** If olive oil is hard for you to take straight, sip it through a straw.

## Pointers for best results from your gallstone cleanse:

- Once stones have passed, concentrate your diet on strengthening the liver/gallbladder area to prevent further stone formation.
- Drink at least eight 8 oz. glasses of bottled water each day.
- Eliminate foods that create an allergy response. Allergenic substances cause swelling of bile ducts, impairing bile flow. Common allergy-causing foods that may induce gallstone symptoms are eggs (very troublesome), pork, onions, milk, citrus, corn, beans and nuts.
- Coffee (including decaf) aggravates gallbladder problems. Avoid coffee until the stones are resolved.

## Benefits you'll notice as your body responds to a gallstone cleanse

Relief signs are quickly apparent. Nausea and abdominal pain stop. The gallbladder plays an important part in the digestion of fats. Digestion of fats and overall digestion will improve. A healthy appetite should return.

## Gallstone cleanse nutrition plan

*This is a 9 day gallstone flush plan.*

### Three day olive oil and lemon juice flush

**On rising:** take 2 tbsp. olive oil and juice of 1 lemon in water. Sip through a straw if desired.

**Breakfast:** have a glass of organic apple juice.

**Mid-morning:** have 2 cups of chamomile or cascara tea.

**Lunch:** take another glass of lemon juice and olive oil in water; and a glass of fresh apple juice.

**Mid-afternoon:** have 2 cups of chamomile tea or cascara tea.

**Dinner:** have a glass of carrot/beet/cucumber juice; or a potassium juice or broth (pages 101).

**Before Bed:** take another cup of chamomile tea.

### Follow with a 5 day alkalizing diet

**On rising:** take 2 tbsp. cider vinegar in water with 1 tsp. honey; or a glass of grapefruit juice.

**Breakfast:** have a glass of carrot/beet/cucumber juice, or a potassium broth or juice.

**Mid-morning:** have 2 cups of chamomile tea, and a glass of organic apple juice.

**Lunch:** take a vegetable drink with Pure Planet Chlorella; Crystal Star Energy Green Drink Mix; a small green salad with lemon-olive oil dressing and a cup of dandelion tea.

**Mid-afternoon:** have 2 cups of chamomile tea, and another glass of apple juice.

**Dinner:** have a small green salad with lemon-oil dressing; add daikon radish shreds as a gentle diuretic flusher and another glass of apple juice.

**Before Bed:** 1 cup chamomile or dandelion tea.

### End with a one day intensive olive oil flush

At 7 p.m. on the evening of the 5th day of the alkalizing diet, mix one pint of olive oil and 10 juiced lemons; take ¼ cup every 15 minutes until it is gone. Lie on the right side for best assimilation

## Herbs & supplements

*Choose 2 to 3 cleansing boosters.*

**Fiber supplements reduce risk of stones:** Fiber absorbs excess cholesterol so it can be eliminated. Fiber is most important in preventing and removing gallstones. Jarrow Gentle Fibers; Futurebiotics Colon Green; Aloe Life FiberMate; All One Whole Fiber Complex.

**Increase bile solubility to reduce cholesterol levels:** Nature's Way enteric coated peppermint oil caps Pepogest; Crystal Star Bitters & Lemon extract to help dissolve bile solids. Herbal Answers Aloe Vera Juice with herbs daily, with milk thistle seed extract drops added to each glass.

**Lipotropics remove fat deposits:** Omega-3 flax seed oil 3x daily; Vitamin A 25,000IU & D 1000IU. Methionine tablets before meals; Vitamin E 400 IU daily.

**Enzyme support:** Enzyme Essentials Lypozyme contains highest amount of lipase found in any product to help break down of gallstones.

**Herbal sediment dissolvers:** Crystal Star Stone-ex caps (with dandelion, gravel root, milk thistle and hydrangea) and Planetary Formulas Stone Free have a long successful history of dissolving sediment. Milk thistle extract increases solubility of the bile to help dissolve gallstones. Hydrangea is a stone solvent for gall and kidney stones. Gymnema sylvestre capsules balance blood sugar to reduce a cause of stones. Turmeric contains curcumin which increases the solubility of bile to keep prevent gallstones from forming and helps eliminate already formed stones, Jarrow Formulas Curcumin-95.

**Peppermint and chamomile tea** helps dissolve gallstones. Peppermint oil in an enteric-coated capsule may also be used between meals.

## Bodywork techniques

*Pick bodywork and relaxation techniques to accelerate and round out your cleanse.*

**Enema:** Take an enema at the beginning of the cleanse to release toxins in the colon and remove undo stress on the gallbladder through backup of colonic toxins. (Enema instructions page 151).

**Apply castor oil packs** to the abdomen daily throughout the cleanse for 1 to 2 hours at a time.

**Take a gallstone essential oil bath:** Add a total of 10 drops of essential oils to your bath. Stir the water briskly to disperse evenly. Use a combination of two or three of the following essential oils: bergamot, lemon, eucalyptus, chamomile, camphor, geranium, hyssop, lavender, or rosemary. Or, put a total of 15 drops of these above essential oils in 1 oz. of jojoba oil and rub on gallbladder area.

**Flower Essence Remedies:** Bach Flower Rescue Remedy or Deva Flowers Crab Apple.

## For your continuing diet

The key to both prevention and control of gallstones is diet improvement. Increase your fresh fruit and vegetable intake for more food fiber. Vegetable proteins from foods like soy, oat bran and sea vegetables help prevent gallstone formation. Reduce your intake of animal protein, especially dairy products (casein in dairy products increases formation of gallstones). Avoid fried foods and sugary foods altogether if you are at risk for gallstones

# detox diet for GERD

GERD (Gastroesophageal reflux disease) is due to leaking of stomach acid back into the esophagus and acid coming up into the throat. GERD also occurs in severe cases of osteoporosis, when the rib cage and upper body collapse to the point where normal food transit is impeded. (My mother suffered from this; it was extremely painful.) People who suffer from acid

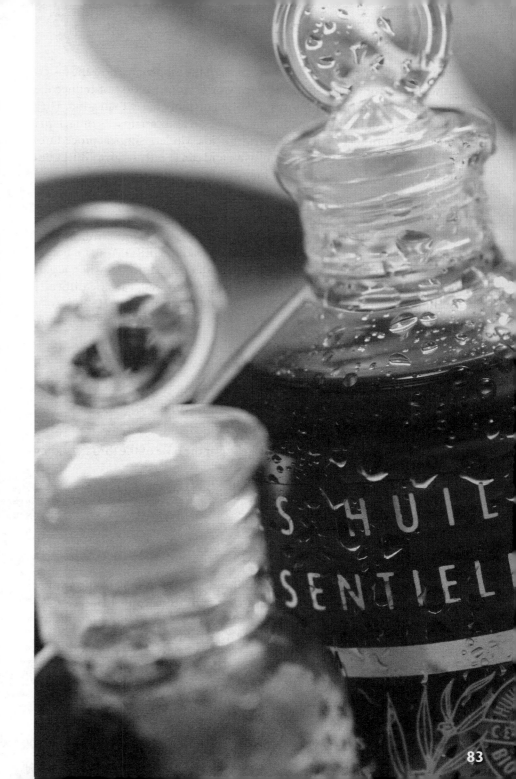

reflux are far more likely to develop cancer of the esophagus, now the fastest growing type of cancer in the western world. Antacids do not reduce the cancer risk, only mask symptoms and often do more harm than good. They don't prevent or cure the underlying condition and can upset stomach pH causing it to produce even more harmful acids. Modern surgical procedures like Laparoscopic are minimally invasive and can greatly reduce GERD, but surgery side effects like diarrhea may be permanent.

What puts you at risk for GERD? Overeating and resulting obesity, enzyme deficiency, constipation from a low residue diet and too many fast foods, fried foods and dairy foods (all acid-forming), prescription drug side effects, and severe osteoporosis can all lead to GERD. A hiatal hernia is another common cause of GERD. A hiatal hernia occurs when a part of the stomach protrudes through the diaphragm wall, causing difficulty swallowing and breathing, burning and reflux in the throat, and great nervous anxiety. Today's American diet habits mean that a hiatal condition is common… and so is GERD.

## Signs you may have GERD

- Chest pains, heartburn and bloating after eating
- Belching, hiccups and regurgitation after eating
- Difficulty swallowing and a full feeling at the base of the throat, leading to chronic hoarseness
- Raised blood pressure usually accompanied by gastro-intestinal bleeding, or a stomach ulcer

## The problem with antacids…

15 million Americans have heartburn daily. Another 50 million suffer heartburn at least once a week severe enough to disrupt their sleep. We spend $1.7 billion on indigestion remedies each year! But antacids are designed to provide only temporary relief. Evidence is piling up that excessive use of over-the-counter antacids may cause long term problems for digestive health. They may even become a health problem themselves because they radically change your digestive chemistry.

## Do any of these antacid side effects pertain to you?

**The tolerance effect:** The more you use antacids, the more you need them. Antacids neutralize stomach HCl (hydrochloric acid), needed for digestion, or they block it, confuse the body and disrupt its normal processes. If you take a lot of antacids, your body overcompensates, producing excess stomach acid.

**Antacids disrupt your pH balance:** Optimum pH is between 7.35 and 7.45. If you take lots of antacids, your GI tract fluctuates between over alkaline and over acid, leading to problems like diarrhea or constipation, gallbladder disorders and hiatal hernia. A friend thought his heartburn symptoms would improve if he doubled his acid blocker dosage. He ended up in the bathroom all night, passing completely undigested food. Disrupting body pH alters bowel ecology, potentially causing dramatic growth of harmful organisms, like candida yeasts.

**Pernicious ingredients:** Many antacids contain aluminum which causes constipation and bone pain. Others overdose you on magnesium causing diarrhea. Some contain both aluminum and magnesium, so you may get alternating constipation and diarrhea. Antacids full of sodium may cause water retention.

**Some drugs interact with antacids:** People on drug therapy for HIV should know antacids can decrease their HIV drug absorption by up to 23%. Oral contraceptives like "the pill" may lose their effectiveness if taken with antacids. People using NSAIDS drugs for arthritis along with antacids suffer 2½ times more serious gastrointestinal complications than those taking a placebo! Antacids not only block drug absorption, they also block your food absorption of nutrients, especially B12, necessary for virtually all immune responses.

**Some antacids build up and impede body processes:** I know a woman who was hospitalized three times for kidney stones. Her physician advised her to stop taking her antacids because the unabsorbed calcium in them was causing her kidney stones.

**By blocking critical stomach acid, your natural line of defense against germs, proton pump inhibiting drugs can lead to serious disease.** The newest research reveals protein-pump-inhibiting drugs, now available over-the-counter, may double the risk of penumonia, especially dangerous for the elderly or those with weakened immune systems.

## Detox diet plan for chronic heartburn or GERD

*Cleanse the digestive system and establish good enzymes.*

Start with a detox, pectin mono diet of apples and apple juice for 2 days. (For people that really suffer, this makes them feel better almost right away.) Then for 4 days, use a diet of 70% fresh foods and brown rice for B vitamins. Take 2 glasses of mineral water or aloe vera juice daily. Add high fiber foods gradually if digestion is delicate. When digestion has normalized, follow a low fat, low salt, high fiber diet.

### Follow with an alkalizing, purifying plant-based diet

- For ongoing relief, drink juices for stomach acid balance at least once daily. Choose from: Carrot juice, or Green Foods Carrot Essence for healing vitamin A; Carrot/cabbage, a stomach healer; Pineapple-papaya for extra enzymes; Liquid chlorophyll, 1 tsp. in water before meals.
- Eat plenty of cultured foods like yogurt, kefir and miso soup, fresh and lightly steamed vegetables, fruits, and enzyme-rich foods like papaya and pineapple. More alkaline-forming foods to add: mineral water, sea veggies, herb tea, miso, brown rice, honey, and most fruits. (Some melons aggravate reflux.)
- Eliminate fried and spicy foods—they slow the rate at which your stomach empties, allowing food to travel back to the esophagus. Eliminate refined carbohydrates and sugary foods—they boost gastric acidity.
- Omit red meats, fatty dairy foods, dried fruits, sodas and caffeine (coffee especially forms acid). Switch to herbal teas, like a green and white tea blend with ginger for better digestion.
- Foods that aggravate a hiatal hernia: coffee, chocolate, red meats, hard alcohol drinks, sodas.
- Frequent bouts of hiccups are very common today—try Wild Cherry tea (sometimes dramatic help).

## Quick Tips:

- If 1 tsp. cider vinegar in water relieves your heartburn, you need more stomach acid.

- If you are bloated, take ½ tsp. baking soda in water to ease distension. (short term)
- If you have flatulence, take a catnip or slippery elm enema for immediate relief.
- If your stomach is sour, settle it with lime juice and a pinch of ginger.
- If you absorb poorly, a glass of wine can offer better absorption.
- At first sign of heartburn, take 2 oz. aloe vera juice.

## These supplements help normalize digestion and smooth out heartburn

**Bitters herbs help the cause of heartburn:** Crystal Star Bitters & Lemon extract each morning as a preventive; Flora Gallexier; Gaia Herbs Sweetish Bitters; Crystal Star GERD Guard caps before and after meals (highly recommended).

**Enzyme therapy:** Crystal Star Dr. Enzyme (between meals for best results); Nature's Plus chewable bromelain; American Health Papaya Chewables; Transformation Digestzyme and Gastrozyme.

**Get to the heart of heartburn:** L-glutamine 1500 mg. daily for long-term relief; Nutricology Perm A Vite if you also have leaky gut syndrome. Lane Labs Nature's Lining to strengthen the stomach wall (highly recommended); Betaine HCl capsules after meals for people over 40.

**Soothe the burn:** Slippery elm tea or lozenges; Marshmallow tea; Hylands homeopathic Indigestion after meals; Umeboshi plum paste. Acute indigestion: Nature's Herbs DGL Power; 2 tbsp. Aloe vera juice.

**For belching and burping:** AkPharma Beano drops; Rainbow Light Advanced Enzyme System.

**Good digestive teas:** Peppermint, spearmint or alfalfa-mint tea; ginger, dill, caraway ease digestion. Catnip-fennel-lemon peel tea; Chamomile tea; Wild Yam tea, especially if you have eaten too much refined sugar.

**Probiotics for friendly flora:** UAS DDS-plus + FOS; Jarrow Jarro-Dophilus.

Bodywork and lifestyle changes do wonders for digestion.

- Avoid all tobacco. Nicotine affects gastric functions.
- Lie on your back and draw knees up to chest to relieve abdomen pressure. To prevent night time reflux, elevate head off bed 6 – 8 inches. Don't eat within two hours of your bedtime.
- Have a chiropractic adjustment to the area or a massage therapy treatment at least once a month. (I have personally seen massage therapy work for many people.)
- NAET (Nambudripad Allergy Elimination Technique) helps eliminate food allergy reflux.
- Try to eat when relaxed. Eat smaller meals. Chew food very well. No liquids with meals. Eat slowly so that you are less likely to swallow air and belch. Don't lie down after eating.

# kidney stone cleanse

Every decade since World War II, the U.S. has seen a steady rise in kidney stone cases. Today 10% of American men and 5% of American women have a kidney stone by the time they're seventy. Kidney stones are directly linked to low dietary fiber, high fat and high calcium (usually from dairy sources), and large amounts of animal protein, refined sugar, alcohol and salt. They parallel the rise of the Standard American Diet, full of fat, fried foods, rich dairy products and sugar. Excessive use of antacids and adrenal exhaustion also contribute to kidney stones. Kidney stones form when minerals that normally float free in the kidney fluids combine into crystals. Too much inorganic mineral waste and too little fluid, means the molecules can't dissolve and form sharp-edged stones. There are three types of kidney stones: those composed of calcium salts, the most common type (75 – 85% incidence), struvite, or non-calcium-containing crystals (10 – 15% incidence), and uric acid crystals (at about 5 – 8%). It takes from 5 to 15 hours of vigorous, urgent treatment to dissolve and pass small stones.

A vegetarian diet, low in proteins and starches, that emphasizes fresh fruits, vegetables and cultured foods to alkalize the system, is the key to avoiding kidney stone formation. This type of diet is high in fiber to reduce urinary calcium waste. It eliminates acid-forming foods, like caffeine-containing foods, salty, sugary and fried foods and soft drinks that inhibit kidney filtering. It avoids mucous-forming foods, like pasteurized dairy products, heavy grains, starches and fats, to relieve irritation and inhibit sediment formation.

## Is your body showing signs that it needs a kidney stone cleanse?

There may be no apparent symptoms at first except a dull ache in the lower back. When the stone(s) become large enough to block the urinary tract, there is excruciating, radiating pain with extremely painful urination. The abdomen becomes distended. A woman may have heavy menstrual bleeding or anemia, signs of a vitamin K deficiency, which can lead to stones. As infection sets in, there are chills, nausea, vomiting and fever.

## Pointers for best results from your kidney stone cleanse

- Dehydration which causes a reduction in urine volume and an increased rate of excretion of stone constituents is a factor relating to kidney stones. Drink 8 – 10 glasses of bottled water each day of your cleanse, so that waste and excess minerals are continuously flushed.
- Use fresh vegetable and fresh fruit juices during your cleanse.

## After your cleanse

- When you begin eating solid foods, make sure you are eating enough fresh fruits and vegetables. Studies have shown that even meat eaters showed a lower incidence of stones when they ate higher amounts of fresh fruits and vegetables.
- Keep salt and protein low for at least 3 weeks.
- Establish a diet with plenty of fiber.

## Kidney stone cleanse  nutrition plan

*Start with this 3 to 5 day nutrition plan.*

**Vitamin K is an important part** of your body's natural inhibitors of kidney stone formation. Spinach and sea vegetables, high in vitamin K, help vegetarians have a lower incidence of kidney stones.

**Take 2 tbsp. olive oil through a straw** every 4 hours to help dissolve stones.

### The night before your kidney stone cleanse...

**Take a cup of chamomile tea.**

### The next 2 – 4 days...

**On rising:** take cranberry juice (from concentrate) in water with 1 tsp. honey; or 2 tbsp. apple cider vinegar in water with 1 tsp. honey; or Crystal Star Green Tea Cleanser; and a cup of chamomile tea.

**Breakfast:** have a glass of cranberry juice, or fresh watermelon juice, or watermelon chunks.

**Mid-morning:** take 1 cup watermelon seed tea. (grind seeds, steep in hot water 30 minutes, add honey); or a green drink (see next column); or dandelion tea, or Crystal Star Bladder Comfort tea.

**Lunch:** have a carrot/beet/cucumber juice, and a spinach salad with cucumbers.

**Mid-afternoon:** have a cup of chamomile tea; and asparagus stalks and carrot sticks with kefir cheese; or fresh apples with kefir or yogurt dip.

**Dinner:** have brown rice with tofu and steamed veggies; or steamed asparagus with miso soup and snipped, dry sea veggies on top; or a baked potato with kefir cheese and a spinach salad; or baked or broiled salmon with rice and baked onions.

**Before Bed:** take a glass of aloe vera juice and another cup of chamomile tea; or miso/ginger soup with sea vegetables sprinkled on top.

## Herbs & supplements

*Choose 2 to 3 cleansing boosters.*

**Kidney stone cleansers:** ascorbate or Ester C powder in water; ¼ tsp. every hour to bowel tolerance until stones pass—about 5000mg daily.

**Mineral balancers to prevent stones:** Flora Vege-Sil caps 2 daily for kidney stone prevention; Solaray Calcium Citrate 4 daily, with QBC to reduce inflammation.

**Vitamin C** 3000mg with bioflavonoids daily for a month to acidify urine and prevent stones;

**Futurebiotics Vital K** or vitamin K 100mcg daily.

**Enzyme support:** Crystal Star Dr. Enzyme (a protease supplement that breaks apart protein-based viscid matter that cements salts into stones) or Enzyme Essentials Excell-zyme (kidney antioxidant).

**Dissolve kidney sediment wastes:** Crystal Star Stone-ex caps; Enzymatic Therapy Acid-A-Cal caps to dissolve sedimentary waste, with bromelain 500mg daily; Trimedica Alkamax.

**Chamomile, rosemary, or dandelion/nettles tea**—about 5 cups a day for one to 2 weeks.

**Jean's Greens P.P.T. tea.**

**Chlorophyll superfood** for vitamin K to inhibit growth of stones: Crystal Star Energy Green, Barleans Greens, Fit For You, Intl. Miracle Greens; Sun Wellness Chlorella 2 pkts. daily.

**Fiber supplements** reduce risk of stones: All One Whole Fiber Complex; Nature's Secret Ultimate Fiber; Aloe Life Fiber Mate.

## Bodywork techniques

*Pick bodywork and relaxation techniques to accelerate and round out your cleanse.*

**Exercise:** Take a daily brisk walk to keep kidney function flowing. Stagnate urine flow is a factor in kidney stone formation.

**Enemas:** Take an enema the first, second and the last day of your kidney cleansing program to help release toxins. Use spirulina, or catnip enemas.

See enema instructions (page 151) in this book.

**Heat therapy:** Apply wet, hot compresses and lower back massage when there is inflammation flare up, especially lobelia or ginger fomentations. Take hot saunas when possible to release toxins and excess fluids, and to flush acids out through the skin.

**Massage therapy:** At least once during your cleanse to stimulate circulation and reduce pain.

**Bladder/Kidney Baths:** Take hot and cold, or Epsom salts sitz baths to stimulate circulation.

**Aromatherapy kidney stress relief:** Add a total of 8 – 10 drops of essential oil to your bath. Stir the water briskly to disperse evenly. Use a combination of two or three of the following essential oils: juniper, cedarwood, sandalwood, lemon, chamomile, eucalyptus or geranium.

**Note:** Avoid antacids for indigestion. They may increase risk for stone formation.

## For your continuing diet

Avoid oxalic acid-forming foods, like cooked spinach, chard or rhubarb, chocolate, black tea, coffee and grapes during your cleanse. Avoid all yeast-containing foods during a kidney stone cleanse… no baked breads. After the cleanse, follow a low salt, low protein, vegetarian diet with 75% fresh foods for 2 weeks. Avoid all refined, fried, fatty foods, cola drinks, salty, sugary foods, and caffeine-containing foods. Eliminate dairy and reduce animal protein for 1 month.

# modified cancer detox

Did you know that cancer used to be extremely rare? Today 200 different diseases fall under the cancer label. Statistics now show that more than one in three Americans will eventually get cancer. Right now, ten million Americans are living with cancer. 1.4 million more will be diagnosed this year. Almost 560,000 Americans are expected to die from the disease this year. Cancer costs the economy $206 billion annually, making it the most expensive disease in the U.S. by far.

Yet, the newest research shows that if we spent more time on cancer prevention rather than treatment, the number of cancer deaths in the U.S. could drop by nearly a third. That translates into 100,000 fewer cancer cases and 60,000 prevented cancer deaths by 2015! But, powerful chemotherapy drugs, radiation and surgery are still the main "approved" cancer therapies, and they come at great cost- often for health and your pocketbook.

Detoxification followed by diet improvement is a major weapon against cancer. Dietary factors are undeniably involved in the vast majority of cancers. Improving your diet directly improves your defenses against cancer. The more fruits and vegetables you eat, the less your cancer risk from colon and stomach cancer to breast, even lung cancer. For many cancers, people who eat plenty of fruits and vegetables have half the risk of people who eat few fruits and vegetables. Most studies show that even small to moderate amounts of fruits and vegetables make a big difference.

What causes cancer? There are many types of cancer, but diet is always the first place to look. Approximately one-third of cancer deaths in the U.S. that will occur this year can be traced back to poor nutrition, obesity and lack of exercise. Hormone-driven cancers like ovarian, breast, uterine, kidney, bladder, prostate and colon cancers are closely related to the kind of protein and fat we eat, especially protein and fat from meats, and oxidized fats from junk foods and fried foods. Dietary factors are also directly linked to cancer of the rectum, stomach, intestines, mouth, throat, esophagus, pancreas, liver and thyroid. Trans fatty acids from fried fast foods and commercial snack foods are especially dangerous. European studies show breast cancer risk is 40% higher in women who have high body levels of trans fatty acids! Make sure to check labels for trans fatty acid content on any snack foods you purchase. Alcohol abuse, too much sugar and red meat (barbecued meat is the most carcinogenic) can also be traced back to cancer development.

Still, there is encouraging evidence that certain dietary factors also act as anti-carcinogens, preventing tumor development and growth, inhibiting tumor metastasis of cancerous growths, and helping to normalize cancer cells. Nutritional therapy for cancer relies on re-establishing metabolic balance. Whole food nutrition allows the body to use its built-in restorative and repair abilities.

A cancer-fighting diet can intervene in the cancer process at many stages, from its inception to its growth and spread. Even if your genetics and lifestyle are against you, your diet can still make a tremendous difference in your cancer odds. For example, we know that certain body chemicals must be "activated" before they can initiate cancer. Antioxidant rich foods can help block the activation process, determining whether a cancer-causing virus or a cancer promoter (like too much estrogen) will turn tissue cancerous. Even after cells mass into benign structures that may grow into tumors, food compounds can intervene to stop further growth. Some actually shrink the patches of precancerous cells, even repair some cellular damage.

Other foods accelerate body detoxification, and prevent the genetic ruin of cells, a prelude to cancer. It's one of the reasons I emphasize a detoxification diet as part of a cancer control program.

Although far less powerful at later stages, diet can still influence the spread of cancer. Wandering cancer cells need the right conditions in which to attach and grow. Food agents can foster a hostile or a favorable environment. So even after cancer is diagnosed, the right foods may help prolong your life.

Two fruits and three vegetable servings a day show amazing anticancer results. People who eat plenty of fruits and vegetables have half the risk of people who eat few fruits and vegetables. Eating fruit twice a day, instead of twice a week, can cut the risk of lung cancer by 75% even in smokers. One National Cancer Institute spokesman said it is almost mind-boggling, that ordinary fruits and vegetables could be so effective against such a potent carcinogen as cigarette smoke. The evidence is so overwhelming that some researchers are beginning to view fruits and vegetables as powerful preventive drugs that could even wipe out the scourge of cancer. What an about-face this has been for cancer study!

## Here are the foods that provide prime nutrition with cancer-fighting and immune-enhancing properties

**Fruits and vegetables, rich in vitamin C, for immune support and antioxidant protection:** citrus fruits, tomatoes, peppers and broccoli.

**Active culture yogurt,** to help neutralize carcinogens, and deactivate enzymes that allow body substances to turn into cancer.

**Antioxidant foods:** wheat germ, soy foods, yellow, orange and green vegetables, green tea, citrus fruits, and olive oil help normalize precancerous cells, and neutralize cancer-causing free radicals. Normal cells multiply with oxygen, and cancer cells multiple without oxygen (anaerobic cell activity).

**Eating plenty of enzyme-rich fresh fruits and vegetables** and using supplemental enzymes offer potent defense in fighting cancer. (See enzyme therapy below.)

**Fiber-rich foods:** whole grains, fruits and vegetables to absorb excess bile and improve healthy intestinal bacteria.

**Phytochemical food elements,** especially those found in cruciferous vegetables, break down carcinogens and remove them from the body. These same vegetable substances also break down excess estrogens responsible for some breast cancers, and inhibit tumor growth.

**Folic acid foods:** whole wheat and wheat germ, leafy vegetables, beets, asparagus, fish, and citrus fruits are critical to normal DNA synthesis so healthy cells do not mutate and turn cancerous.

**A modified macrobiotic diet** switches the reliance on animal proteins and fats over to vegetable proteins like grains, beans, sprouts and sea vegetables. (Red meat and other animal proteins have not only the undesirable baggage of unhealthy saturated fats, but are also laden with pesticides, hormones, and various body-polluting substances.) Essential Fatty Acids replace the unhealthy fats, such as saturated fats (typically from animal sources), or "hydrogenated" oils, such as found in margarine. The process of hydrogenating an oil is what transforms unsaturated fat into an unhealthy "trans fat." Healthy fat choices include olive oil, flaxseed oil, perilla oil and evening primrose oil. This modified macrobiotic diet also switches the reliance on highly processed foods to enzyme and antioxidant-rich foods such as fresh, raw vegetables and fruits. The traditional macrobiotic diet consists of 50 to 60% grains, 20 to 30% vegetables; fruit and eggs is a tiny percent.

A macrobiotic diet's greatest benefit is that it is cleansing and strengthening at the same time. Those who advocate macrobiotics for serious diseases like cancer also believe that the high percentage of enzyme-rich vegetables and fruits in the modified macrobiotic diet are the most potent cancer fighters. Cancer cells grow because there is an absence of enzymes to fight them off. The fiber (fibrin) around a cancer cell is made of protein. Proteolytic enzymes digest this protein coating which allows the body's white blood cells to attack and destroy the cancer cell. At the same time, the enzymes also reduce the stickiness of the cancer cell, the mechanism the cell uses to attach itself and form tumors. The more cancer cells—the more enzymes the body needs. Protease is a proteolytic enzyme available in supplement form.

**Enzyme therapy** has earned a special position as a rational and highly promising preventive measure for cancer, especially in preventing the formation of cancer cells. Even though this is not always possible, European scientists, who have been in the vanguard of enzyme therapy, feel the goal should be to combat new cancer cells from being formed when the cancer is still at the single-group stage, or has made only small metastases with small numbers of cells into the blood or lymph vessels. Enzyme therapy has been effective prophylaxis for metastatic spread. Enzyme therapy is also recommended before and after cancer surgery in order to help compensate for the weakening of the immune system which accompanies surgical intervention. A significant number of European oncologists now use enzymes for their cancer patients in hospitals.

European physicians also use enzyme therapy as an adjunct to traditional treatments. Recent radiotherapy studies show that when enzymes are administered along with radiation, lower radiation doses can produce the same effect. The enzymes also protect against radiation sickness and side effects. Patients regain their appetite, and feel more alive, both physically and mentally.

## Is your body showing signs that it needs a modified cancer cleanse?

*Are you at risk? Start protective therapies early if you're alerted by these early warning signs.*

1. a change in bowel or bladder habits, especially blood in the stool.
2. chronic indigestion, bloating and heartburn, especially difficulty swallowing.
3. unusual bleeding or discharge from the vagina.
4. lumps or thickening of the breasts or testicles.
5. a chronic cough or constant voice hoarseness; bloody sputum.
6. growth or changes in warts or moles, or scaly skin patches that never go away, especially if they become inflamed or ulcerate.
7. unusual weight loss or fatigue.

**Important note:** Please see a qualified health professional if you have any of these signs.

## Pointers for best results from your modified cancer cleanse

- Drink 8 – 10 glasses of bottled water each day of your cleanse, including herbal teas. Water lubricates and flushes wastes and toxins from all cells, accelerating the cleansing program.

- Use green superfoods like chlorella, spirulina and barley grass. They are rich in every known cancer-fighting nutrient—chlorophyll, phytochemicals, antioxidants, vitamins, minerals, enzymes, and more. Superfoods are also powerful immune builders.

- Cancers are opportunistic, attacking when immune defenses and bloodstream health are low. Chronic colds, cold sores and herpes outbreaks are signs your defenses are low. Promote an environment where cancer and degenerative disease can't live—where inherent immunity can remain effective. These diseases do not seem to grow or take hold where oxygen and nutrients are high in the vital fluids. The cleansing and quality nutrients of this cleanse boost the immune system and create an unfavorable environment for cancer cells. Persist with your efforts to change unhealthy eating habits and incorporate healthy ones.

## Benefits that you may notice as your body responds to the modified cancer cleanse

- Most people notice an increased sense of well-being.
- Since this diet is non-mucous forming, low in fat foods and high in vegetable fiber, most body congestion will begin to clear.

• Circulation improves due to the stimulating effect on the heart and circulatory system from foods like miso, green tea, and shiitake mushrooms.

## Modified cancer cleanse nutrition plan

*Start with this 3 to 7 day nutrition plan.*

### The night before your cancer cleanse…

**Have a green leafy salad** for dinner to give your bowels a good sweeping.

**Before each meal (wait 20 minutes before eating), and before bed: take 2 oz. Herbal Answers Herbal Aloe Force in water.**

### The next day…

**On rising:** take 2 fresh squeezed lemons, 1 tsp. maple syrup and 8 oz. of water; or a restorative broth like Crystal Star Systems Strength.

**Breakfast:** have Pulsating Parsley Juice: 6 carrots, 1 beet, 8 spinach leaves and ¼ cup fresh parsley; or have a mixed fresh fruit salad; or fresh wheatgrass juice.

**Mid-morning:** take a cup of Crystal Star Cleansing & Purifying Tea or Daily Detox by M.D. or a mixed vegetable juice; or Sun Wellness Chlorella, Green Foods Green Magma, or fresh wheat grass juice. Or take an herb tea, like pau d'arco, Natural Energy Plus Caisse's Tea, Essiac Tea, or a glass of fresh carrot juice.

**Lunch:** have a Super V-7 veggie juice: 2 carrots, 2 tomatoes, handful each of spinach and parsley, 2 celery ribs, ½ cucumber, ½ green bell pepper. Add 1 tbsp. of a green superfood: Crystal Star Energy Green; NutriCology Pro-Greens; Fit for You, Intl. Miracle Greens; Barleans Greens. Or have steamed broccoli or cauliflower with brown rice; or have a big fresh green salad.

**Mid-afternoon:** have a fresh carrot juice; or a recovery broth like Crystal Star Systems Strength; or a cup of miso soup with fresh ginger and sea greens crumbled on top.

**Dinner:** have brown rice and steamed vegetables with maitake or shiitake mushrooms. Maitake's unique natural killer cells are powerful against tumors and boost interleukin, an immune protein that fights cancer. Sprinkle on dry, chopped sea vegetables, 1 tbsp. flax or olive oil, and nutritional yeast.

**Before Bed:** have green tea or Crystal Star Green Tea Cleanser. Green tea exhibits anticancer and cancer chemoprotective effects.

**Note:** In order for the macrobiotic balance to work correctly with your body, avoid the following foods: Red meat, poultry, preserved, smoked, cured meats of all kinds, and dairy foods except occasional eggs. Coffee and carbonated drinks. All refined, frozen, canned, processed foods; white vinegar, and table salt. Nightshade plants: tomatoes, potatoes, peppers, eggplant; and hot spices. (Modified macrobiotic diets may use these foods sparingly.)

## Herbs & supplements

*Choose 2 to 3 cleansing boosters.*

**Detoxify:** Crystal Star Blood Detox caps, Green Tea Cleanser or Flora Floressence tea each morning. Give yourself a weekly vitamin C flush (also relieves pain)—up to 10g daily (until stool turns soupy). Una da gato, if liver fluke parasites are involved-many cancers; Calcium D-Glucarate 400mg daily, promotes glucuronidation to help eliminate toxins. Daily Detox by M.D.

**Mushroom therapy improves ability to fight cancer:** Maitake mushroom extract or Grifron Maitake D-fraction extract stimulate cancer cell death. Agaricus mushroom stimulates interferon. Shiitake mushroom, or Lane Labs Noxylane 4 from shiitake mushroom (triples natural killer cell activity.) Reishi or Maitake Products Reishi caps detoxify, disperse toxins. Cordyceps especially for breast cancer.

**Anti-angiogenesis blocks tumor support:** Lane Labs shark cartilage, or Phoenix Biologics Bovine tracheal cartilage. Lane Labs AngioPM, 6 caps daily for one month (highly recommended fresh bindweed leaf extract. Not during pregnancy, surgery, heart disease or a healing wound).

**Natural anti-neoplastons reduce tumors:** Green or white tea; folic acid 800mcg; vitamin E 800IU. EFA's and Omega-3 oils: Evening Primrose oil 4000mg daily; fish or flaxseed oil, 1 oz. daily for cancer. NutriCology Pro-Greens with EFAs.

**Antioxidants fight cancer/elevate T-cell levels:** Glutathione 150mg daily; Lipoic acid, or Jarrow Alpha Lipoic Acid 600mg daily; Rosemary essential oil; Astragalus extract. Allergy Research Glutathione with vitamin C; NutriCology Laktoferrin with colostrum and Total Immune formula; Flora Vegesil or Eidon Silica Mineral Supplement; Indiumease (indium).

**Enzyme support:** Protease enzyme taken between meals helps dissolve the fibrin coating on cancer cells, and helps shrink tumors by stimulating removal of abnormal tissue. Purifies the blood by breaking down protein invaders. Consider Crystal Star Dr. Enzyme with Protease & Bromelain.

**Immune support:** Herbs: panax ginseng, echinacea, ashwagandha, jiaogulan, Siberian eleuthero, goldenseal, licorice, astragalus, ligustrum, suma, dandelion and cayenne. Supplements: Allergy Research Thiodox (lipoic glutathione); NutriCology Laktoferrin and Total Immune; Flora Vegesil; Eidon Silica Mineral Supplement.

**Green Superfoods:** Crystal Star Energy Green; Pure Planet Chlorella or Spirulina; Fit for You Miracle Greens with barley grass.

## Bodywork techniques

*Pick bodywork and relaxation techniques to accelerate your cleanse.*

**Enema:** Enemas are a specific for cancer detoxification: Take an enema the first, second and the last day of your cleansing program to help release toxins out of the body. Irrigate: Or have a colonic once a week for more thorough elimination.

**Exercise:** Regular exercise is almost a "cancer defense" in itself. Exercise acts as an antioxidant to enhance body oxygen use and boost immune response; it accelerates waste passage out of the body. Exercise alters body chemistry to control fat retention, a key involvement with cancer.

**Rest:** Immune power builds the most during sleep—essential to long-term recovery from cancer.

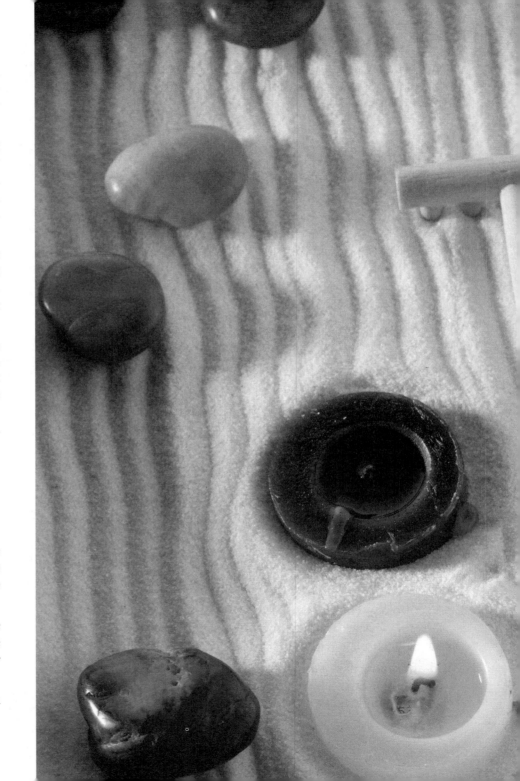

**Overheating therapy:** highly effective against cancer. See page 146 for an in-home method.

**Guided imagery:** effective in helping the immune system to work better, and the hormone system to stop producing abnormal cells.

**Deep Breathing Exercise:** Deep, relaxed breathing removes stress, composes the mind, improves mood and increases energy levels. It's the simplest form of concentration—a basic principle of yoga meditation.

1. Shift your focus away from your racing mind or stressful emotions to focus attention on your breath.

2. Consciously take slow, deep, regular breaths, the mind will become calm.

3. Recall a pleasant past experience.

4. Physically feel thankfulness or love about the good things and people you have in your life.

5. Sincerely question your inner intuition to help find your health solution, or a more efficient response to the situation, one that will minimize future stress.

## For your continuing diet

The best chance for cancer isn't drugs or surgery—it's diet and lifestyle choices you make yourself. Cancers live and grow in unreleased fatty waste and mucous deposits. Fat intake is the key dietary risk factor linked to cancer. Avoid unhealthy fats—add essential fatty acids. Organic fruits and vegetables are essential to a successful cancer program. Refined sugars and junk foods have a direct effect on cancer growth. Have at least one daily drink of a green superfood.

# parasite infection detox
## intestinal worms, amoebic dysentery, giardia

The human body is a host to over 130 different types of parasites! As many as 85% of North Americans have had at least one type of parasite. Worm and parasite infestations can range from mild and hardly noticeable to serious, even life-threatening. As many as 50 million American children are infected with parasitic worms. Pin worms are extremely common in kids and very contagious. Medical treatment is effective, but preventive therapy works best. Make sure the entire family washes their hands after using the rest room. (20% of parents catch parasites from their infected kids!) Make sure small children don't eat non-food items like dirt.

Amoebas are protozoans usually contracted from parasite infested water or food which cause dysentery. Cryptosporidium parvum, the most common water borne parasite in the U.S., causes watery diarrhea, nausea, cramps, fever, and is not killed by chlorination. Some estimate that up to 50% of the U.S. water supply is contaminated with Giardia lamblia, another protozoan that is also chlorine-resistant. 2.5 million cases of Giardia are reported by the CDC every year. Giardia survives especially well in cold mountain streams and frequently infects backpackers and hikers. Other parasites move all over the body, including the brain, weakening the entire system.

**Nutritional therapy is a good choice for thread and pin worms, but not for heavy infestations.** Short term conventional medical treatment is more beneficial for masses of hook and tape worms and blood flukes. (Research shows that liver flukes may be a cause of cancer.) In cases of immunosuppression like AIDS, parasite infection can be serious, even life threatening. Pregnant women should also take care to avoid parasite triggers to avoid pregnancy complications and increased miscarriage risk.

## Do you have parasite signs?

**Pin worms:** generally not serious, but can cause itching, perineal, perianal and vaginal irritation. Very active at night, common in young children, and can often be spotted as white, thready worms in and around the anus.

**Round worms:** fever, intestinal cramping.

**Hookworms:** 2nd most common parasite infection in America: anemia, abdominal pain, diarrhea, lethargy.

**Tapeworms:** intestinal obstruction (even from a single worm). Tapeworm eggs in the liver have been mistaken for and treated as if they were cancer.

**Blood fluke (Schistosomiasis):** lesions on the lungs, hemorrhages under the skin, liver problems, abdominal pain,, diarrhea, and vomiting. Protozoa (amoebae): arthritis-like pain, leukemia-like symptoms, dysentery, pain, and dehydration.

**Giardia:** Look for the following symptoms which present after a 1 – 2 week incubation period: diarrhea, nausea, abdominal pain and cramps, fatigue, weight loss.

## Are you at risk for parasites?

Nationwide research conducted by the Centers for Disease Control over the last 25 years reveals that one in every six people selected at random had one or more parasites. Most kissed and slept with their pets. Many frequently ate raw or smoked fish, or prosciutto or homemade sausages. (**Note:** Use toilet seat covers in public restrooms.)

## Nutritional therapy plan

A strong immune system is the best defense for parasites, many of which have become drug-resistant: low nutrition = low immunity.

1. Go on an apple and apple juice mono diet for 4 days. (1 day for a child). Take 8 garlic caps daily during the fast and chew fresh mango or papaya seeds mixed with honey. On the 3rd day, add papaya or cranberry juice with 1 tbsp. wormwood tea, and 1 tbsp. molasses. On the 4th day, add 2 cups senna/peppermint tea with 1 tbsp. castor oil, and eat raw pumpkin seeds every 4 hours (boosts the body's ability to fight parasites by 21%).

2. Herbal fast to expel tapeworms: Mix 4 oz. cucumber juice with honey and water. Take only this mixture for 24 hours. Follow with 3 cups senna/pumpkin seed tea. Drink down at once. Drink at least 8 glasses water a day to flush out dead parasites.

3. For amoebic dysentery: Take a carrot/beet/cucumber juice daily for a week to clean the kidneys. Take a lemon juice/egg white drink each morning. Take 2 tbsp. epsom salts in a glass of water to purge the bowels. Then eat a high vegetable protein diet with cultured foods like yogurt, and bile stimulating foods like dandelion greens, artichokes, radishes.

## Herbs & supplements for your parasite detox

**Release and cleanse the parasites:** Crystal Star Parasite Purge with wormwood (a broad spectrum anti-parasitic, wormwood produces clinical results against pinworms and hookworms, even malaria), or Nature's Secret Parastroy; Herbal Magic Parasite Kit; Arise & Shine Worm Squirm liquid or Farmacopia Immun-neem capsules, 4 daily with 2 garlic caps, or 8 Cayenne/Garlic capsules, after every meal for 2 weeks, and 4 cups fennel tea daily. (Or take garlic oil capsules in the morning. Refrain from eating or drinking until bowels have moved. Repeat for 3 days.) Then take Crystal Star Bitters & Lemon extract or Enzymedica Purify caps each morning. Ayurvedic Trikhatu tablets; Uni-Key Verma Plus. Proteolytic enzymes can fight parasite infestation: Dr. Enzyme, 6 daily between meals

**Anti-infectives:** Crystal Star Anti-Bio caps 4 daily as a lymph flush; Black walnut hull or Myrrh extract is a specific for liver flukes (clinical tests) and schistosomiasis (flat worm); Una da gato caps 6 daily for a month; Basil tea; Oregano Oil caps 600mg for 6 weeks (good test results, but not during pregnancy); Witch hazel leaf tea or dandelion tea, 4 cups daily. Uni-Key Para System or East Park Olive Leaf Extract, (a potent parasiticide); Ginger caps, tea or extract, 3 – 4 times daily (all 42 components in ginger essential oil kill roundworms and other parasites).

**Remove putrefactive fecal matter and mucous build-up:** Solaray Garlic/black Walnut caps; Nature's Way Herbal Pumpkin; Ayurvedic Concepts

Bitter Melon; AloeLife Aloe Gold juice daily. Homeopathic Ipecac. Relax bowels: Valerian caps 4 daily; Slippery elm tea 2 cups daily; Magnesium 400 – 800mg daily.

**For giardia:** Nutribiotic Grapefruit Seed extract internally (read directions carefully); black walnut or myrrh extract, 10 drops under the tongue every 4 hours, or tea tree oil, 4 drops in water 4x daily, or goldenseal extract for 10 days.

**Immune enhancers against parasites:** Floradix Herbal Iron liquid for strength during healing; Beta carotene 50,000IU daily as an anti-infective; B-complex 50mg daily.

**Probiotics are important to re-establish intestinal health:** American Health fermented soy-based Acidophilus liquid; UAS DDS-plus with FOS; Nutricology Symbiotics powder, ½ tsp. 3x daily. Garden of Life Primal Defense contains Homeostatic Soil Organisms—"prebiotics."

## Bodywork

- A purged stool test is helpful for diagnosing parasitic infections.
- Follow with a high resistance diet to prevent recurrence. Eat lots of onions and garlic.
- Avoid all sweets, dairy foods and junk foods.
- 3 tbsp. amaranth or rice each morning helps remove parasites.
- Eat a daily green salad.
- Drink only bottled water.

## Prevention

Practice good hygiene. Wash your hands with warm water and soap after you use the bathroom. Wash hands before meals, too. If you have children, make sure they do the same.

- Apply zinc oxide to anal opening. Then take a warm sitz bath using 1½ cups epsom salts per gallon of water. Repeat for 3 days. Worms often expel into the sitz bath.
- For crabs and lice—apply one of the following around anus: Thyme or sassafras oil, (dilute either with a carrier oil), tea tree oil, (or myrrh

extract and tea tree oil mixed).

- Garlic enemas or a high colonic irrigation helps clean the colon fast and address fungal infections, or yeast overgrowth conditions.

---

# detox for weight loss, weight control

The latest statistics are shocking. One out of every three Americans is overweight! This doesn't count kids who are rapidly becoming an overweight generation. Right now, two-thirds of Americans are trying to lose weight. Amazingly, of those, only 20% are actually reducing their calories or exercising. Next to smoking, obesity is a leading preventable cause of death in the United States, contributing to in excess of 320,000 deaths each year. Still, there is no question that many people are trying very hard to lose weight, without results. Sometimes diet and exercise really isn't enough.

Weight control today is a strategy of prevention lifestyle—an attitude of keeping weight down. Even though Americans are still looking for the "miracle magic bullet" for slimness, everyone is slowly realizing that a good diet has to be front and center for health and body tone. Long term weight control is always the result of a sound nutritious eating plan, rather than a try at the latest fad diet. One of the great advantages of achieving weight loss through a cleansing program is the extra energy you feel from the fresh juices, superfoods, herb teas and healing broths. Most weight loss diets have little nutrition to offer so they leave you feeling tired and lifeless. In the end, even if you lose weight, your body feels so deprived that it starts ravenous cravings for foods that put the weight right back on.

A cleanse is one of the best ways to jump start a new health program. Unhealthy fats, like saturated fats in meats and dairy foods, trans-fats like those in many dairy foods, hydrogenated or partially hydrogenated oils like those in margarine, shortening and many snack foods, and oxidized fats, like those in all fried foods, collect into excess body fat. Sugary foods and highly processed foods (like fast foods) are so devoid of digestive enzymes that they end up collecting as excess fat, too. Further, if you are congested, your body tries to dump its metabolic wastes to get them out of the way—one of the places that receives metabolic wastes is excess fat.

## Watchwords

Everybody knows yo-yo dieting doesn't work. Did you know it increases the risk of gallstones, too? For the best results, start slowly on your weight loss program and stick with it. The five keys to an effective weight control diet: low fat, high fiber, stress control, regular exercise, lots of water.

Fat isn't all bad. It's your body's chief energy source. Most overweight people have too high blood sugar and too low fat levels. This causes constant hunger; the delicate balance between fat storage and fat utilization is upset; and your ability to use fat for energy decreases. Eating fast, fried, or junk foods aggravates this imbalance. You wind up with empty calories and more cravings. Fat becomes non-moving energy; fat cells become fat storage depots. But don't replace fats with fat substitutes like Olestra. Fake fats fool your tastebuds, not your stomach. In one study, people who replaced 20% of their fat with fake fats were still hungry at the end of the day and they ate twice as much food as normal! Fake fats are nutrition thieves. Eating a one ounce portion of olestra potato chips on a daily basis reduces blood carotene levels by 50%! Diet soda is another diet downfall. The newest research suggests that diet soda drinkers actually consume more calories at the end of the day and are more likely to be obese.

Changing fat composition in your diet is the key. The importance of cutting back on saturated fat cannot be overstated. Saturated fats are hard for the liver to metabolize. Focus on healthy fats from seafood, sea greens, nuts and seeds which curb cravings by initiating a satiety response levels.

Water can get you over diet plateaus. Dehydration slows resting metabolic rate (RMR), so waste products like ketones build up in tissues. Drink juices or green tea each morning to wash out wastes.

A little caffeine after a meal raises thermogenesis (calorie burning) and boosts metabolic rate. Fat burning spices like ginger, cinnamon, garlic, mustard and cayenne in your recipes work, too.

High fiber fruits and veggies are a key to successful body toning. Have an apple every day!

## A 2 – 3 week detox diet for weight loss

Making a healing diet change and losing excess weight is one of the best things you can do for your health. The rewards are high—a longer, healthier life—and control of your life.

**On rising:** Squeeze 2 lemons in a glass of water, and drink for a quick liver flush.

**Breakfast:** Have a poached or baked egg with bran muffins or whole grain toast with ghee or a healthy jam; or have low fat yogurt and some whole grain cereal.; or Try All One's Weight Loss formula meal replacement shake.

**Mid-morning:** Have a green veggie drink, or natural V-8 juice or peppermint tea; or a cup of miso soup with sea greens snipped on top; or crunchy raw veggies with yogurt cheese dip.

**Lunch:** Have fresh leafy green salad with a lemon/oil or yogurt dressing with baked tofu; or miso soup, with steamed veggies and a light sauce.

**Mid-afternoon:** Have a bottle of mineral water, or a cup of peppermint tea, or apple or cranberry juice; or have a superfood drink like Wakunaga Harvest Greens, Crystal Star Energy Green drink, or Aloe Life Daily Greens.

**Dinner:** Have a stir-fry with lots of greens, onions, mushrooms, with clear soup and brown rice; or baked/broiled fish or seafood with some steamed veggies, brown rice or millet.

**Evening snack:** Have some un-buttered spicy popcorn. It's good for you and its airiness will fill you up and keep you from wanting heavier or "habit" foods.

## Herbs & supplements

*Choose 2 to 3 cleansing boosters.*

**Stimulate BAT (brown adipose tissue) thermogenesis:** Crystal Star Thermo Thinner caps; Gaia Diet Slim; Prince of Peace Green Tea Extract Diet Support with ginseng; Source Naturals Diet Phen with hoodia extract capsules; Nature's Secret Ultimate Weight Loss; Health from the Sun Lean For Less program.

**Deficiencies can lead to food binges:** B-complex with extra B-6 200mg (boosts serotonin and metabolizes carbohydrates); lack of minerals can lead to sugar craving: Crystal Star Ocean Minerals or Eidon Zinc liquid; or Trace Mineral Research Concentrace.

**Raise serotonin to control food cravings:** Crystal Star Tummy Control with St. John's wort, a serotonin stimulant or Will Power caps with hoodia, an appetite suppressant; Try chromium picolinate 400mcg, L-glutamine 2000mg or gymnema sylvestre for sugar cravings. Spirulina and bee pollen for energy proteins and blood sugar balance. Rainbow Light Garcinia Max Diet System. All One Weight Loss Formula low glycemic, relieves cravings. Ginkgo biloba extract 2 – 3x a day to help reduce stress linked to weight gain around the middle (not if you are taking Warfarin).

**Natural fat blockers:** Crystal Star Fat & Sugar Detox for a quick cleanse. Then, fat digesting enzymes, like Transformation Lypozyme; or garcinia cambogia in formulas like Planetary Triphala Garcinia. Now Foods Cider Vinegar Diet Formula with lecithin if cholesterol is also high.

**Boost metabolism:** Jump start weight loss with calcium, about 1600mg daily. Genesis Today 4 Weight Control to help regulate thyroid or Enzymatic Therapy Thyroid/tyrosine caps. For compulsive eating, tyrosine 1000mg with zinc 30mg daily. Ayurvedic guggulsterone, like Solaray Guggul caps; Crystal Star Thyroid Meta Max caps; or Now Foods 7-keto Lean; CoQ-10 (200mg daily turns fat into energy); Bromelain 1500mg 3x daily for maximum metabolism (works amazingly well).

## Bodywork techniques accelerate and round out your cleanse

- Daily exercise releases fat from cells. A brisk walk burns calories and cuts cravings. An outdoor walk in winter raises low serotonin levels. Exercise early in the day raises metabolism as much as 25%! Exercising before breakfast helps the body dip into its fat stores for quick energy and curbs the munchies all day. Even if eating habits just slightly change, you can still lose weight with a brisk hour's walk or 15 minutes of aerobic exercise.

- One pound of fat represents 3500 calories. A 3 mile walk burns up 250 calories. In about 2 weeks you'll lose a pound of real extra fat. That's 3 pounds a month and 30 pounds a year without changing your diet. It's easy to see how cutting down even moderately on fatty, sugary foods in combination with exercise can provide the look and body tone you want. Exercise promotes an afterburn effect, raising metabolic rate from 1.00 to 1.05 – 1.15 per minute up to 24 hours afterwards. Calories are burned at an even faster rate after exercise.

- Weight training increases lean muscle mass, replacing fat-marbled muscle with lean muscle. Muscle tissue burns calories; the more lean muscle you have, the more calories you can burn… important as aging decreases muscle mass. Exercise before a meal raises blood sugar levels and decreases appetite, often for several hours afterward. Deep breathing exercises increase metabolic rate and reduce stress.

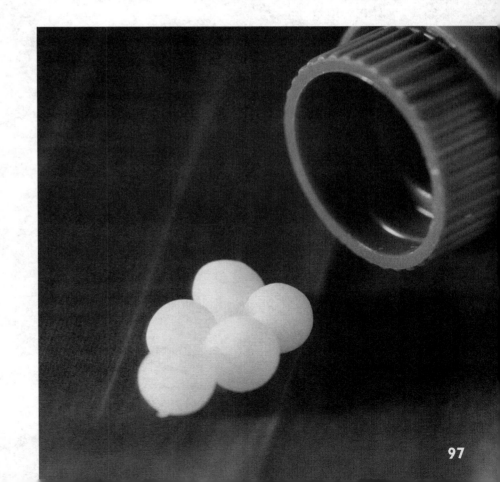

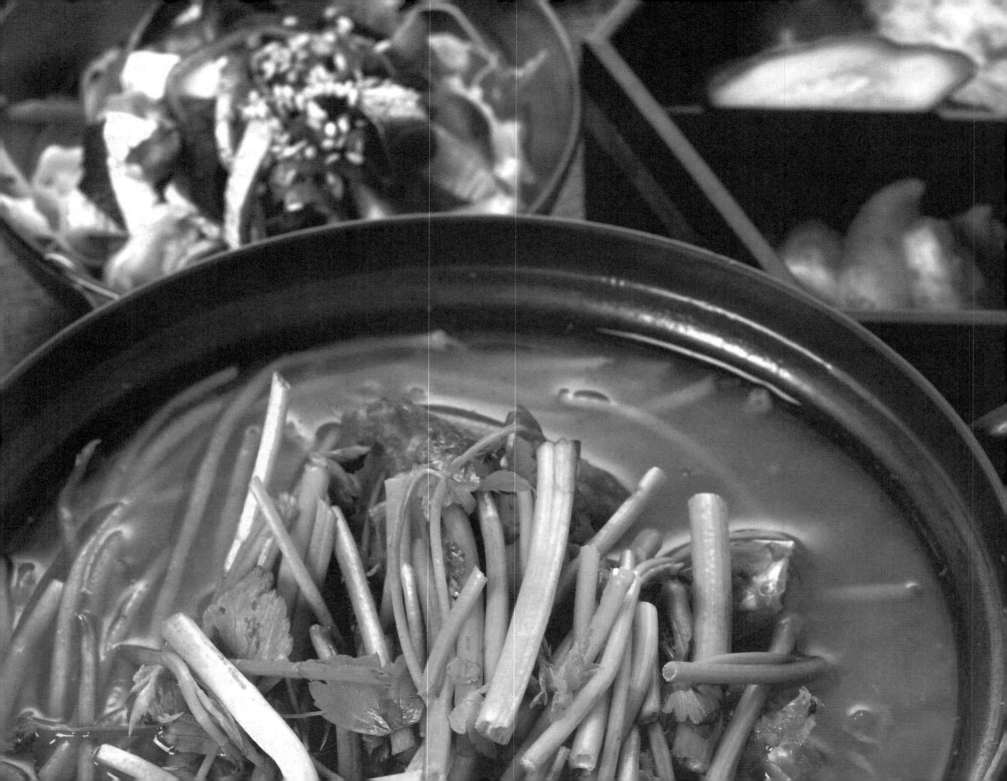

# green cuisine
# cleansing & detox recipes

**WHAT IS GREEN CUISINE? THE RECIPES IN THIS** section have been carefully targeted and tested for a wide variety of cleansing, purifying and detoxification needs.

Each recipe is designed to help you cleanse, thrive and heal, naturally! Many are high in vitamins C, B-complex and minerals to neutralize the effects of pesticides, environmental pollutants and heavy metals, as well as toxins from drugs, caffeine and nicotine.

Cleansing foods should be organically grown and eaten fresh for best results. Only fresh foods and juices retain the full complement of nutrients and plant enzymes that Mother Nature offers.

- **Fruits and fruit juices** eliminate wastes quickly and help reduce cravings.
- **Fresh vegetable juices** carry off excess body acids, and are rich in vitamins, minerals and enzymes that satisfy the body's nutrient requirements with less food.
- **Chlorophyll-rich foods,** like leafy greens and green superfoods like spirulina, chlorella, and barley grass help stabilize and maintain the acid/alkaline balance of the body and also have anti-infective properties. Since chlorophyll has a molecular structure close to our own plasma, drinking them is like giving yourself a mini transfusion. They especially help clear the skin, cleanse the kidneys, and build the blood.
- **Herb teas and mineral drinks** provide energy and gentle cleansing action at the same time, without having to take in solid food for fuel.
- **Sea plants act as the ocean's purifiers** and they perform much the same for the human body, also largely made up of salt water. Sea plant chemical composition is so close to human plasma, that it can help balance your body at the cellular level. Sea vegetables alkalize and purify the blood from the effects of a modern diet. They strengthen the body against illness caused by environmental toxins. Their benefits for a healing diet against serious disease rival the healing powers of land-based vegetables like broccoli and cabbage. They reduce stores of excess fluid and fat, and work to transform toxic metals (including radiation), into harmless salts that the body can eliminate. In fact, the natural iodine in sea vegetables reduces radioactive iodine-131 in the thyroid by almost 80%.

Sea vegetables have superior nutritional content. As one of nature's richest sources of proteins, complex carbohydrates, minerals and vitamins, they transmit those nutrients to your body. Ounce for ounce, sea vegetables are higher in vitamins and minerals than any other food group except herbs. They are almost the only non-animal source of vitamin B12, necessary for cell development and nerve function. Sea vegetables are a superior source of vegetable protein. They provide full-spectrum concentrations of all the carotenes, chlorophyll, enzymes, amino acids and fiber. Their mineral balance is a natural tranquilizer for sound nerve structure and good metabolism. The distinctive salty taste is not just "salt," but a balanced, chelated combination of sodium, potassium, calcium, magnesium, phosphorus, iron and trace minerals. They convert inorganic ocean minerals into organic mineral salts that combine with amino acids (an ideal way for our bodies to get nutrients for structural building blocks). In fact, sea vegetables contain all the necessary trace elements for life, many of which are depleted in land-based soil.

## How do you use green cuisine?

Our bodies are designed to be self-healing organisms. Healing is allowed to occur through cleansing. Cleansing foods and juices can optimize your detox program. In fact, they are crucial to its success in three ways:

- These recipes keep your body chemistry balanced and your body processes stable while you detox, so you don't become uncomfortable. Don't forget that you're cleaning house during a detox program. Mild headaches, slight nausea and weakness may occur as your body purges. (These reactions are usually only temporary and disappear along with the waste and toxins. Drinking more water can curtail most unpleasant detox symptoms.)

- Healthy green cuisine recipes regulate the speed of your detox so your body doesn't cleanse too fast or dump too many toxins into your bloodstream all at once that your body can't handle. Green cuisine recipes keep you from re-poisoning yourself during the detox process.

- They support your nutrition and energy levels while you detox, so you don't become too hungry or too tired. New healthy tissue starts building right away when the detoxification juices are taken in. Gland secretions stimulate the immune system during a cleanse to set up a disease defense environment.

## Diet watchwords

- The day before you begin your detox, eat green salads and fresh fruits, and drink plenty of healthy liquids, so that the upcoming body chemistry changes will not be uncomfortable. A gentle herbal laxative taken the night before can be beneficial.

- Avoid all dairy products and cooked foods during a juice fast.
- Drink 6 to 8 eight oz. glasses of bottled water daily to keep your body continually flushing out the toxins your tissues are releasing.

# detoxification drinks

Detoxification drinks have a powerful effect on the body's recuperative powers because of their rich, easily absorbed nutrients. Fresh juices contain proteins, carbohydrates, chlorophyll, mineral electrolytes and healing aromatic oils. But most importantly, fresh juice therapy makes available to every cell in our bodies large amounts of plant enzymes, an integral part of the healing and restoration process.

Nothing gets done in our bodies without enzymes. They are the activity components of life. Digestive function, assimilation and elimination are all instigated or assisted by enzymes. Enzymes cause every chemical reaction in our bodies. They play a vital part in breaking down foreign matter (like toxins) as well as food. Enzymes and mineral electrolytes (which restore peristaltic bowel activity) are major contributors to moving toxins out of the body instead of building up and poisoning us. When your diet is full of cooked foods without enzymes, or low residue, processed foods (which have a higher tendency to stagnate and putrefy), the process of internal decay develops far more rapidly.

## Should you get a juicer?

Juicers are expensive appliances, but they can really boost the nutrient power of your cleansing drinks. A good juicer essentially predigests fresh fruits and vegetables for almost immediate assimilation by your body. Fresh juices can accelerate your cleanse and noticeably boost your energy level. A juicer can juice all of a fruit or vegetable (even rinds, stems, peels, seeds) to give you up to 95% of the plant's food and nutritive value. Champion, JuiceMan and Acme are all good juicers for a detox program.

# potassium juice

*This is the single most effective juice for cleansing, neutralizing acids and rebuilding the body. It is a blood and body tonic that provides rapid energy and system balance.*

**Makes:** one 12 oz. glass

| | |
|---|---|
| 3 carrots | 3 stalks celery |
| ½ bunch spinach | ½ bunch parsley |

Juice all ingredients. Add 1 to 2 tsp. Bragg's Liquid Aminos if desired.

# potassium essence broth

*If you don't have a juicer, make a potassium broth in a soup pot. While not as concentrated, it is still an excellent source of energy, minerals and electrolytes.*

**Makes:** a 2 day supply

Cover with water in a soup pot:

| | |
|---|---|
| 3 to 4 carrots | 3 stalks celery |
| ½ bunch parsley | 2 potatoes with skins |
| ½ head cabbage | 1 onion |
| ½ bunch broccoli | |

Simmer covered 30 minutes. Strain and discard solids. Add 2 tsp. Bragg's Liquid Aminos or 1 tsp. miso. Store in the fridge, covered.

# cleansing fruit drinks

Fruit juices are like a quick car wash for your body. Their high water and sugar content speeds up metabolism to release wastes quickly. They're fast alkalizers and help reduce cravings for sweets. Still, because of their fast assimilation, pesticides, sprays and chemicals on fruits can enter your body rapidly. So, eat organically grown fruits whenever possible, and wash fruit well if commercially grown. Fruits and fruit juices have their best nutritional effects when taken alone. Eat them before noon for best energy conversion and cleansing benefits.

# acne fighter

*Enzyme-rich blend to clear breakouts.*

**Makes:** 1 drink

Juice:

| | |
|---|---|
| 2 slices pineapple | ½ cucumber, |
| ½ apple | ¼-inch slice ginger root |

# arthritis & bursitis relief

*Anti-inflammatory aid.*

**Makes:** 1 drink

Juice:

| | |
|---|---|
| 2 to 3 oranges, peeled | ¼ pineapple |
| ½ apple, seeded | |

# ginger/lemon cleanse for allergies

*Fast relief.*

**Makes:** 2 drinks (a day's supply)

Juice:

| | |
|---|---|
| 1-inch slice fresh ginger root | 1 fresh lemon |
| 6 carrots with tops | 1 apple, seeded |

## stomach cleanse & breath refresher

*Delicious & refreshing.*

**Makes:** 2 drinks

Juice:

1 bunch grapes                     1 basket strawberries
3 apples, cored                    4 sprigs fresh mint

## diuretic melon mix

*A good morning drink. Take on an empty stomach, 3x daily.*

**Makes:** 1 quart

Juice:

3 cups watermelon cubes            2 cups cantaloupe cubes
2 cups honeydew cubes

## apple cleanse for mucous congestion

*Help for colds and flu.*

**Makes:** 1 drink

Juice:

2 large apples, seeded             ½ tsp. grated horseradish

## bladder infection cleanser

*Clear pathogens while enjoying a healthy drink.*

**Makes:** 2 drinks

Juice:

3 to 4 apples                      ½ cup cranberries

## healthy veins tonic

*Tighten and tone tissue.*

**Makes:** 1 drink

Juice:

1 cup cherries, pitted             1 bunch green grapes
¼ pineapple                        ½ apple, cored and seeded
¼-inch slice ginger root

## ginger aid for prostate enlargement

*Ginger is one of the best herbs for prostate health.*

**Makes:** 2 drinks

Juice:

½ lemon                            ½-inch slice fresh ginger root
1 bunch green grapes

Divide between two tall glasses, and fill to the top with sparkling water.

## blood builder

*A healthy blood purifying drink.*

**Makes:** 4 large drinks:

Juice:

2 bunches grapes                   6 oranges
    (or 2 cups grape juice)            (or 2 cups orange juice)
8 lemons, peeled
    (or 1 cup lemon juice)

Stir in:

2 cups water                       ¼ cup honey

# constipation cleanser

*Relieve bloating and irregularity.*

**Makes:** 1 drink

Juice:
| | |
|---|---|
| 1 firm papaya | ¼-inch slice ginger root |
| 1 pear | |

# circulation stimulant

*Revitalize your circulatory system with this herbal broth.*

**Makes:** 4 drinks

In a saucepan, simmer for 15 minutes the following ingredients:

| | |
|---|---|
| 1 cup cranberry juice | 1 cup orange juice |
| 2 tbsp. honey | 6 cloves |
| 6 cardamom pods | 1 cinnamon stick |
| 4 tbsp. raisins | 4 tbsp. almonds, chopped |
| 1 tsp. vanilla | |

Remove cloves, cardamom and cinnamon stick. Serve hot.

# other good cleansing fruit juices include

- black cherry juice for gouty conditions
- cranberry juice for bladder and kidney infections
- grape and citrus juices for high blood pressure
- celery for nerves
- cantaloupe for allergies

# energizing morning protein drinks

Morning nutrients are more than just early fuel. They are a key factor in a healing diet. Ideally, the body should get about one third of its daily nutrients in the morning. The nutrients you take on rising, at breakfast and mid-morning, lay the foundation for the day's improvement in body chemistry balance. Healing progress can be noticeably accelerated through conscious attention to the nutritional content of the foods you eat before noon.

## Here's why

- Detoxification and blood purification can be stimulated for the next 24 hour period.
- Your liver can be better encouraged to metabolize fats and form healthy red blood cells.
- The body's glycogen supply can be maximized in the morning hours for better sugar tolerance and energy use. If you have hypoglycemia, a good solid breakfast is almost a must.
- Broad spectrum enzyme production can be established through the pancreas for increased assimilation of nutrients and better tolerance of food sensitivities.
- Brain and memory functions make maximum use of fuel in the morning, especially after a restful night.
- Morning is the day's best opportunity to get high fiber foods like whole grains and fruits, for regularity and body balance.
- Metabolism is at its highest in the morning to burn up calories. A low-fat, high energy morning drink can help keep you away from junk foods and unconscious nibbling all day.

## My personal favorite

I especially like brown rice in the morning. It is an efficient source of protein and B vitamins that work particularly well for a brown rice cleanse or a spring cleanse.

I always sprinkle my brown rice with at least 2 tablespoons (usually more) of chopped dry sea vegetables. I usually top it with about a cup of fresh shredded carrots and romaine lettuce. I often stir in about 2 tbsp. sesame seeds and add a little tamari sauce. It's my perfect breakfast.

# non-dairy morning protein drink

*You must have protein to heal. The new breed of light, vegetarian protein drinks like this one are a wonderful way to get protein without meat or bulk or excess fat. These drinks obtain protein from several sources.*

**Makes:** 2 drinks

In a blender, purée until smooth:

| | |
|---|---|
| 1 cup strawberries or kiwi | 1 banana, sliced |
| 1 cup papaya or pineapple, cubed | |
| 1 cup Amazake Rice Drink or 8 oz. soft tofu | |
| 2 tbsp. maple syrup | 1 cup organic apple juice |
| 1 tsp. vanilla | 1 tbsp. wheat germ, toasted |
| ½ tsp. ginger powder | 1 tbsp. crystallized ginger |

# morning meal replacement

*Effective non-dairy protein.*

**Makes:** 2 drinks

In a blender, purée until smooth:

| | |
|---|---|
| 1 cup strawberries or kiwi | 1 banana, sliced |
| 2 tbsp. sweet cloud syrup or barley malt | |
| 1 cup papaya, cubed | 1 cup pineapple/coconut juice |
| 8 oz. soft tofu or 1 cup Amazake rice drink | |
| 2 tsp. vanilla | 2 tbsp. wheat germ, toasted |

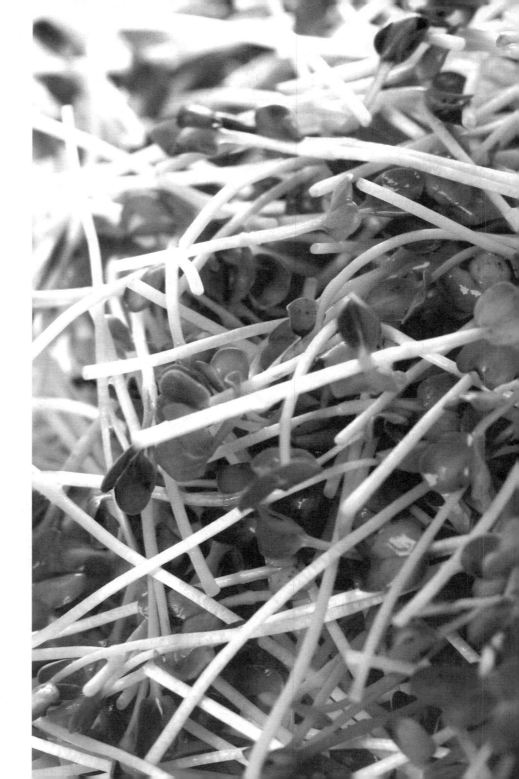

# morning protein immune enhancer

*A good choice for athletes or persons wanting to increase their muscle mass.*

**Makes:** 1 drink

In a blender, blend:
- 3 pineapple rings
- 1 banana
- 4 oz. soy milk (or ½ cup almonds and ½ cup water)
- 3 tbsp. protein powder or 1 tbsp. nutritional yeast

# morning orange shake

*High vitamin C and protein for healing.*

**Makes:** 2 drinks

In a blender, purée until smooth:
- 2 oranges, peeled (leave a small amount of rind on the fruit)
- 1 banana, frozen and sliced
- 2 tbsp. yogurt
- ¼ cup orange juice
- 1 tsp. vanilla

# morning fiber drink

*Also good to take in the evening for morning regularity. Make up the dry mix, then take 1 heaping teaspoon in water or juice in the morning and at bedtime. Store airtight.*

In a blender or coffee grinder, mix together:
- ½ cup oat or rice bran
- ⅓ cup flax seed
- 3 tbsp. psyllium husk powder
- 2 tbsp. fennel seed
- 2 tbsp. acidophilus powder

# de-stress morning shake

*Start your day centered and well nourished.*

**Makes:** 2 drinks

In a blender, blend:
- 1 pint strawberries
- 1 pint, blackberries
- 1 banana
- ½ pear
- 2 oz. tofu
- 1 tbsp. nutritional yeast

# green drinks, vegetable juices & blood tonics

I believe green drinks are critical to the success of every cleansing program. The molecular composition of chlorophyll is so close to that of human hemoglobin that these drinks can act as tonics for the blood, and tonics for the brain and immune system. They are an excellent nutrient source of vitamins, minerals, proteins and enzymes. They contain large amounts of vitamins C, B1, B2, B3, pantothenic acid, folic acid, carotene and choline. They are high in minerals, like potassium, calcium, magnesium, iron, copper, phosphorus and manganese. They are full of enzymes for digestion and assimilation, some containing over 1,000 of the known enzymes necessary for human cell response and growth. Green drinks also have anti-infective properties, carry off acid wastes, neutralize body pH, and are excellent for mucous cleansing. They can help clear the skin, cleanse the kidneys, and purify and build the blood.

Green drinks and vegetable juices are potent fuel in maintaining good health, yet don't come burdened by the fats that accompany animal products. Those included here have been used with therapeutic success for many years. You can have confidence in their nutritional healing and regenerative ability.

## Chlorophyll is the key to green therapy

One of the most therapeutic ingredient of all fresh green plants and green superfoods (like chlorella and spirulina), is chlorophyll. Chlorophyll is the pigment that plants use to carry out the process of photosynthesis—absorbing light energy from the sun, then converting it into earth and plant energy. This energy is transferred into our cells and blood when we eat chlorophyll-rich greens.

Chlorophyll is the basic component of the "blood" of plants. The chlorophyll molecule is also remarkably similar to human plasma, except that it carries magnesium in its center instead of iron. Green foods help human bodies build red blood cells. In essence, eating any of the chlorophyll-rich foods is almost like giving yourself a little transfusion to help treat illness, enhance immunity and sustain well-being. They have a synergistic effect when added to a normal diet. The green superfoods are valuable in all of the healing diets.

Chlorophyll is a primary aid for organ detoxification, particularly the liver. It helps to neutralize and remove drug deposits from the body, purify the blood, and counteract acids and toxins in the system. Even the medical community is seeing chlorophyll as a possible means of removing heavy metal build-up, because it can bind with several heavy metals and help eliminate them. Because of its detoxifying and anti-bacterial qualities, chlorophyll has proven to be a valuable remedy in the treatment of colds, rhinitis, inner-ear infections and inflammation.

A new U.S. Army study reveals that a chlorophyll-rich diet can double the lifespan of animals exposed to lethal radiation. Chlorophyll is now being considered (since the days of Agent Orange and Gulf War Syndrome) as a health protector against some chemical warfare weapons.

# daily carrot juice cleanse

*Highly nutritious daily cleanser.*

**Makes:** 2 large drinks

Juice:

| | |
|---|---|
| 4 carrots | ½ cucumber |
| 2 stalks celery with leaves | |

# personal best v-8

*A high vitamin/mineral drink for normalizing body balance. A good daily blend even when you're not cleansing.*

**Makes:** 6 glasses

Juice:

| | |
|---|---|
| 6 to 8 tomatoes | 3 to 4 green onions with tops |
| (or 4 cups tomato juice) | ½ green pepper |
| 2 carrots | 2 stalks celery with leaves |
| ½ bunch spinach, washed | ½ bunch parsley |
| 2 lemons, peeled (or 4 tbsp. lemon juice). | |

Add 2 tsp. Bragg's Liquid Aminos and ½ tsp. ground celery seed.

# healthy mary tonic

*A virgin mary is really a healthy green drink when you make it fresh.*

**Makes:** 4 drinks

Juice:

| | |
|---|---|
| 3 cups water | ½ green bell pepper |
| 2 large tomatoes | 2 celery stalks with leaves |
| 1 green onion with tops | 1 handful fresh parsley |

Add 1 tsp. crumbled, dry sea veggies, (any kind), or 1 tsp. kelp powder.

## cleansing energy tonic

*A good afternoon pick-me-up juice during a 3 to 7 day cleanse.*

**Makes:** 2 drinks

Juice:

4 cups mixed sprouts (esp. alfalfa, buckwheat, sunflower, mung)
1 large carrot · 1 stalk celery with leaves
½ cucumber · 1 green onion
2 tbsp. raw sauerkraut.

## kidney flush

*A purifying kidney cleanser and diuretic, with high potassium and other minerals.*

**Makes:** 4 drinks

Juice:

4 carrots with tops · 1 cucumber with skin
4 beets with tops · 1 handful spinach leaves
4 celery stalks with leaves

## immune enhancer

*Drink this at first sign of cold or flu.*

**Makes:** 2 drinks

Juice:

½ bunch parsley · 1 garlic clove
6 carrots · 3 stalks celery with leaves
1 large tomato · 1 red bell pepper
a dash of hot pepper sauce · 4 romaine leaves
  (or cayenne pepper) · 1 stalk broccoli

Add 1 tsp. miso paste mixed with a little water.

## candida yeast cleanser

*Healthy juice with anti-yeast activity.*

**Makes:** 2 drinks

Juice:

1 bunch parsley · 2 cloves garlic
6 carrots · 2 stalks celery
3 kale or collard leaves

Add 1 tsp. miso paste mixed with a little water.

## blood tonic

*This is an amazingly simple, but effective Chinese medicine restorative for women after childbirth, people with anemia, or those suffering blood loss from surgery.*

**Makes:** 8 drinks

Simmer in 8 cups of water:

35 black dates · 5 slices fresh ginger

Stir in:

1 tsp. royal jelly (or 1 tbsp. royal jelly mixed with honey)
1 tbsp. sesame tahini

Sip throughout the day for several weeks.

## intense parsley cleanse

*Flush out toxins and release water weight.*

**Makes:** 2 drinks (a day's supply)

Juice:

1 bunch parsley · 6 carrots with tops
½ apple, seeded

# alkalizing apple broth

*This broth alkalizes body pH, gives a spicy energy lift and helps lower serum cholesterol.*

**Makes:** 4 drinks

| | |
|---|---|
| ½ red onion, chopped | 2 cloves garlic, minced |
| 1 tsp. canola oil | 1 small red bell pepper |
| 2 tart apples, cored | 1 lemon, partially peeled |
| 2 tbsp. parsley | 2 cups Knudsen's Very Veggie (or any good spicy tomato juice) |

Sauté the onion and garlic in the canola oil until soft.

While sautéing, purée the remaining ingredients in the blender. Add onion mix to blender and purée. Pour back into the pot and bring to a simmer before removing from heat.

# prostate sediment cleanser

*Support a healthy prostate.*

**Makes:** 2 drinks (a day's supply)

Juice:
2 large handfuls mixed dark green leaves (especially spinach, kale, collards and dandelion leaves)
3 large tomatoes

# skin cleansing tonic

Deep greens to cleanse, nourish and tone skin tissue from the inside.

**Makes:** 1 drink

Juice:

| | |
|---|---|
| 1 cucumber with skin | ½ bunch fresh parsley |
| 1 4 oz. tub alfalfa sprouts | 3 to 4 sprigs fresh mint |

# excess body fluid/water retention cleanser

*Great for relieving excess water weight fast.*

**Makes:** 1 large drink

Juice:

| | |
|---|---|
| 1 cucumber | 1 beet |
| ½ apple, seeded | 4 carrots with tops |

Add a 2-inch piece fresh daikon radish or soak a few slivers of dried daikon and add.

# high blood pressure reducer

*A targeted juice can support balanced blood pressure.*

**Makes:** 1 large drink

Juice:

| | |
|---|---|
| 2 garlic cloves | 1 handful parsley |
| 1 cucumber | 4 carrots with tops |
| 2 stalks celery with leaves | |

# remove the cobwebs brain booster

*Wake up your brain.*

**Makes:** 1 large drink

Juice:

| | |
|---|---|
| 1 bunch parsley | 4 carrots |
| 1-inch piece fresh or preserved burdock or ginseng root | |
| 2 stalks celery | |

# arthritis relief detox

*Ease painful symptoms, support recovery.*

**Makes:** 1 large drink

Juice:

large handful spinach          large handful parsley
large handful watercress          5 carrots with tops
3 radishes

Add 1 tbsp. Bragg's Liquid Aminos.

# hemorrhoid & varicose vein drink

*Vitamin C, calcium and bioflavonoids boost collagen production which helps new more elastic tissue to form.*

**Makes:** 2 drinks (a day's supply)

Juice:

3 handfuls of dark greens (kale, parsley, spinach, or watercress)
5 carrots with tops          1 green bell pepper
2 tomatoes

# reduce high cholesterol

*Healthy heart support.*

**Makes:** 2 drinks

Juice:

1 large handful parsley          5 carrots with tops
2 apples          ½ tub alfalfa sprouts

# diabetes balancer

*Green beans offer potent protection against diabetes.*

**Makes:** 1 large drink

Juice:

3 romaine lettuce leaves          3 carrots with tops
3 handfuls fresh green beans          2 brussels sprout heads

Add 1 tsp. miso paste dissolved in water and stir.

# gentle cleanse for Crohn's Disease & Colitis

*Take a small cup daily to help strength return.*

**Makes:** 4 small drinks

Juice:

3 handfuls greens (1 spinach, 1 parsley, and 1 kale or collard)
3 beets with tops          5 carrots
½ green pepper          ½ apple, seeded

# overweight detox

*Use as part of a fat/cellulite detox program.*

**Makes:** 1 large drink

Juice:

1 large handful dark greens like spinach, kale or parsley
1 stalk celery with leaves          1 carrot
1 bell pepper          1 tomato
1 broccoli floweret

Add 1 tsp. dry sea veggies (any type).

# diverticulitis detox

*Use as part of colon/bowel healing program.*

**Makes:** 2 drinks (a day's supply)

Juice:

| | |
|---|---|
| 1 large handful parsley | ¼ head green cabbage |
| 2 large tomatoes | 4 carrots with tops |
| 1 garlic clove | 2 stalks celery with leaves |

# stress cleanse

*Use as part of a stress cleanse.*

**Makes:** 1 large drink

Juice:

| | |
|---|---|
| 1 small handful each, parsley and watercress | |
| 2 stalks celery | 1 carrot |
| ½ red bell pepper | 1 tomato |
| 1 broccoli floweret | |

# constipation cleanse

*Fast relief.*

**Makes:** 2 drinks (a day's supply)

Juice:

| | |
|---|---|
| ¼ head green cabbage | 3 stalks celery with leaves |
| 5 carrots with tops | |

# psoriasis & eczema cleanse

*Cleanse and tone your skin.*

**Makes:** 1 large drink

Juice:

| | |
|---|---|
| 1 tomato | 1 cucumber |
| 2 stalks celery | 1 handful each, parsley and watercress |

# magnesium migraine cleanse

*Relax and relieve.*

**Makes:** 1 large drink

Juice:

| | |
|---|---|
| 1 garlic clove | 1 handful parsley |
| 5 carrots | 2 stalks celery, with tops |

# revitalizing tonic

*A good drink for an addiction purifying program or any kind of hangover. Effective hot or cold. Works every time.*

**Makes:** 8 drinks:

In the blender, purée:

| | |
|---|---|
| 1 ½ cups water | 1 cup chopped onions |
| 2 stalks celery chopped | 1 bunch parsley chopped |
| 2 tbsp. chopped basil | 2 tsp. hot pepper sauce |
| 1 tsp. rosemary leaves | ½ tsp. fennel seeds |
| 2 tsp. Bragg's Liquid Aminos | |

Pour into a large pot with 48 oz. Knudsen's Spicy Veggie Juice. Bring to a boil and simmer for 30 minutes. Use hot or cool.

# herb teas for detoxification

Herb teas and high mineral drinks during a liquid diet can provide energy and cleansing without having to take in solid proteins or carbohydrates for fuel. Herbal teas are the most time-honored of all natural healing mediums. Essentially body balancers, teas have mild cleansing and flushing properties, and are easily absorbed by the system. The important volatile oils in herbs are released by the hot brewing water, and when taken in small sips throughout the cleansing process, they flood the tissues with concentrated nutritional support to accelerate regeneration, and the release of toxic waste. In general, herbs are more effective when taken together in combination than when used singly.

## How to take herbal teas for best results in your detox program

1. Use a glass, ceramic or earthenware pot. Stainless steel is acceptable, but aluminum negates the herbal effects, and the metal may wash into the tea and into your body.

2. Pack a small tea ball with loose herbs.

3. Bring 3 cups of cold water to a boil. Remove from heat. Add herbs, and steep covered (10 to 15 minutes for a leaf and flower tea, 20 to 25 minutes for a root and bark tea).

4. Keep lid tightly closed during steeping and storage. Volatile herbal oils are the most valuable part of the drink, and will escape if left uncovered.

5. Drink teas in small sips over a long period of time rather than all at once, to allow the tissues to absorb as much of the medicinal value as possible.

6. Take 2 to 3 cups of tea daily for best medicinal effects.

## A few combinations

**A tea combination for cleansing and purifying the body:** green tea, white tea, dandelion leaf/root, burdock, gotu kola and red sage.

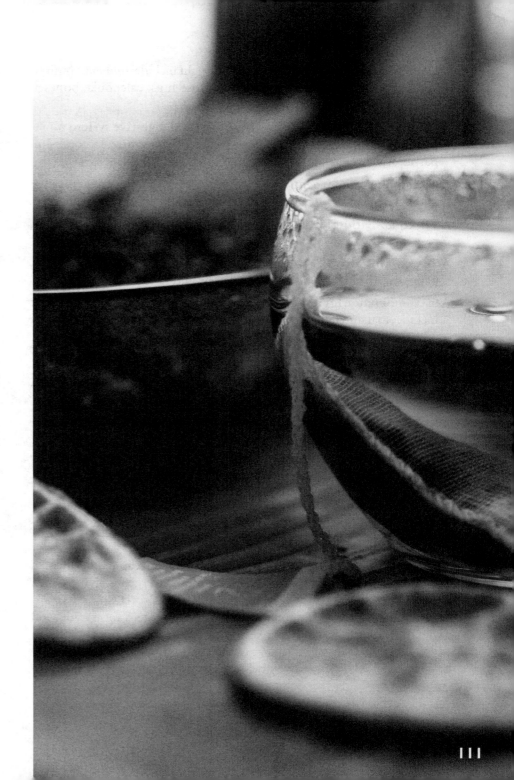

**A tea combination for mucous cleansing** might include: mullein, comfrey, green tea, marshmallow, pleurisy root, rose hips, calendula, boneset, ginger, peppermint and fennel seed.

**A tea combination for cleansing the bowel and digestive system** might include: senna leaf, papaya leaf, fennel seed, peppermint, lemon balm, parsley, calendula, hibiscus and ginger.

**A tea combination for gentle bladder and kidney flushing** might include: cranberries, cat's claw, uva ursi, juniper berries, ginger and parsley.

**A tea combination for clearing sinuses** might include: marshmallow, rose hips, mullein and fenugreek.

**A tea combination for relieving stress** might include: rosemary, peppermint, chamomile, catnip, feverfew and kava root.

**A tea combination for removing congestion from chest and sinuses** might include: marshmallow root, mullein, rose hips and fenugreek seed.

**A tea combination for rebuilding body energy** might include: gotu kola, peppermint, red clover and cloves.

**A tea combination for female fertility** might include: damiana, licorice, red raspberry, ho shou wu, ashwagandha, ginger and scullcap.

**A tea combination for warming against aches and chills** might include: wild cherry bark, licorice root, rose hips and cinnamon.

**A tea combination for restoring bowel and colon regularity** might include: fennel seed, flax seed, fenugreek seed, licorice root, burdock root and spearmint.

**A tea combination for cleansing the liver:** white tea, dandelion root, burdock root, watercress, yellow dock and red sage

I think my favorite herb tea for a good detox is green tea, an unfermented tea rich in flavonoids with antioxidant and anti-allergen activity. Green tea has a long history in the Orient as a beneficial body cleanser. Its antioxidant polyphenols do not interfere with iron or protein absorption, and as with other plant antioxidants, like beta carotene and vitamin C, green tea polyphenols work at the molecular level, combatting free radical damage to protect against degenerative disease.

# rootbeer revitalizer

*Here's the old-fashioned version of a popular favorite. Decidedly delicious medicine for cleansing and digestion.*

Combine in a large bowl:

| | |
|---|---|
| 3 oz. dry sassafras bark, broken | 2 tsp. fresh grated ginger root |
| 2 oz. dry sarsaparilla root | 1 tbsp. ground cinnamon |
| 1 oz. dry dandelion root | 2 tsp. orange peel |
| 1 oz. dry burdock root | |

Mixture can be kept dry and stored until you are ready to use. To prepare, add 4 tbsp. dry mixture for each quart of water, simmer for 15 to 20 minutes, strain and chill.

# homemade ginger ale for cleansing & digestion

*This is an original nineteen-twenties home remedy tea for both children and adults. It works amazingly well to settle the stomach, and help elimination during a cold, flu or fever. I like it better than today's ginger ale. Use it as part of your liquid intake during a detox.*

**Makes:** 1 quart

| | |
|---|---|
| 3 cups water | 2 tsp. fresh grated ginger root |
| 1 tsp. dry red raspberry leaves | 1 tsp. dry sassafras root, chopped |
| 1 tsp. dry sarsaparilla root | |

Bring water to a boil, add ginger, raspberry leaves, sassafras and sarsaparilla, and simmer for 5 minutes. Take off of heat and let steep for 15 minutes. Strain and add 1 cup sparkling water just before serving. Add fresh lemon slices if desired.

# enzyme therapy

Plant enzymes are the key to longterm results from detoxing with fresh plant juices. Enzymes are the cornerstone of health because they are the foundation elements of the immune system. Plant enzymes allow our bodies to use the full array of plant nutrients, including the main components of anti-aging—antioxidants to fight free radicals, and keep immunity strong.

## Enzymes operate on both chemical and biological levels

Chemically, they are workhorses that drive metabolism to use the nutrients we take in.

Biologically, they are our life energy. Without enzyme energy, we would be a pile of lifeless chemical substances.

Each of us is born with a battery charge of enzyme energy at birth. As we age, our internal enzyme stores are naturally depleted. A new study shows that a 60 year old has 50% fewer enzymes than a 30 year old. The faster you use up your enzyme supply—the shorter your life. Much of the anti-aging research in the natural healing world is about boosting enzyme supply to delay the aging process.

## There are three categories of enzymes:

1. Metabolic enzymes, which repair cells and tissues and are involved in the healing process, are needed for every chemical reaction that takes place in the human body.

   **Note:** Enzyme supplements taken in between meals (when there isn't food to digest), function as metabolic enzymes, absorbed directly into the body to repair and heal.

2. Our own digestive enzymes assimilate our food and nutrients. Human digestive enzymes are stronger than any of the body's other enzymes, and more concentrated than any other enzyme combination found in nature. A very good thing, since our processed, over-cooked, nutrient-poor diets demand a great deal of enzymatic work!

3. Fresh plant enzymes start food digestion and enhance our own digestive enzymes. All foods in their natural state contain the enzymes required to digest them. All food, whether plant or animal, has its own enzymes that serve it in life. When eaten, these become the property of the eater and are now its food enzymes, and begin immediately to work for the eater's digestive benefit. Humans cannot independently assimilate food—our bodies must have the help of the food itself. Only whole food enzymes give your body what it needs to work properly. The best plant enzyme sources for humans are bananas, mangos, sprouts, papayas, avocados, ginger and pineapples.

## How does plant enzyme therapy work?

Enzyme therapy uses metabolic enzymes to stimulate immune response. The link between enzymes and our immune system comes from lymphocytes, or white blood cells. Immune organs, like the thymus and lymph nodes, keep a constant level of white blood cells circulating through the body to attack foreign invader cells. When body toxins are detected, white blood cells attack them and essentially digest them by secreting enzymes on their surfaces.

Some diseases, such as cancer, leukemia, anemia and heart disease can even be diagnosed by measuring the amount and activity of certain enzymes in the blood and body fluids.

So far, enzyme therapy has been most helpful in conditions like heart disease, tumor malignancies, skin problems, low and high blood sugar, stomach and colon pain, eye diseases and headaches. Some enzymes clean wounds, dissolve blood clots and control allergic reactions to drugs.

Plant enzymes help us to heal faster. Certain enzymes, particularly proteolytic enzymes or proteases, shorten the inflammatory process during healing by breaking up debris in the injured area and stimulating our own healing enzyme activity without suppressing the immune system (unlike cortisone or hydrocortisone drugs). Proteolytic enzymes, like bromelain from pineapples, are used as anti-inflammatory agents for sports injuries like sprains, and respiratory problems where they help unclog. They can also boost healing from degenerative diseases and surgery, reducing swelling and pain for a more rapid recovery.

Fresh plant juices in a detox program are especially important for protease enzyme deficiency. Protease digests unwanted debris in the blood including certain bacteria and viruses. Protease deficient people are usually immune compromised, making them susceptible to bacterial, viral and yeast infections, and a general decrease in immunity. A protease deficiency sets up an environment for arthritis, osteoporosis and other calcium-deficient diseases. Since protein is needed to carry protein-bound calcium in the blood, a first sign of protease deficiency would be unusual anxiety and insomnia.

Protease deficiency also leads to inadequate protein digestion which leads to hypoglycemia resulting in moodiness, mood swing and irritability.

## Do you have enough enzymes?

Enzyme depletion, lack of energy, disease and aging all go hand in hand. The first signs of enzyme deficiency are fatigue, premature aging and weight gain. Unless we do something to stop the one-way-flow of enzyme energy out of the body, our digestive and eliminative capacities weaken, obesity, and chronic illness set in and lifespan shortens.

Most nutrient deficiency problems as we age result not from the lack of the nutrients themselves, but from the body's inability to absorb them. Eating junk foods and overcooked foods without enzymes means the pancreas and the liver have to use their enzyme stores. As a result, reserve enzymes for metabolic processes are pulled from their normal work, to digest your food.

But even this substitute measure doesn't make up for the missing enzymes that should be in the food, because the body needs that food's enzymes to break itself down correctly so it can deliver its own nutrients (Nature provides for everything).

Enzyme deficiency means we end up with undigested food in the blood. So, white blood cell immune defenses are pulled from their jobs to take care of the undigested food and the immune system takes a dive. It's a perfect environment for disease. Eating enzyme-rich foods takes care of this unhealthy cascade of reactions before it ever starts.

## How can we maximize daily enzyme benefits?

I believe Nature intended us to eat a largely plant-based diet with fresh foods that have plenty of plant enzymes. It is not necessary to always eat raw foods. But it is important to have a large percentage of your overall diet be enzyme-rich. Clearly, as you increase consumption of fresh foods, the enzymatic activity within your body also increases.

**WARNING:** Enzyme protection and enzyme therapy are dramatically affected by the use of a microwave oven because high heat destroys enzymes. Enzymes are extremely sensitive to heat. Even low degrees of heat can destroy food enzymes and greatly reduce digestive ability. Heat above 120° F. completely destroys them. Enzymes are also destroyed by substances like tobacco, alcohol, caffeine, fluorides, chlorine in drinking water, air pollution, chemical additives and many medicines.

## golden enzyme drink

*A drink specifically for healing enzyme properties.*

**Makes:** 2 drinks

Juice:
    1 fresh pineapple, skinned/cored
    1 tsp. honey                4 carrots

## ever green enzyme drink

*A personal favorite for taste, mucous release and enzyme action.*

**Makes:** 1 drink

Juice:
    1 apple, cored             1 tub (4 oz.) alfalfa sprouts
    3 small handfuls fresh mint     1 tsp. spirulina granules
    ½ fresh pineapple, skinned/cored

# good digestion punch

*Natural sources of papain and bromelain for enzymes, and enzyme-rich ginger to break up stomach acids.*

**Makes:** 2 drinks

Juice:
| | |
|---|---|
| 1 papaya, peeled/seeded | 1 fresh pineapple, skinned/cored |
| ¼-inch fresh ginger, peeled | |

# enzyme cooler

*An intestinal cleanser to help lower cholesterol and allow better assimilation of foods.*

**Makes:** 2 large drinks

Juice:
1 apple, cored (½ cup apple juice)
2 lemons, peeled (¼ cup lemon juice)
1 pineapple, skinned and cored (or 1 ½ cups pineapple juice)

# fruit & aloe stomach & digestive cleanser

*Gentle cleanser, especially helpful for IBS.*

**Makes:** 1 drink

Whirl in the blender
| | |
|---|---|
| 1 apple, cored | 2 tbsp. aloe vera juice |
| ¼ tsp. ground ginger | |

Add enough water to make 8 oz.

# vegetable & vinegar stomach/digestive cleanser

*Boost stomach activity and natural cleansing activity.*

**Makes:** 1 drink

Juice:
| | |
|---|---|
| ½ cucumber with skin | 2 tbsp. apple cider vinegar |
| ¼ tsp. ground ginger | |

Add enough water to make 8 oz.

# constipation-cleansing enzyme salad

*High fiber for optimum colon/bowel health.*

**Makes:** 2 salads

Mix together lightly in a bowl:
| | |
|---|---|
| 1 firm papaya, cubed | 3 tbsp. minced crystallized ginger |
| 1 pear, cubed | 1 cup raspberries |
| ½ cup raspberry vinegar | ½ cup water |

# mineral-rich cleansing broth

*A body rebuilding recovery tonic.*

**Makes:** 6 cups of broth

Add to a large soup pot:
| | |
|---|---|
| 1 ½ qts. water | 1 large onion, chopped |
| 3 sliced carrots | 2 potatoes, cubed |
| 1 cup fresh parsley, chopped | 2 stalks celery with tops |

Bring to boil; reduce heat; simmer 30 minutes. Strain; add 1 tbsp. Bragg's Liquid Aminos.

# mineral-rich aminos drink

*A complete, balanced food-source vitamin/mineral electrolyte drink—rich in greens, amino acids and enzyme precursors. Use for detoxification, or after illness or a hospital stay.*

**Makes:** 8 drinks

| | |
|---|---|
| 4 – 6 packets miso soup powder | 2 tbsp. fresh parsley leaf |
| ½ cup soy protein powder | 1 packet instant ginseng tea |
| 2 tbsp. bee pollen granules | 1 tsp. spirulina/chlorella granules |
| 1 tbsp. nutritional yeast flakes | 1 tsp. acidophilus powder |
| 1 tbsp. crumbled dry sea vegetables | |

Mix ingredients in the blender, then add about 2 tbsp. of the powder into 2 cups of hot water for 1 drink. Let flavors bloom for 5 minutes before drinking. Sip over a half hour period for best assimilation. Add 1 tsp. Bragg's Liquid Aminos to each drink if desired.

# chinese weight management soup

*A detox recipe for a weight loss liquid diet. Take 2 to 4 cups daily to eliminate congested fluids, break down blood fats and activate the intestines.*

| | |
|---|---|
| 2 oz. astragalus | 2 oz. poria |
| 2 oz. fresh chopped ginger | 12 – 18 pitted red dates |
| ½ cup barley | 7 cups vegetable stock |
| 3 celery stalks, diced | 3 beets, diced |
| 3 cloves garlic, minced | 12 shiitake mushrooms, sliced |
| ½ cup fresh watercress leaves or sunflower sprouts | |

Tie the astragalus, poria and ginger in a muslin bag. Simmer with the barley and dates for one hour in the vegetable stock

Add the celery, beets, garlic and shiitake mushrooms, and simmer for another 20 minutes. Remove herb bag. Add watercress leaves or sunflower sprouts and serve.

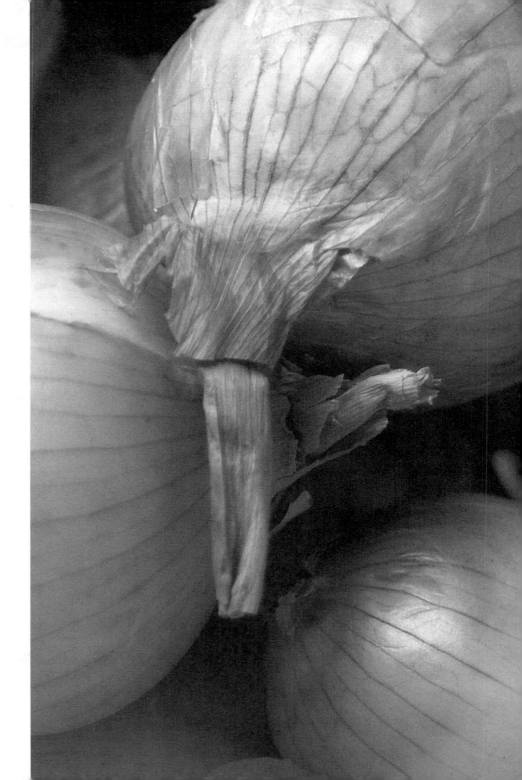

# pineapple/papaya enzyme salad

*Heal your body with powerful enzyme therapy.*

**Makes:** 4 large salads

Toss together:
    half a pineapple peeled and cubed
    1 cup strawberries        1 cup blackberries
    1 cup raspberries        1 cup blueberries

Use the enzyme dressing below if desired.

## enzyme dressing

*A healthy, low fat, enzyme-rich salad dressing.*

**Makes:** enough for 4 large salads

In the blender, blend:
    1 cup lemon or plain yogurt, or kefir cheese
    1 tbsp. lime juice        1 tbsp. lemon juice
    1 tsp. ginger syrup, or ½ tsp. ginger powder
    ¼ tsp. tamari

# purifying daikon & scallion broth

*A clear drink with bladder/kidney cleansing activity.*

**Makes:** one bowl
    4 cups vegetable broth        2 scallions, with tops
    6-inch piece daikon radish, peeled and cut in matchstick pieces

In a saucepan, heat all ingredients gently together for 5 minutes.

Stir in:
    1 tbsp. tamari or 1 tbsp. Bragg's Liquid Aminos
    1 tbsp. fresh cilantro leaves        ½ tsp. pepper.

# spring cleaning enzyme soup

*Use as part of a spring cleanse.*

**Makes:** 8 cups soup

Simmer washed and chopped greens in pot with 2 cups water:
    2 cups fresh nettle tops        1 cup fresh watercress leaves
    ½ cup fresh dandelion leaves

Have ready:
    1 large minced onion        2 tbsp. olive oil
    2 carrots, diced        2 turnips, diced
    3 tbsp. miso paste        6 cups water
    1 cup sunflower sprouts

Sauté onion in the olive oil, and add to the simmering greens. Add carrot, turnips, miso paste and 6 cups water. Simmer 30 minutes. Add sunflower sprouts.

# after dinner enzyme digestive tea

*Eases bloating and gas.*

Steep:
    2 parts peppermint        2 parts hibiscus
    1 part papaya leaf        1 part rosemary

# high protein sprout cocktail

*This high protein juice is particularly good for ending a fast.*

**Makes:** 2 drinks

Juice:
    3 cored apples with skin        1 tub (4 oz.) alfalfa sprouts
    6 sprigs fresh mint

117

# spring bitters salad

*Healthy cleansing support.*

**Makes:** 6 salads

Toss together:

| | |
|---|---|
| ½ cup dandelion leaves | ½ cup spinach leaves |
| 4 cups red leaf lettuce | ½ cup fresh parsley |

1 cup mixed wild greens like chicory, borage, violet leaves, sorrel, and beet greens

½ cup mixed tips of chives, fennel, mint, tarragon and yarrow

Add:

| | |
|---|---|
| 1 tomato, chopped | 1 cup alfalfa sprouts |
| 1 leek, white portion chopped | |

# cleansing soups & hot tonics

Broths are a very satisfying form of nutrition during a cleansing fast. They are simple, easy, inexpensive, can be taken hot or cold, and provide a means of "eating" and being with others at mealtime without going off a liquid detox program. This is more important than it might appear, since solid food, taken after the body has released all its solid waste, but before the cleanse is over, will drastically reduce your diet's success. Broths are also alkalizing and help balance body pH.

Hot tonics are neither broths nor teas, but unique hot combinations of vegetables, fruits and spices with purifying and energizing properties. The ingredients provide noticeable synergistic activity when taken together—with more medicinal benefits than the single ingredients alone. Take them morning and evening for best results.

# purifying broth

*Rich in potassium and minerals.*

**Makes:** 6 cups

Sauté in 2 tbsp. canola or olive oil:

| | |
|---|---|
| ¼ cup chopped celery | ¼ cup daikon radish |
| ¼ cup chopped leeks | ½ cup broccoli, chopped |

Add:

| | |
|---|---|
| 6 cups rich vegetable stock | 2 tbsp. fresh grated lemon peel |
| 2 tsp. Bragg's Liquid Aminos | ¼ cup chopped parsley |
| ¼ cup grated carrots | |

Simmer for 1 minute, then serve hot.

# rice purifying soup

*A good start to a macrobiotic cleansing diet.*

**Makes:** 6 cups

Toast in a large pan until aromatic (about 5 minutes):

| | |
|---|---|
| ⅔ cup lentils | ⅔ cup split peas |
| ⅔ cup brown rice | 2 cloves garlic, minced |

Add:

| | |
|---|---|
| 1 onion, chopped | 1 carrot, chopped |
| 1 stalk celery, chopped | 3 cups onion or veggie broth |
| 3 cups water | 1 tsp. cayenne pepper |
| ½ tsp. lemon pepper | ½ tsp. ginger powder. |

Simmer over low heat for 1 hour, stirring occasionally.

# onion & miso broth

*A therapeutic broth with antibiotic and immune-enhancing properties.*

**Makes:** 6 small bowls of broth

| | |
|---|---|
| 1 chopped onion | ½ tsp. sesame oil |
| 1 stalk celery with leaves | 1 qt. vegetable stock |
| 4 tbsp. miso | 2 green onions with tops |

Sauté onion in the sesame oil for 5 minutes. Add celery, sauté for 2 minutes. Add vegetable stock, cover and simmer 10 minutes. Add miso and green onion. Remove from heat; purée in blender.

# miso, green tea and mushroom broth

*Delicious, nutritious and balancing.*

**Makes:** 2 large servings

| | |
|---|---|
| 2 tbsp. green tea leaves | 2-inch piece lemongrass |
| 2 tbsp. sea vegetables | 1 cup water |
| 3 cups dry shiitake mushrooms | 1 large garlic clove, minced |
| ½ small onion, diced | 1 tsp. olive oil, |
| 1 tsp. sesame oil | 3 cups vegetable stock |
| ¼ cup shredded carrots | 1 tbsp. miso paste |
| cayenne pepper | |

Soak the shiitake mushrooms in a bowl of cool water, just enough to cover, for 20 minutes or until soft. Then slice thinly, saving the soaking water.

In a different bowl, steep the green tea (place in an infuser for easy removal), lemongrass and sea vegetables in 1 cup near-boiling water. Allow to steep for 5 minutes, then discard the tea leaves and lemongrass. Add the sliced shiitake mushrooms.

In a soup pot, lightly sauté the garlic and onion with the olive oil and sesame oil. Add the vegetable stock, bring to a boil and add carrots, miso paste, mushroom soaking water and cayenne pepper to taste. Cook five minutes. Add tea/mushroom mixture, reduce heat and simmer gently for five more minutes.

# immune protection broth

*Drink during high risk seasons for added protection.*

**Makes:** 6 large servings (a week's supply)

| | |
|---|---|
| 1 oz. dry reishi mushrooms | 1 oz. dry shiitake mushrooms |
| 4 tbsp. dry sea vegetables | 1 oz. astragalus bark |
| 1-inch piece ginger root | |

In a bowl, soak above ingredients in water to cover. When soft, sliver mushrooms (save soaking water); discard astragalus and ginger.

In a soup pot, add mushrooms, 8 cups water, the soaking water, plus:

| | |
|---|---|
| 4 tbsp. organic pearled barley | 4 tbsp. organic brown rice |
| 2 cups chopped organic vegetables (any kind) | |

Simmer 30 minutes.

# chinese medicine deep detox stew

*A traditional stew to enhance immunity, reduce cholesterol and regulate blood pressure.*

**Makes:** 4 bowls

| | |
|---|---|
| 15 shiitake mushrooms | 1 oz. black fungus |
| 3 cloves garlic | 2 leeks |
| 4 tbsp. sesame seeds | 2 tbsp. sesame oil |
| 2 burdock roots, chopped | 2 oz. dry hijiki seaweed |
| 1 bunch bok choy, chopped | 1 small can lycii berries |
| 6 tbsp. white miso | |

Soak the shiitake and black fungus in a bowl of cool water, just enough to cover, for 20 minutes or until soft. Then slice thinly, saving the soaking water.

In a soup pot, sauté the garlic, leeks and sesame seeds in the sesame oil for 5 minutes. Add the burdock and hijiki and sauté for 5 minutes more.

Add mushrooms, fungus, soaking water, another 6 cups water and bring up to a simmer. Then add the bok choy, lycii berries, and white miso. Let simmer for several minutes to allow the flavors to blend.

**119**

# immune booster soup

*Enjoy this soup as part of your healing diet.*

**Makes:** 4 bowls

| | |
|---|---|
| 2 tbsp. olive oil | 1 leek |
| ½ cup scallions, sliced | ½ cup fennel, diced |
| 6 garlic cloves, minced | 6 cups vegetable stock |
| 1 cup green cabbage, chopped | 1 cup broccoli florets |
| 2 cups frozen peas | 4 cups dark green leaves |
| ½ cup fresh parsley |   (kale, collards, spinach, chard) |
| 2 tsp. astragalus extract | 4 tbsp. sea vegetables |
| cayenne to taste | |

Sauté the olive oil, leek, scallions, fennel and garlic for 5 minutes or until aromatic. Add vegetable stock, green cabbage and broccoli, and simmer for for another 10 minutes. Add peas, dark green leaves, parsley and astragalus extract. Simmer 5 minutes, add sea vegetables and season with cayenne to taste.

# herb & vegetable immune enhancing broth

*Alkalizing and nutritious.*

**Makes:** 4 cups of broth

| | |
|---|---|
| 3 cups vegetable stock | 2 tbsp. miso dissolved in 1 cup water |
| 1 tbsp. nutritional yeast flakes | 2 tbsp. green onions, chopped |
| ½ cup tomato juice | ½ tsp. dry basil |
| ½ tsp. thyme | ½ tsp. savory |
| ½ tsp. marjoram | |

In a soup pot, bring the vegetable stock to a simmer. Add the remaining ingredients and bring back to a simmer before removing from heat.

# women's blood tonic

*This Chinese herb blood-nourisher is a long term tonic for menopausal women. The herbs can be bought in a health food store.*

**Makes:** 6 large bowls

| | |
|---|---|
| 8 cups vegetable stock | 1 oz. dong quai root |
| 1 oz. astragalus | ½ oz. poria mushroom |
| 1 oz. wild yam root | 8 black dates |
| 16 red dates | 2 tbsp. tamari or |
| |   Bragg's Liquid Aminos |

In a soup pot, bring the vegetable stock to a simmer. Add the remaining ingredients (except for the tamari) and simmer for 30 minutes. Discard herbs and add the tamari.

# spring cleanse carrot soup

*Use as part of a spring or liver cleanse.*

**Makes:** 6 bowls

| | |
|---|---|
| 1 large onion, minced | 2 tbsp. olive oil |
| 8 cups water | 1 cup dry nettles or watercress |
| ½ cup dry yellow dock root | ½ cup fresh dandelion leaves |
| 4 carrots, diced | 3 tbsp. white miso. |

In a soup pot, sauté the onion in the olive oil until translucent. Add the water, nettles, yellow dock, dandelion leaves, carrots and miso. Bring to a simmer and cook 30 min.

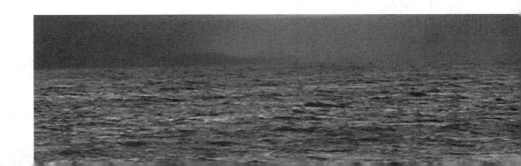

# mineral balance soup

*This detox soup from Japan has anti-viral, anti-diabetic and anti-aging properties.*

**Makes:** 2 bowls

| | |
|---|---|
| ¼ daikon radish, chopped | ¼ large burdock root |
| 1 carrot, sliced | 2 shiitake mushrooms, sliced |

In a soup pot, combine all ingredients, then add just enough water to cover. Simmer for one hour. Discard burdock root.

# sea vegetable tonics

Sea vegetables and marine superfoods like spirulina and chlorella are a veritable medicine chest of premium nutrition. Ounce for ounce sea vegetables are higher in essential nutrients than any other food group. They are vigorous sources of proteins, enzymes, antioxidants and amino acids with whole cell availability. Sea plants offer your body basic building blocks for acid/alkaline balance, regulate body fluid osmosis, strengthen nerves synapses, digestive and circulatory activity, help reduce cholesterol and regulate blood sugar levels.

They are especially rich in minerals like iodine and potassium (with all forty-four trace minerals), and chlorophyll, have substantial amounts of beta carotene, B vitamins (the only vegetarian source of measureable B-12), essential fatty acids, octacosanol for tissue oxygenation and soluble fiber.

# mineral-rich energy green

*Helps build strong teeth, bones, nails and hair. A good choice for weight loss.*

**Makes:** 4 drinks

In a blender, combine:

| | |
|---|---|
| ½ cup Amazake Rice Drink | ½ cup oats |
| 2 tbsp. bee pollen granules | 1 packet instant ginseng tea |
| 2 packets barley grass or chlorella granules | 2 tbsp. gotu kola herb, |
| | 2 tbsp. alfalfa leaf |
| 1 tbsp. dandelion leaf | 1 tbsp. crumbled dulse |
| 1 tsp. vitamin c crystals with bioflavonoids | |

Then mix 2 tbsp. into 2 cups of hot water per drink. Let flavors bloom for 5 minutes before drinking. Add 1 tsp. lemon juice or 1 tsp. Bragg's Liquid Aminos if desired.

# basic sea veggie miso special

*Two tablespoons dry sea veggies daily is a therapeutic dose.*

**Makes:** about 4 bowls

| | |
|---|---|
| 4 cups water | 4 tbsp. white miso |
| 2 chopped green onions | 8 oz. firm tofu (small cubes) |
| 6 tbsp. dry crumbled wakame | ½ cup soy mozzarella (small cubes) |
| 3 tsp. nutritional yeast flakes | |

Bring the water to a simmer. Add miso, green onions, tofu and wakame. Simmer for 2 minutes. Remove from heat and add soy mozzarella cheese. Sprinkle with the nutritional yeast flakes. Let flavors bloom 30 seconds and serve.

# mineral-rich alkalizing enzyme soup

*An exceptional source of minerals, trace minerals and enzymes for good assimilation.*

**Makes:** about 4 bowls

Put the following vegetables in a pot with 1 ½ quarts of cold water:

| | |
|---|---|
| 2 potatoes, cubed | 1 onion, chopped |
| 2 carrots, sliced | 1 stalk celery with leaves, sliced |
| 1 cup fresh parsley | 4 tbsp. chopped dry dulse |

Simmer for 30 minutes. Strain and take hot or cold. Add 2 tbsp. soaked flax seed or oat bran if there is chronic constipation. Add 1 tsp. Bragg's Liquid Aminos to each bowl if desired.

# fresh corn and arame soup

*Whole body cleanser.*

**Makes:** 6 servings

In a blender, combine with 1 cup water:

| | |
|---|---|
| 4 cups fresh corn kernels | 1 tsp. garlic powder |
| 1 cup chopped almonds | 1 avocado |
| 4 tbsp. chopped, dry arame | ½ bunch fresh cilantro, chopped |
| 3 tsp. cumin seeds | 1 tbsp. lemon pepper |

Warm gently in a saucepan and serve.

# recipes to clear congestion, and cold/flu infection

These drinks are specifically designed to help clear toxins and infective organisms from your system. They work extremely well—in some cases almost immediately. Use them when you're feeling toxic or run down, or to help you recover from a "hanging on" illness.

# garlic tonic broth

*Use especially at the onset of flu symptoms.*

**Makes:** *6 cups broth*

| | |
|---|---|
| 6 cups water | 2 small heads garlic |
| 1 large onion, chopped | 2 stalks celery, diagonal cut |
| ½ tsp. curry powder | 1 bay leaf |
| 1 pinch saffron | ½ cup fresh parsley, chopped |
| ½ tsp. dry sage | dry sea vegetables to taste |

Add all ingredients to a soup pot, bring to a boil, lower heat and simmer for 20 minutes. Let cool slightly, remove bay leaf and purée in blender.

# cold defense cleanser

*Make this broth the minute you feel a cold coming on. Drink in small sips.*

**Makes:** 2 drinks

In a saucepan, gently simmer:

| | |
|---|---|
| 1 ½ cups water | 1 tbsp. honey |
| 1 tsp. garlic powder | ½ tsp. cayenne |
| 1 tsp. ground ginger | 1 tbsp. lemon juice. |

Remove from heat, and add 3 tbsp. brandy.

# colds & flu congestion tonic

*This tonic really opens up nasal and sinus passages fast. Very potent.*

**Makes:** 2 bowls

Toast in a pan until aromatic:

| | |
|---|---|
| 4 cloves minced garlic | ½ tsp. cumin seeds |
| ¼ tsp. black pepper | ½ tsp. hot mustard powder. |

Stir in 1 tbsp. flax oil, toast a little more and add:

| | |
|---|---|
| 1 cup water | 1 cup cooked split or frozen peas |
| 1 tbsp. fresh cilantro | 1 tsp. turmeric |
| ½ tsp. sesame salt | ½ tsp. ground coriander. |

Simmer gently 5 minutes and serve.

# chinese healing chicken soup

*All over the world, people find that chicken soup really works to speed recovery from colds.*

**Makes:** 2 large bowls of soup

Bring to a simmer:

| | |
|---|---|
| 3 – 4 cups chicken broth | ½ cup bean sprouts |
| 1 cup shredded chicken | ½ cup carrots, diced |
| 2 thin slices of ginger | 2 tbsp. tamari |

Add above ingredients to a soup pot and simmer for 10 minutes.

Add:

| | |
|---|---|
| ½ cup fresh pea pods | ½ cup shredded cabbage |

Simmer for another 3 minutes.

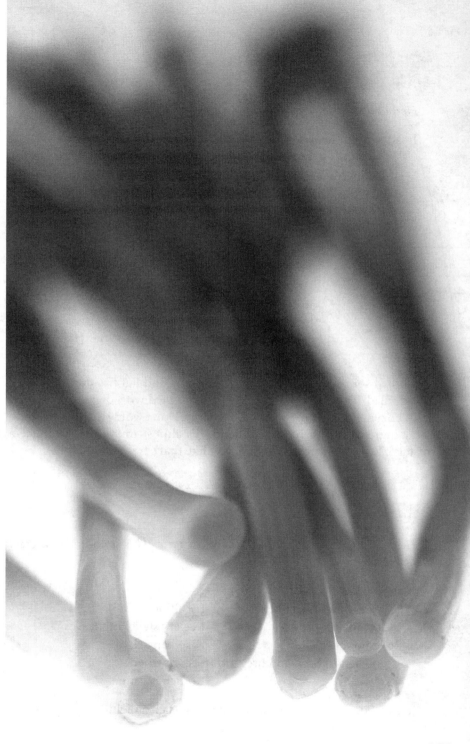

# anti-rhino cold-fighting tea

*Herbal teas are a great addition to any cold/flu fighting program.*

In a teapot of near-boiling water, allow to steep:
1 teaspoon chamomile flowers.
1 dropperful each of echinacea and goldenseal extract
2-inch piece ginger root, skinned and sliced thinly

Steep for ten minutes before straining.

# cold spring and summer soups for easy cleansing

Chilled soups are easy to make, refreshing and light… they're really a liquid salad. They are ideal for cleansing, packed with digestion-friendly plant enzymes for nourishment and energy. Don't worry if you don't have every ingredient in a recipe on hand. It's almost impossible to make a mistake. Just substitute something you like that's fresh and handy.

# gazpacho

*Healthy, low sodium, with all the great taste. This soup makes a great salad dressing, too.*

**Makes:** 2 bowls

| | |
|---|---|
| 2 large tomatoes, cubed | 1 scallion |
| 1 cup alfalfa sprouts | 1 celery stalk with leaves |
| ½ lemon, peeled, | 1 tsp. tamari, |
| 1 pinch each basil and oregano (fresh or dried) | |
| ½ avocado | 1 pinch cayenne |

In a blender, purée ingredients enough to retain a slightly chunky texture.

# high-mineral soup

*Low calorie and delicious.*

**Makes:** 2 bowls

In a blender, purée the following with just enough water to thin:

| | |
|---|---|
| 1 large tomato | 2 stalks celery, chopped |
| 3 green cabbage leaves | ½ small cucumber |
| 6 large spinach leaves | ¼ small beet |
| 1 small green onion | 1 tsp. vegetable salt |

Top with 1 tbsp. crumbled, toasted dulse or crunchy sea palm.

# high-energy soup

*A refreshing, high-energy tonic*

**Makes:** 2 to 3 large bowls

In a blender, purée all ingredients:

| | |
|---|---|
| 4 carrots, chopped | ½ bunch spinach |
| 1 small jicama, peeled/chopped | 1 large tomato |
| 1 stalk celery, chopped | 4 oz. tub alfalfa sprouts |
| 1 handful fresh parsley | |

Add a little water to thin and a dash of hot pepper sauce to spice.

# carrot almond soup

*Very high vitamin A and E for faster recovery.*

**Makes:** 2 to 3 large bowls

In a blender, purée all ingredients:

| | |
|---|---|
| 3 cups carrot juice | 1 cup almonds |
| 1 red bell pepper | ½ bunch dill weed |
| 1 tsp. lemon juice | ¼ tsp. garlic powder |

# high-protein soup

*An excellent choice for high vegetable-source protein.*

**Makes:** 2 to 3 large bowls

In a blender, purée all ingredients:

| | |
|---|---|
| 1 cup mixed nuts and seeds | 1 cup mung or alfalfa sprouts |
| 1 cup grated veggies (squash, zucchini, carrots, celery, peas, etc.) | |
| 3 tbsp. onion, minced | ½ tsp. garlic powder, |
| 1 tsp. tamari | ¼ tsp. cayenne pepper |
| 1 to 2 cups water to thin to desired consistency | |

# infection stopper soup

*A potent therapeutic soup, especially for the flu.*

**Makes:** 2 bowls

| | |
|---|---|
| 2 to 3 garlic cloves | 1 tbsp. balsamic vinegar |
| 1 cup chopped mixed kale, collards and spinach leaves | |
| 1 large tomato, chopped | 2 stalks celery, chopped |

Sautée the garlic in a little olive oil until fragrant, then add remaining ingredients to the pan and gently simmer for a few minutes over low heat. Purée in a blender and refrigerate before serving.

# watermelon diuretic soup

*Release water weight and feel better fast.*

**Makes:** 6 bowls

In a blender, purée all ingredients:

| | |
|---|---|
| 1 6-lb. watermelon | 1 lime, peeled |
| 1 lemon, partially peeled | ⅔ cup blueberries |
| ½ cup fennel bulb, diced | ½ cup mint, chopped |
| 1-inch piece fresh ginger, peeled and sliced | 1 red chile pepper |

# arthritis relief asparagus soup

*This soup is excellent to release congestive wastes and crystalline deposits that lead to joint pain.*

**Makes:** 4 bowls

In a blender, purée all ingredients:

| | |
|---|---|
| 1 cup whole almonds | 2 cups fresh asparagus |
| 1 small handful parsley | (save tips for topping) |
| 2 cups leafy salad greens | 2 stalks celery |
| 1 clove garlic | |

Garnish each bowl with the reserved asparagus tips.

# antioxidant ginger broth

*Anti-aging, antioxidant benefits.*

**Makes:** 4 drinks

| | |
|---|---|
| 3 tbsp. olive oil | 2 tbsp. garlic, minced |
| 2 tbsp. ginger root, minced | 2 onions, chopped |
| 2 lbs. carrots, chopped | 4 cups vegetable stock |
| 1 tbsp. grated orange zest | 1 ½ cups orange juice |
| cayenne pepper | crumbled sea vegetables to taste |

Sauté olive oil, garlic, ginger and onions for 5 minutes or until aromatic. Add carrots and vegetable stock. Simmer for 40 minutes. Remove solids with a slotted spoon. Purée in the blender and return them to the pot with other liquid. Add zest and orange juice. Season with cayenne and sea vegetables to taste.

# simple raw salads & dressings for cleansing

A simple fruit or vegetable salad is the best way to begin and end a liquid detox diet. A small salad the night before prepares your body and starts the cleansing process. A salad on the last night of a fast begins the enzymatic and healthy digestive peristalsis. Use the following salads any time you want to put less strain on your digestive system.

## Fruit salads to take until noon

Fruits are wonderful for a quick system wash and cleanse. Their high natural water and sugar content speeds up metabolism to release wastes rapidly. Fresh fruit has an alkalizing effect in the body, and is high in vitamins and nutrients. The way that you eat fruits is as important as which fruits you eat. Eat fruits alone or with other fruits for their best healing and nutritional effects. With a few exceptions, eat fruits before noon to take advantage of your body's best energy conversion and cleansing benefits.

# morning fresh fruits & yogurt

*High fiber for body system cleansing.*

**Makes:** 4 salads

Mix together lightly in a bowl:
| | |
|---|---|
| 1 banana, sliced | 1 peach or pear, sliced |
| 1 apple, cored and cubed | ¼ fresh pineapple, sliced |
| 1 orange, peeled and sectioned | 2 tbsp. raisins |
| 2 tbsp. toasted sunflower seeds | ½ cup lemon/lime yogurt |

Top with 2 tbsp. granola if desired

# pineapple enzyme sundae

*Serve as breakfast or a healthy dessert.*

**Makes:** 6 salads

Mix together lightly in a bowl:
3 cups fresh pineapple or mango, cubed
3 cups apples or apricots, chopped
12 fresh strawberries or cherries
6 tbsp. almonds, finely chopped

# mid-morning fruit treat

*Deliciously satisfying.*

**Makes:** 4 salads

Mix together lightly in a bowl:
| | |
|---|---|
| 4 bananas, sliced | 2 pears, sliced |
| 3 cups green grapes | 2 peaches, sliced |
| 4 nectarines, sliced | |

To top with a delicious sauce: in a blender, purée 2 cups of fresh fruit with 1 cup raisins. Top fruit treat with 4 tbsp. shredded coconut.

# morning melon salad

*For best digestion, activity and cleansing results, eat melons alone.*

**Makes:** 4 salads

Mix together lightly in a bowl:
1 honeydew melon, cubed (rind removed)
½ casaba, cubed (rind removed)
½ cantaloupe, cubed (rind removed)

If desired, use a blender to make a sauce with a portion of the melon mix and pour over salad.

# spring cleanse salad

*Excellent as part of a spring or arthritis detox.*

**Makes:** 2 salads

Mix together lightly in a bowl:

| | |
|---|---|
| 1 peach, peeled, cubed | 1 nectarine, peeled, cubed |
| 1 apricot, peeled, cubed | 12 cherries, pitted |

# morning citrus mix

**Makes:** 2 salads

Mix together lightly in a bowl:
2 oranges, peeled and sectioned

| | |
|---|---|
| 2 cups fresh pineapple, cubed | 1 grapefruit, cubed |
| 1 kiwi, peeled and cubed | 2 cups red & black seedless grapes |

Keep sauces and dressings simple for body cleansing fruit salads. I make them in the blender and pour them over the fruit just before I'm ready to eat.

# basic fruit creams

*I use variations of this in so many recipes!*

**Makes:** 2 servings

In a blender, blend:
1 or 2 small pieces of any fruit you used in a salad
1 tbsp. honey

For a thin sauce, add about ½ cup water. For thicker sauce, add 1 banana or ½ avocado.

# apple-avocado cream

*Full of fiber and essential fats.*

**Makes:** 2 cups

In a blender, blend:

| | |
|---|---|
| 2 golden delicious apples | 1 – 2 avocados |
| ½ cup apple juice | 1 tbsp. honey |

# pineapple whip dressing

*High vitamin C and potassium.*

In the blender, blend:

| | |
|---|---|
| ¼ fresh pineapple, cubed | 2 – 3 bananas, sliced |

# A fresh vegetable salad is one of mother nature's "superfoods"

Massive new research is validating what natural healers have known for decades. The more fruits and vegetables you eat, the less your risk of disease. For example, people who eat plenty of vegetables have half the risk of developing cancer as people who eat few vegetables.

Most studies show that even moderate amounts of vegetables make a big difference. Eating certain fresh vegetables twice a day, instead of twice a week, can cut the risk of lung cancer by 75%, even in smokers. The evidence is so overwhelming that some researchers are beginning to view fruits and vegetables as powerful preventive "drugs" that could substantially wipe out the scourge of cancer. What an about-face this has been for cancer study!

The healing power of vegetables works both raw and cooked. It is not always true that raw vegetables are better. Even though several fragile anticancer agents, like indoles and vitamin C, are destroyed by heat, a little heat makes beta carotene more easily absorbed. I frequently recommend

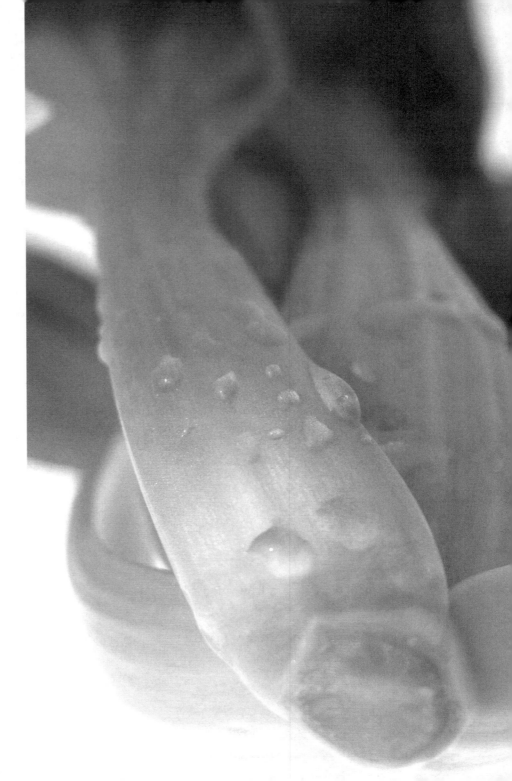

lightly cooked vegetables because their action is gentler, especially if your body is very ill or your digestion is impaired.

What is a serving of fresh vegetables? One serving is about ½ cup of cooked or chopped vegetables, 1 cup of leafy vegetables, or 6 ounces of vegetable juice. Only 10% of Americans eat that much every day.

## shredded salad supreme

*To me, grated or shredded veggies have much more flavor—more of their nutritious, flavorful juices are released during the grating process.*

**Makes:** 1 large salad

Mix together in a bowl:
| | |
|---|---|
| 1 cup carrots, grated | 1 cup cabbage, shredded |
| 1 cup zucchini, shredded | 2 green onions, cut in matchsticks |
| 1 handful fresh parsley | top with toasted sesame seeds |

Use with Mustard Garlic Sauce (page 132), if desired.

## evergreen salad

*High chlorophyll for cleansing.*

**Makes:** 2 salads

Mix together in a bowl:
2 cups mixed greens (romaine, endive, chicory, spinach), chopped
1 small handful watercress leaves, parsley and chives, minced
2 cups green onions, minced

For the dressing, mix together and pour over salad:
| | |
|---|---|
| juice of ½ lemon | 1 tbsp. dijon mustard |
| 1 tbsp. sesame seeds | 1 tbsp. toasted sesame oil |

# lettuce & lemon potpourri

*Tangy and nutritious.*

In a bowl, make a mix of your favorite lettuces. Then, add:

| | |
|---|---|
| 2 tbsp. fresh lemon juice | 1 tbsp. fresh lime juice |
| 1 tsp. honey | 1 tsp. Italian herbs |
| a pinch of cracked pepper | 1 tbsp. olive oil |

Toss with the lettuces until they're coated.

# cucumber body flushing salad

*A great choice for weight control.*

**Makes:** 3 large salads

Slice and divide on salad plates:

| | |
|---|---|
| 2 large cucumbers, peeled | 3 large tomatoes |
| ½ cup celery, chopped | 1 red pepper, finely chopped |

For a topping, mix in a small bowl:

| | |
|---|---|
| 1 clove garlic, minced | 2 tbsp. fresh chives, chopped |
| juice of ½ lemon | 2 tsp. dry sea vegetables (any type), minced |

# guacamole salad

*Use as a dip for baked corn chips or eat by itself.*

**Makes:** 2 to 4 salads

In a bowl, mix:

| | |
|---|---|
| 1 ripe avocado, mashed | juice of 1 fresh lemon |
| 1 tsp. granulated dulse | 2 tomatoes, diced |
| ½ red pepper, diced | 1 tbsp. red onion, minced |

# fresh goulash salad

*A new twist on the dinner salad.*

**Makes:** 4 salads

In a bowl, toss together:

| | |
|---|---|
| 1 cup tomatoes, diced | 1 cup zucchini, shredded |
| 1 cup fresh corn kernels | ¼ cup bell pepper, chopped |
| ¼ cup green onion, finely chopped | |
| A few pinches of thyme, oregano and marjoram | |

Top with a fresh goulash sauce:

In a blender, blend:

| | |
|---|---|
| 1 tomato | 1 pinch cayenne pepper |
| 4 tbsp. sunflower seeds | juice of ½ lemon |

Pour over the salad.

# spinach & sprout salad

*An excellent protein and greens salad to end a detox cleanse. Serve chilled.*

**Makes:** 2 salads

Toss together in a large bowl:

1 small bunch fresh spinach leaves, washed
8 oz. fresh mung bean sprouts
2 cakes tofu, diced (or 4 oz. fresh sliced mushrooms)

For a healthy dressing, mix and top with:

| | |
|---|---|
| 2 tbsp. toasted sesame oil | 2 tbsp. brown rice vinegar |
| 2 tsp. tamari | 2 tsp. crystallized ginger, minced |
| 1 tsp. sesame salt | |

# mushrooms and greens

*Toss all ingredients and add a dressing of your choice. Dark, chlorophyll-rich greens are delicious with mushrooms. Try watercress and mushrooms, too.*

**Makes:** 2 to 4 salads

In a bowl, toss together:
- 2 cups spinach leaves, washed and sliced
- 4 tbsp. green onions, minced
- 4 tbsp. balsamic vinegar
- 2 beets with tops, diced in matchsticks
- 2 cups mushrooms, thinly sliced

# sprouts galore

*High vegetable protein and Vitamin K source.*

**Makes:** 6 salads

In a large bowl, mix together:
- 4 cups mung and lentil bean sprouts
- 4 tbsp. tamari or Bragg's Liquid Aminos
- 2 tbsp. green onions, finely chopped
- ½ clove garlic, minced
- 2 tbsp. olive oil
- 2 tsp. kelp

# sprouts plus

*A tasty variation on the sprout salads.*

**Makes:** 2 salads

In a bowl, mix:
- 1 tub alfalfa sprouts
- 1 cup celery, chopped
- 2 cups carrots, grated

# sesame-mushroom medley

*Chill for 1 hour before serving.*

**Makes:** 6 salads

In a large bowl, mix together:
- 1 lb. mushrooms, sliced
- 1 bunch scallions, sliced
- 2 tbsp. toasted sesame oil
- 3 tbsp. each toasted black and white sesame seeds
- 1 red bell pepper, diced
- 1 tsp. coriander
- 1 pinch cayenne pepper

For a healthy dressing, mix and top with:
- 1 tbsp. tamari
- 1 tbsp. mirin or sake wine
- juice of 2 limes

# four mushroom immune-boost

*Medicinal mushrooms are some of the most potent healing foods available.*

**Makes:** 6 salads

In a large saucepan, sautée in 1 tbsp. olive or sesame oil for 4 minutes:
- 2 garlic cloves, minced
- 3 oz. oyster mushrooms
- 3 oz. reishi mushrooms
- 2 tbsp. balsamic vinegar
- 2 tsp. pickled ginger, minced
- 3 oz. shiitake mushrooms
- 3 oz. portobellas (or maitake)

Add and simmer 2 minutes:
- ¼ cup tamari
- ¼ cup seasoned stock

Set aside mushroom mix.

In a large bowl, toss:
- 1 head belgian endive, finely sliced
- ½ head red leaf lettuce, chopped
- ½ head endive, chopped
- 1 head raddichio, chopped

Divide between salad plates and top with mushroom mix.

## make a rainbow salad

*Prepare each vegetable separately. Then, serve this salad on a round platter with each veggie in concentric "rainbow color arcs."*

**Makes:** 6 salads

> 2 cups purple cabbage, thinly sliced
> 2 cups broccoflower, thinly sliced
> 3 small crookneck squash, grated
> 2 large beets, grated
> 4 carrots, grated
> 3 small zucchini, grated

For a healthy dressing, mix and toss salad with:

| | |
|---|---|
| 3 tbsp. toasted sesame seeds | 3 tbsp. toasted sesame oil |
| 2 tbsp. tamari | 1 tsp. garlic powder |

## wild spring herb and flower salad

*An excellent liver cleanser.*

**Makes:** 6 salads

In a large bowl, mix:

> ½ head romaine lettuce, chopped
> ½ head red leaf lettuce, chopped
> ½ head frisée lettuce, chopped
> ⅓ cup young nasturtium leaves
> ¼ cup fresh dandelion leaves, chopped
> 2 tbsp. dried sea vegetables, toasted (any type)

| | |
|---|---|
| ½ cup arugula leaves | ¼ cup sweet violet flowers |
| ⅓ cup sweet violet leaves | ¼ cup orange mint leaves |
| ¼ cup lemon balm leaves | 1 tbsp. fresh dill weed, chopped |

Top salad with 3 tbsp. olive oil and 2 tbsp. balsamic vinegar.

## sweet & sour cucumbers

*Use as part of a spring cleanse or anytime the mood strikes you.*

**Makes:** one salad

In a bowl, mix:

| | |
|---|---|
| 1 cucumber, thinly sliced | ¼ cup red onion, chopped |

For a healthy dressing, blend and top with:

| | |
|---|---|
| 2 tsp. olive oil | 2 tsp. honey |
| 3 tsp. raspberry vinegar | |

Chill for 2 hours. **Optional:** Before serving top with 1 tablespoon of plain or lemon yogurt.

## sweet & sour mixed salad

*A healthy alternative to sweet and sour dishes served at restaurants.*

**Makes:** one large salad

In a bowl, mix and set aside:

> 1 cucumber, thinly sliced
> ½ green or red bell pepper, thinly sliced

In a sauce pan, sauté until aromatic:

| | |
|---|---|
| 3 thin slices red onion | 1 tsp. honey |
| ¼ cup tarragon vinegar | 1 tsp. daikon radish |

Mix with veggies. Serve over lettuce.

For a healthy dressing, blend and top with:

| | |
|---|---|
| 6 tbsp. olive oil | 4 tbsp. lime juice |
| 4 tbsp. tomato juice | 1 tsp. sesame salt |

# carrot & lemon salad

*A good digestive health recipe.*

**Makes:** 2 salads

In a bowl, mix:
- 2 cups carrots, grated
- 2 tsp. fresh mint, minced
- 2 tbsp. raisins

For a healthy dressing, blend and spoon over carrots:
- 2 tbsp. lemon juice
- ¼ tsp. 5 spice powder
- 1 pinch stevia leaf
- 1 ½ tbsp. canola oil
- 2 tsp. fresh parsley, diced

# carrot & cabbage slaw

*A cabbage lover's delight.*

**Makes:** 2 salads

In a food processor, mix and set aside:
- ½ head Chinese cabbage
- 1 carrot

Then, make a healthy dressing. In s small bowl, blend:
- 2 tsp. honey
- 1 tsp. crystallized ginger
- 1 green onion, minced
- 3 tbsp. tarragon vinegar
- ¼ tsp. sesame salt

Toss with veggies, and chill to marinate.

# simple sauces & dressings for your cleansing veggie salads

Make fresh, right before serving if you can for best taste and nutrition.

# basic vegetable dressing

*Almost every vegetable, or mix of veggies, can be blended with seasonings to make a low fat, cleansing dressing for salads. Options: Use avocado to bind after liquefying other ingredients. Add a little water into blender to help blend mixture.*

**Makes:** 2 servings

In a blender, mix:
- 1 veggie (your choice), chopped
- 1 tbsp. tamari
- 1 tbsp. granulated dulse
- 1 tbsp. olive oil

**Optional:** Add 1 tsp. powdered garlic, ginger or mustard.

# mustard garlic sauce

*One of my personal favorites.*

**Makes:** 2 servings

In a blender, blend:
- ½ cup walnuts, chopped
- 1 tbsp. dijon mustard
- 1 tsp. garlic, minced
- 2 tbsp. tahini
- 1 lemon, peeled
- 1 tsp. tamari

Add a little water to thin slightly.

# low-fat northern italian

*Healthy and delicious.*

**Makes:** 2 servings

In a bowl, whisk together:

| | |
|---|---|
| 1 tbsp. fresh parsley, chopped | 2 tsp. wine vinegar |
| a pinch garlic/lemon seasoning | 2 tsp. lemon juice |
| 2 tsp. olive oil | 1 tbsp. water or white wine |

# avocado dressing

*Rich in essential fats for skin health and beauty.*

**Makes:** 4 servings

In a blender, mix:

| | |
|---|---|
| 3 avocados | ½ cup celery, chopped |
| ½ cup red bell pepper, diced | ½ lemon, peeled |
| ½ cup scallions, minced | ½ cup parsley flakes |
| 1 tsp. garlic herb seasoning | a little water to blend |

# zucchini sauce

*A chunky, fiber-rich sauce.*

**Makes:** 4 servings

In a food processor, mix:

| | |
|---|---|
| 1 medium zucchini, grated | 1 small jicama, peeled |
| ½ medium tomato, chopped | ½ avocado |
| 2 scallions, finely chopped | ½ red bell pepper, chopped |
| 1 tbsp. fresh basil, minced | 1 clove garlic, minced |
| 1 tbsp. olive oil | ½ tsp. vegetable seasoning |
| 1 tbsp. tamari | 4 tbsp. water |

# tahini & lemon dressing

*Healthy and with an Asian flaire.*

**Makes:** 4 servings

In a small bowl, blend:

| | |
|---|---|
| 1 cup tahini | 1 lemon, peeled |
| 1 clove garlic | 1 tbsp. honey |
| 1 sprig each fresh basil and thyme | |

# cool mint dressing

*Eases digestive distress, too.*

**Makes:** 2 servings

In a small bowl, mix:

| | |
|---|---|
| 8 mint leaves, minced | 2 tsp. lemon juice |
| 1 cucumber, diced | 2 tbsp. sesame oil |
| 1 tbsp. tamari | |

# herbs & lemon dressing

*I'm a big fan of cooking with herbs. A healthy dressing is a good place to start.*

**Makes:** 1 serving

In a mixing bowl, whisk:

| | |
|---|---|
| 1 tsp. raspberry vinegar | 1 tsp. lemon juice |
| 1 tbsp. fresh parsley, diced | 2 tbsp. olive oil |
| ¼ tsp. dijon mustard | 1 tsp. fresh basil, minced |
| ¼ tsp. lemon pepper | ¼ tsp. dry tarragon |
| ¼ tsp. dry oregano | ¼ tsp. honey |

# ginger-flaxseed dressing

*A good source of essential fats and vitamin E.*

**Makes:** 2 cups

In a blender, mix:

| | |
|---|---|
| 1 cucumber, chopped | ½ cup sunflower seeds |
| 1 tbsp. flax seeds | 1 tbsp. fresh grated ginger |
| 1 tsp. sesame oil | 1 ½ cups water |

# sunflower seed cream

*A good alternative to salty soy sauce.*

**Makes:** 2 servings

In a blender, mix all ingredients with 2 – 4 tbsp. water:

| | |
|---|---|
| 1 cup sunflower seeds | ½ lemon peeled |
| ½ tsp. tamari | ½ tsp. dulse |
| 1 sprig fresh basil | 1 sprig fresh sage |

# immune-enhancing vinegar

*This vinegar, rich with immune-boosting herbs, strengthens your system as it adds zip to salads. Both fresh and dried herbs work. Warm the vinegar to help to release the herbal benefits. Except for the peppers, amounts of individual herbs aren't important; just fill the jar with what you have on hand. Use as you would any vinegar.*

Pack a clean jar with:

| | |
|---|---|
| echinacea leaves | shiitake mushrooms |
| astragalus chips | thyme |
| basil | sage leaves |
| 6 garlic cloves | 2 whole dry cayenne peppers |

Pour brown rice vinegar or apple cider vinegar over herbs to cover. Let stand 4 – 6 weeks.

# no-oil tamari lemon

*A good choice for people who need to be on very low fat diets.*

**Makes:** one serving

In a bowl, whisk:

| | |
|---|---|
| 2 tbsp. lemon juice | 1 tbsp. tamari |
| 1 tbsp. honey | 1 tsp. sesame seeds |
| 1 tsp crystallized ginger, minced | |

# honey/mustard dressing

*Chill before serving. Use as a nutritious dip, too.*

**Makes:** one serving

In a small bowl, blend:

| | |
|---|---|
| 2 tbsp. olive oil | 1 tsp. dijon mustard |
| 1 tbsp. cider vinegar | 1 tsp. dried dill |
| 1 tsp. honey | ¼ tsp. lemon pepper |

# ginger lemon/lime dressing

*Creamy, but without the fat of milk.*

**Makes:** 4 servings

In a mixing bowl, whisk:

| | |
|---|---|
| 1 cup lemon yogurt | 1 tbsp. lime juice |
| 1 tbsp. lemon juice | ½ tsp. ginger powder |

# salads with sea vegetables

Sea vegetables are natural cleansing superfoods. Their high antioxidant qualities make sea vegetables effective toxin scavengers that can help detoxify both the digestive and eliminative tracts. I try to eat them every day, and since I believe in a green salad every day, too, sea veggies and salads have become a staple combination in my lifestyle. Dried sea vegetables can be soaked in water and reconstituted before adding to a salad. Roasted nori or dulse flakes are a tasty, crunchy sprinkle on a salad before serving. They are also wonderful as part of a low-fat, nutritious salad dressing.

## sesame sea veggie vinaigrette

*Delicious homemade sesame seed dressing.*

**Makes:** 3 servings

In a small mixing bowl, blend together:

| | |
|---|---|
| ¼ cup tamari | 3 tbsp. brown rice vinegar |
| 1 tsp. each black sesame seeds, white sesame seeds | |
| 1 tbsp. toasted sesame oil | 1 tbsp. sake |
| 2 tsp. honey | a pinch granulated dulse |

## wakame salad pickles

*Use this recipe as an appetizer or as a "pickle" garnish for any salad.*

**Makes:** 4 servings

Soak 1 cup or ½ oz. dried wakame in water on a small plate until tender. Drain. Cut into quarter-inch strips. Set aside.

To make the dressing, mix in a small bowl :

| | |
|---|---|
| ½ tsp. toasted sesame oil | ¼ cup red onion, thinly sliced |
| 1 tsp. honey | 1 tsp. crystallized ginger, minced |

Top wakame with dressing. Chill for 4 hours and serve.

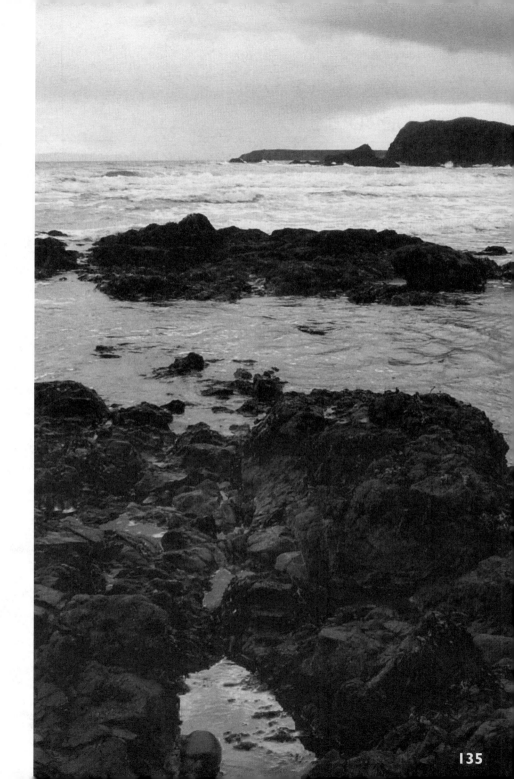

# marinated sea palm with roasted red peppers

*A perfect topper for salads, vegetables, grains, grilled salmon and swordfish.*

**Makes:** 4 servings

Soak 1 oz. dry sea palm fronds on a small plate with water until tender. Drain and set aside.

In a small bowl, mix:
2 roasted red bell peppers, thinly sliced (bottled okay)
2 tbsp. fresh mixed herbs, minced (like rosemary, basil and thyme)
4 tbsp. balsamic vinegar       2 tsp. lemon pepper
4 cloves garlic, minced        ½ cup sesame oil
3 tbsp. honey                  2 tbsp. crystallized ginger root

Pour over sea palm and marinate for about 4 hours before serving.

# sea veggie soup and salad sprinkle supreme

*This blend is a flavor enhancer, and a nutritional part of any recipe. Crumble into a bowl; then just barely blend in the blender, so that there are still sizeable chunks of the sea vegetables. They expand in any recipe with liquid, and when heated, return to the beautiful green color they had in the ocean. Use freely as a seasoning on salads, soups and rice.*

Heat in a dry pan:
¾ cup dried dulse, chopped
½ cup dried nori or sea palm, chopped
¼ cup dried wakame, chopped
¼ cup dried kombu, chopped
¼ cup toasted walnuts, chopped
½ cup toasted sesame seeds

# watercress and herb salad

*I love to use watercress in my recipes. Try this one out!*

**Makes:** 1 to 2 servings

In a large salad bowl, mix:
2 tbsp. dried nori or sea palm, finely chopped
2 tbsp fresh marjoram leaves, minced
1 bunch watercress sprigs      1 bunch fresh parsley
1 tsp. garlic, minced          1 cup fresh basil leaves, chopped
2 tbsp. fresh tarragon, minced 1 tbsp. fresh sage leaves, minced
2 tbsp. olive oil              ¼ tsp. cayenne pepper
1 tbsp. fresh lemon juice      1 ½ tbsp. water

# sesame nori no-oil dressing

*A delicious recipe to introduce sea vegetables—as a condiment for a low-fat diet.*

**Makes:** 4 servings

Combine in a jar and shake well to blend:
1 cup toasted nori, chopped    4 tbsp. brown rice vinegar
3 tbsp. sesame seeds, pan roasted
1 cup onion or mushroom broth
1 tsp. tamari or Bragg's Liquid Aminos

Serve over vegetable or rice salads, or ramen noodles.

# sea vegetable main dishes for a detox diet

Modern science is validating many of the traditional benefits of sea plants, especially in relation to their algin content. In fact, the alginic acids in sea vegetables perform a dual miracle. First, algin absorbs toxins from the digestive tract in much the same way that a water softener removes the hardness from tap water. It binds with the ions of toxic heavy metals which are then converted to harmless salts. The salts are insoluble in the intestine and are excreted, so less toxins enter the circulatory system. Second, algin also chelates radioactive matter present in the human body and binds it for elimination via the large intestine. Algin compounds are also thought to be responsible for much of the success of seaweeds in the treatment of obesity, asthma, atherosclerosis and blood purifying.

Still, even though scientists know that algin compounds in seaweeds directly counteract carcinogens, most researchers believe that sea plants primarily boost the body's immune system, allowing it to combat the carcinogens itself.

Sun-dried, packaged sea vegetables retain almost all of their health advantages. The recipes here can be used over a lifetime as part of your immune-boosting detox maintenance plan.

I can't think of a seaweed I don't like… so I've offered a sampling to give you an idea of their great variety and taste. They're good in soups, with cooked vegetables, over hot rice, even in sandwiches.

# nori

The popularity of sushi has introduced many Americans to the sweetness of nori. But this delicate sea vegetable with its distinctive nutty taste is far more versatile. Nori (and its American cousin, laver) is the highest in B-complex vitamins, as well as vitamin C and E.

Nori, and its American counterpart laver, is easy to roast. Spread the dried plant on a baking sheet, sprinkle with teriyaki sauce and bake at 300° for 5 to 8 minutes until crisp but not burned.

## sushi main dish salad

*California maki in a bowl—with the same great taste of sushi rolls.*

**Makes:** 4 salads

In a dry saucepan, toast:
    1 cup brown rice (or a wild and brown rice mix)

Add in:
    2 cups water or light miso broth

Bring to a boil, cover and simmer 30 minutes until all liquid is absorbed. Remove from heat. Set aside.

In a mixing bowl, toss:

| | |
|---|---|
| 1 avocado, chopped | 3 scallions, minced |
| 1 cup crab pieces | 2 tbsp. brown rice vinegar |
| a pinch wasabi powder | |

Blend with the cooked rice. Crumble a toasted nori sheet over the top.

Optional: serve with a dab of the following Hot Mustard Dressing

## hot mustard dressing

In a small bowl, mix:

| | |
|---|---|
| 4 tsp. Chinese hot mustard | 1 tbsp. tamari |
| pinch wasabi powder | 2 tbsp. toasted sesame oil |

## high protein sprouted nori rolls

*This borrows on the principles of macrobiotics and is an excellent adjunct to any healing diet. Add a little water if needed to blend.*

**Makes:** 6 – 8 servings

In a blender, prepare a nut and seed mixture:

2 cups almonds              1 cup sunflower or sesame seeds
½ tsp. sesame oil           1 lemon, peeled
1 tbsp. fresh or pickled ginger, chopped
3 tbsp. tamari

Lay out 6 to 10 toasted nori sheets. Spread nut-seed mixture over sheets. Then, spread 3 cups alfalfa or sunflower sprouts across nut and seed mix, forming a line down the edge of the sheet.

Then, cut into long thin sticks and place lengthwise across nori:

1 carrot                    1 avocado
1 cucumber

Roll up like a burrito. Then eat like a burrito, or cut in 2″ thick rolls. Optional: decorate with fresh basil leaves, sweet-hot mustard or a dab of wasabi.

## sea palm

Sea palm is an ocean vegetable that looks like a miniature palm tree attached to the rocks on the California coast. It lives in the pounding surf of the shoreline, bending and waving in the tides instead of the winds. It has become very popular in California healthy food recipes for its sweet taste and versatility.

Sea palm is delicious. Mix Sea Palm Fronds in a bowl with chopped Almonds or Sunflower or Pumpkin Seeds and 2 tbsp. Teriyaki Sauce. Roast in a 325° oven for 8 to 10 minutes until dry and crunchy. Then sprinkle the mix over a pizza or rice and roast it in. Yum!

## sea palm & tofu casserole

*Finally a tasty casserole without all the cheese!*

**Makes:** 6 servings

Soak 1 oz. dried sea palm fronds in water. Drain and cut in 2-inch lengths. Place in a pan with a little water, cover and simmer for 20 minutes until tender.

Mix in:

1 lb. tofu, mashed          1 tsp. dry basil
1 tsp. dry oregano

Then, sauté in 2 tbsp. canola oil or onion broth for 10 minutes:

1 large onion, diced        1 ½ lbs. carrots, diced

Remove from heat and purée in the blender with 3 tbsp. umeboshi paste or sweet and sour sauce. Toss with sea palm/tofu mix. Heat gently in a skillet.

Then, make the topping. Purée in a blender:

⅓ cup toasted sesame seeds   1 tsp. tamari
6 sprigs fresh parsley       water to make a thick sauce

Spread the topping on the tofu mixture in the skillet, and cook for 5 more minutes to heat. Serve hot.

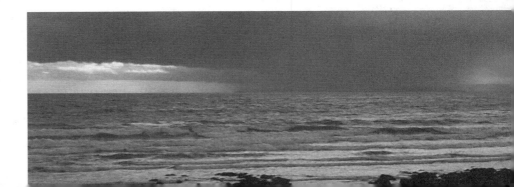

# ocean ribbons

Ocean ribbons are a brown sea plant, thin and delicate like Japanese Kombu, but noticeably sweeter and more tender. They grow on the outermost reaches of the rocky intertidal zone among sea palm and mussel beds, looking like a glistening miniature willow trees overhanging the water at low tide. You can watch ocean ribbons keep the environment clean. Branching off the woody trunk of a mature ocean ribbon plant, over 500 blades sweep its rock face clear of other organisms in the thrashing tidal surges. I like ribbons best with vegetables, in light soups and as a pickled side dish or topping for rice.

## ocean ribbons pickles

*A very unique Asian snack.*

**Makes:** 4 servings

Soak 6 strips ocean ribbons in cold water for 15 minutes. Drain, then chop in 3-inch pieces. Set aside.

In separate bowls, have prepared:
    1 red onion, thin sliced in crescents
    1 long European cucumber, thin sliced

Layer veggies and ocean ribbons in a flat bowl and cover with equal parts mirin, tamari and ume plum vinegar. Press with a weight for 3 hours. Toss and serve.

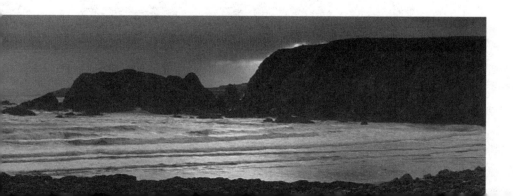

# deep detox stew

*This is a variation on a Traditional Chinese Medicine immune-supporting stew. It helps reduce cholesterol, regulate blood pressure and aid fat digestion.*

**Makes:** 6 bowls

In a pan, soak in 6 cups water until soft, about 20 minutes:
    18 dried shiitake mushrooms, thinly sliced
    1 ½ oz. dried black fungus or reishi mushrooms, thinly sliced
    2 oz. dried ocean ribbons seaweed, thinly sliced

Strain mushrooms and seaweed and set aside. Save soaking water.

Make the miso-sesame paste. In a dry skillet, roast:
    ¼ cup black sesame seeds          ¼ cup white sesame seeds

Then, combine with:
    ⅓ cup miso soup          3 tbsp. of the mushroom-seaweed
                                               stock

And set aside.

In separate bowls, have prepared:
    2 leeks, white and green parts, sliced thinly
    1 fresh burdock root, cut in matchsticks
    1 daikon radish, cut in matchsticks
    1 bunch bok choy, sliced thinly
    3 cloves garlic, minced

Make the stew:

In a large saucepan, sauté the leeks with the garlic in 2 tbsp. sesame oil for several minutes until aromatic. Add the burdock, daikon roots and mushroom-seaweed soaking water. Cover, and let stew 10 minutes until burdock is tender. Mix in the miso-sesame paste, and add the bok choy, mushrooms and ocean ribbons. Cover and cook a few minutes until bok choy is tender. Season with 1 tbsp. tamari.

# wakame

Wakame and its American cousin alaria, are mild and smooth, excellent with rice, black beans and cous cous. Wakame's heavyweight minerals, enzymes and fiber, but lightweight texture and flavor, make it perfect for cleansing soups and salads.

I like to roast wakame before I use it in a grain or pizza recipe. Just chop bite-sized pieces and roast for 3 to 5 minutes at 300°. Use right from the package for soups. Blanch wakame for 20 minutes in hot water before using in a salad. Then, cut out midribs and toss with your greens. Pan-fry as a snack in a little toasted sesame oil and tamari until dark green and crisp.

## millet salad with wakame

*A great way to add more whole grains into your diet.*

**Makes:** 4 salads

In a dry pan, roast 1 cup millet until aromatic. Then, add 2 ½ cups water. Cover. Cook 25 minutes. Remove from heat and fluff with a fork. Set aside.

In a saucepan, add ½ cup wakame pieces, chopped, to hot water. Blanch 3 minutes. Remove with a slotted spoon.

Keep hot and mix in:
½ cup carrots, diced          ¼ cup celery,  diced
⅓ cup daikon radish, diced

Blanch 5 minutes and drain. Season with lemon pepper.

Add:
½ cup fresh parsley, chopped     ½ cup cucumber, diced
handful of dry roasted almonds

Toss all together with millet, and serve on lettuce with the following Sesame Miso Dressing.

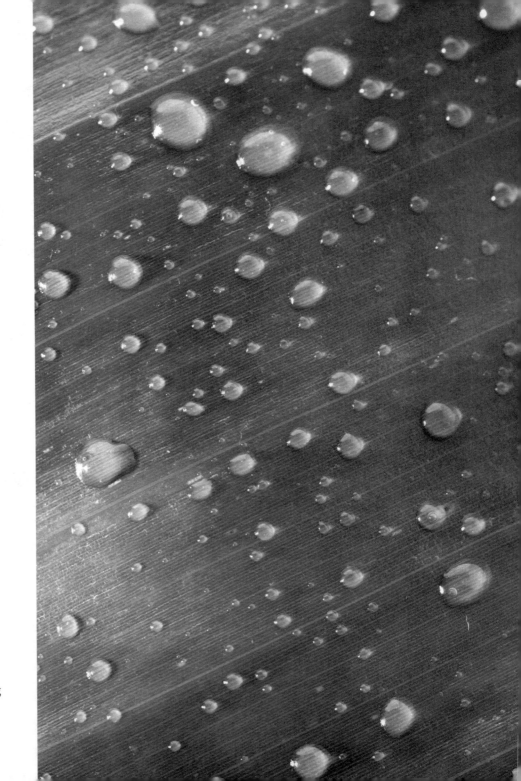

## sesame miso dressing

**Makes:** 1 ½ cups dressing

In a bowl, blend:

⅓ cup plain sesame oil

2 tbsp. toasted sesame oil

½ tsp. vegetable seasoning

3 tbsp. sesame seeds, toasted

1 pinch cayenne or hot pepper sauce to taste

1 tbsp. light miso

2 tbsp. brown rice vinegar

1 tbsp. lemon juice

# kelp and kombu

Kelp and kombu are all-purpose sea veggies. They are delicious in soups in place of chicken or beef stock—especially if you're on a cleansing diet. Just put a strip in for flavor as you make the soup. Then, remove or chop in when the soup is ready. You don't have to add salt if you use kelp. Its minerals provide a salty flavor by themselves. Kelp and kombu are extra good with beans because natural glutamates tenderizes them.

# kelp & honey bits snack

*One of my favorite sweet snacks.*

**Makes:** a dozen snacks

Soak dried kelp or kombu pieces in water in a small bowl. Drain and chop into bite size pieces to fill ½ cup. Set aside.

In a saucepan, bring to a boil ¼ cup honey and ½ cup water.

Reduce heat, add sea vegetables and simmer until liquid is evaporated, about a half hour. Set aside.

On a baking sheet, spread 1 cup sesame seeds or ground almonds

Arrange the sea vegetables on top, turning with tongs to coat. Bake in a 300°F oven for 30 minutes.

# couscous, red lentils & kelp

*A delicious low fat, high protein cleansing meal.*

**Makes:** 6 servings

In a large saucepan, bring 1 ¼ cups water to a boil.

Add:

1 cup couscous

5-inch piece of kelp

2 tbsp. canola oil

Stir, cover and remove from heat. Allow to stand 5 minutes. Remove kelp. Fluff with a fork. Then, sauté with:

2 tbsp. onion broth

½ cup leeks, (white parts only) chopped

1 cup red lentils

1 tsp. tamari

1 tsp. garlic/lemon seasoning

2 cups vegetable stock

1 tomato, chopped

1 tsp. basmati vinegar

a pinch cayenne

Reduce heat, cover and simmer for 20 minutes.

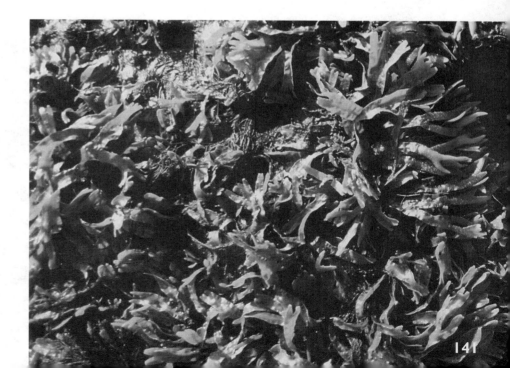

# kombu salad with vinegar sauce

*Use as part of brown rice cleanse or a macrobiotic healing diet.*

**Makes:** 4 salads

    1 handful of dried of kombu (or wakame), in 1-inch lengths

Soak for 1 hour in rice vinegar or lemon juice. (Acidity tenderizes the sea vegetables). Rinse, drain, set aside.

Then, cut into matchsticks:

    1 European-type cucumber, peeled and halved

Sprinkle with sea salt and put in a colander over a pan to drain for 30 minutes. Squeeze out any remaining excess water. In a salad bowl, toss cucumber and kombu with 8 oz. corn niblets and then top with the following Vinegar Sauce.

Serve on tiny appetizer plates.

## vinegar sauce

In a small bowl, blend:

    1 tbsp. brown rice vinegar      1 clove garlic, mashed
    1 tsp. chili powder (or 2 – 3 dashes of hot pepper sauce)
    1 tbsp. honey      1 tbsp. pan-roasted sesame seeds
    ½ bunch green onions with tops, finely chopped

# dulse

Dulse has a nutty, bacon-like taste, so it's great in dips, sandwiches, soups, salads and stir-fries. A rich red seaweed, it's a good source of iron, B vitamins, plant protein and fiber. Cooking with dulse is a treat. You can pan-fry it in a oil-sprayed pan until the pieces turn brownish and crisp like chips. You can dry-roast the pieces in a 300° oven until they turn greenish—not black (burned). Then crumble the crispy pieces onto grains, soups, pizza and popcorn.

I love roasted dulse ground in the blender with walnuts, dried tomatoes and dry basil. Mmmmmm—I use it as a condiment on lots of steamed veggie dishes.

Dulse can be used like bacon bits in sandwiches, chip dips, soups and stir fries.

# brown rice, dulse & tofu

*The protein complementarity of brown rice, dulse and tofu is good for a healing diet.*

**Makes:** 8 servings

In a pan filled with water, soak:

    8 dried shiitake mushrooms
    a small handful dried dulse

When soft, thinly slice mushrooms and dulse, and set aside. Save soaking water.

In a saucepan, dry roast 1 ⅓ cups brown rice. Then, cook in 2 ½ cups water (yields 4 cups cooked). Set aside.

In a skillet, sauté in 2 tbsp. sesame oil:

    2 cakes tofu, cubed      2 cloves garlic, minced
    1 onion, chopped      1 tsp. nutritional yeast flakes
    1 tsp. cumin powder      1 tsp. sesame seeds
    ¼ tsp. lemon pepper

Mix blend into rice. Set aside.

Sauté in 2 tbsp. sesame oil until color changes:

    2 carrots, chopped      2 celery stalks, chopped
    2 zucchini, chopped      1 green bell pepper, sliced thinly
    plus the mushrooms and dulse

Add mushroom soaking water and steam-braise for 5 minutes. Vegetables should be just tender/crisp, not completely cooked. Add to rice and tofu. Season with herb salt and serve.

# brown rice, dulse & greens classic

*I often have this as my healthy breakfast.*

**Makes:** 6 main dish servings

Have prepared:
> 4 cups cooked brown rice.

In a 300° oven, roast for 8 minutes and set aside:
> ½ cup walnuts, chopped     ¼ cup dulse, chopped
> 2 tbsp. sesame seeds

Have ready:
> 1 cup romaine lettuce, shredded
> 1 cup Chinese napa cabbage, finely chopped
> ½ cup bean sprouts or sunflower sprouts
> 1 cup bok choy     1 cup spinach leaves
> 1 carrot, diced     1 slice of onion, chopped
> ½ tsp. fresh ginger, minced     1 garlic clove, minced

Preheat a large wok with 3 – 4 tbsp. sesame oil. Heat the ginger and garllic until fragrant. Add the carrots and onion and sauté for 5 minutes. Mix in the greens and cook just until color changes. Add the sprouts, brown rice, and dulse and seed mix. Blend and heat briefly. Turn off heat. Make a well in the center and add a raw egg (optional). Toss for 3 minutes until hot and set. Turn onto large serving platter. Sprinkle with 1 tbsp. tamari.

# black-bean & dulse chili

*A vegetarian, mineral rich chili alternative.*

**Makes:** 6 bowls

In a pan filled with water, soak:
> ½ oz. dried shiitake mushrooms
> ½ oz. dried black fungus mushrooms
> ½ oz. dry dulse

Drain and thinly slice mushrooms and dulse. Set aside.

Have ready:
> 2-inch piece daikon radish, finely chopped
> ½ cup black beans (uncooked)
> 1 clove garlic, minced     1-inch fresh ginger
> 6 cups vegetable stock

In a large saucepan, simmer the black beans, the mushrooms, dulse and herbs in the vegetable stock.

Add:
> 1 tsp. ground chili negro     1 tsp. herb salt
> 1 cup fresh string beans

Cook on medium low for one hour until bubbly and fragrant.

Top with:
> ½ cup toasted pumpkin seeds     ½ cup fresh minced cilantro

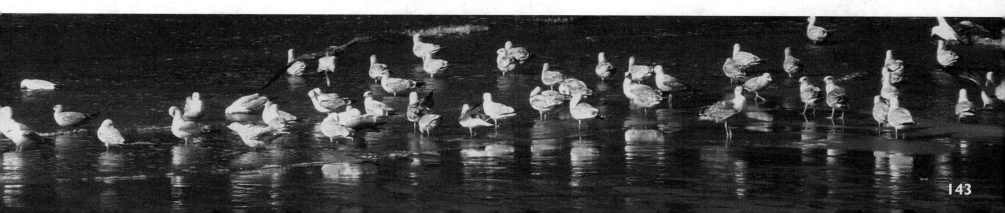

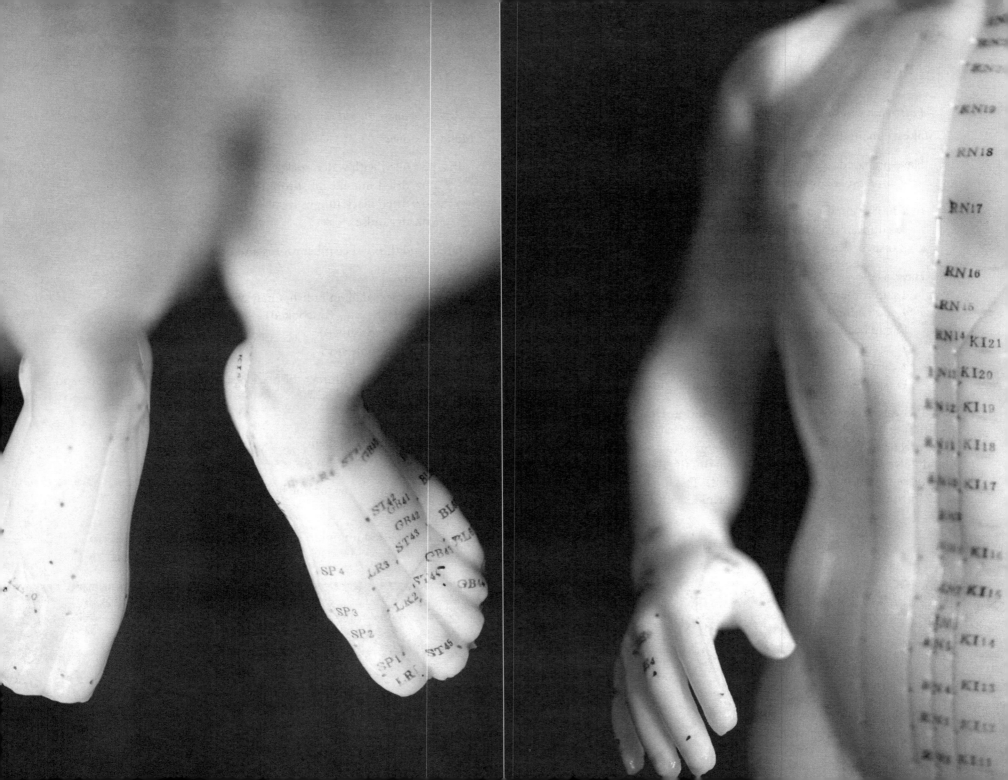

# bodywork for detoxification

## exercise has significant influence on detoxification

**E**XERCISE SPEEDS UP REMOVAL OF TOXINS THROUGH perspiration. Sweating helps expel toxins through the skin, your body's largest organ of elimination. Exercising to the point of perspiration offers overheating therapy benefits, too. Tests show that when athletes sweat, for example, they excrete potential cancer causing elements, like heavy metals and pesticide PCBs from their bodies through perspiration.

**Exercise stimulates removal of toxins through deep breathing.** Low impact aerobics help build a stronger diaphragm and lungs.

**Exercise stimulates metabolism,** especially before you eat, to aid in weight loss. Exercise uses up stored body fat. Calories are burned at a greater pace for several hours after you exercise.

**Exercise stimulates the circulatory system,** lowering blood pressure and preventing heart disease by increasing blood flow. New heart endurance tests show exercise strengthens your circulatory system right down to your capillaries… even forming new ones!

**Exercise stimulates the lymphatic systems.** Blood is pumped through your body by your heart, but lymphatic fluid depends solely on exercise for circulation. Lymph function is critical to your body's ability to cleanse itself.

**Exercise reduces stress by increasing body oxygen levels.** It improves your mood while you purify. Endorphins, the body's "feel good" hormones, are released into the brain by vigorous exercise, explaining the "high" people often experience after exercise.

**Exercise prevents disease.** We know disease often results from an underactive body. Almost any kind of exercise transports oxygen and nutrients to your cells while it carries away toxins and wastes to your elimination organs. Evidence shows good results for: cancer prevention, diabetes management, weight loss, heart and circulatory health, healthy muscle tissue/joints, depression relief, bone building, and memory.

Here are my exercise recommendations for your cleanse:

1. During initial, heavy cleansing: simple, body-balancing, stretching exercises.

2. During the rest of your cleanse: low-impact, aerobic exercise, like a walk or an easy swim for better circulation and lymph activity.

3. For your maintenance program, strengthening exercise (like a daily walk, swim or equipment workout). A moderate exercise program that raises your heart rate for a period of 20 to 30 minutes offers the most benefits.

# overheating therapy is an ancient cleansing technique

Overheating therapy, or hyperthermia as a healing technique, has been known throughout history, from ancient Greek physicians (who raised body temperature as an immune defense against infection), to the elaborate bath complexes of the Romans, to the sweat lodges of the American Indians and the steam baths of the Scandinavians.

Today, high heat procedures, like overheating baths, saunas and steam rooms are experiencing new popularity as people realize their enormous benefits for health. Slightly raising body temperature speeds up metabolism, inhibits the growth of harmful viruses or bacteria, and literally burns out invading organisms. Overheating your body stimulates a slight fever. Fever is a traditional powerful healing tool against disease—a natural defense and healing force created by the immune system to rid the body of harmful pathogens. A high temperature increases metabolism, inhibits viral and bacterial growth, and speeds up natural detoxification.

Ancient herbalists used heat-producing herbs as protective healing measures against colds and simple infections, even against serious degenerative diseases like cancers. Today, artificially induced fevers are used in many bio-holistic clinics for treating acute infectious diseases, arthritic conditions, skin disorders and leukemia. The newest research indicates that AIDS and other virus syndromes respond to blood heating.

Despite skepticism by conventional medicine, supergerms like the HIV virus, that have no effective counteractive drug therapies, mean that other methods must be tried. In 1997, CNN Health News reported on a blood-overheating procedure for AIDS in treating Kaposi's sarcoma, a cancer that produces severe skin lesions in HIV-infected patients. The sores vanished in about four months after the therapy, along with other symptoms. Since then, many AIDS sufferers with sarcoma have undergone overheating therapy with success. In some cases, the blood has even tested negative for the HIV virus! (Researchers warn that even if the blood tests free of HIV, the virus may still be in the bone and resurface.)

## Here's how overheating therapy works as a detoxification mechanism

When exposed to heat, blood vessels in the skin dilate to allow more blood to flow to the surface, activating the sweat glands, which then pour the water onto the skin's surface. As the water evaporates from the skin, it draws both heat and toxins from the body, becoming a natural detoxification treatment as well as a cooling system.

Modern health care professionals are finding that a non-life-threatening fever can do exceptional healing work. Simple overheating therapy can even be effectively practiced in your home, via either a dry sauna or an overheating bath. Both are able to stimulate the body's immune mechanism without the stress of fever-inducing drugs.

## Here's how to take an overheating bath

1. Do not eat for two hours before treatment. Empty your bladder and colon if possible.

2. Get a good thermometer so that your water temperature can be correctly measured. I recommend monitoring bath temperature at all times.

3. Use a large tub if possible. Plug the emergency outlet to raise the water to the top of the tub. You must be totally immersed for therapeutic results—with only nose, eyes and mouth left uncovered. Start slowly running water at skin temperature. After 15 minutes raise temperature to 100°F, then in 15 minutes to 103°F. Even though the water temperature is not high, heat cannot escape from your body when you are totally covered, so body temperature will rise to match that of the water, creating a slight healing fever.

4. A therapeutic bath should be about 45 minutes. If you experience any discomfort, sit up in the tub for 5 minutes.

5. Gentle massaging with a skin brush during the bath stimulates circulation, brings cleansing blood to the surface of the skin, and relieves the heart from undue pressure.

A sauna is another way to use overheating therapy principles. Sauna therapy was developed in Finland, but today it is used all over the world by alternative physicians and clinics to help people release environmental toxins like pesticides and heavy metals. A 30 to 40 minute sauna induces a healing, cleansing fever, and also causes profuse therapeutic sweating. A good sweat uses the skin as a "third kidney" to eliminate body wastes through perspiration. Finish each sauna with a cool shower and a brisk rubdown to remove toxins that have been eliminated through the skin.

Like an overheating therapy bath, a sauna speeds up metabolism, and inhibits the replication of pathogenic organisms. It stimulates vital organs and glands to increased activity. It dramatically increases by profuse sweating the detoxifying and cleansing capacity of the skin. (For optimum skin cleansing and restoration, take a sauna once or twice a week.) Immune response is enhanced and its healing functions are accelerated.

## Here's a quick overview of the cleansing benefits of a dry sauna

- It creates a fever that inhibits the replication of pathogenic bacteria and viruses.
- It increases the number of leukocytes in the blood to strengthen the immune system.
- It provides a prolonged, therapeutic sweat that flushes out toxins and heavy metals.
- It accelerates cardiovascular activity and reduces high blood pressure.
- It stimulates vasodilation of peripheral blood vessels to relieve pain and speed healing of sprains, bursitis, arthritis and muscle pain.
- It promotes relaxation and a feeling of well-being.

Steam baths go back to prehistoric steaming hot springs of our first ancestors. Early man, like primates today in both Japan and Russia, used hot springs to clean and warm themselves, and to remove parasites.

Just as with dry heat saunas, ancient Greeks and Romans used them to sweat for health. But the benefits for a steam bath are different than for a sauna. Hot steam particularly helps respiratory diseases and rheumatic pain. The humid heat of a steam bath is ideal for skin tone and texture.

A steam bath works quicker than a sauna, cleansing the body in about 15 minutes compared to 30 to 40 minutes in a sauna. The powerful detoxification, healing process of hyperthermia does not take place until the body reaches $101 - 103°$ F. In a dry heat sauna, your body's cooling mechanism retards hyperthermia by natural evaporation. In a steam bath, evaporation is not possible so there is no loss of body heat. In fact, steam condensation actually becomes the heat transfer mechanism on the body.

**Note:** Overheating is one of the most effective treatments in natural healing. Inducing a "fever" is a natural, constructive means the body also uses to heal itself. Yet, heat methods are powerful and should be used with care. If you are under medical supervision for heart disease or high blood pressure, a heart and general vitality check is advisable. If you are ill, or have been recently, supervision is necessary during an overheating bath and reactions must be monitored closely. The pulse should not go over 130 or 140. In addition, some people who are seriously ill lose the ability to perspire; this should be known before using overheating therapy. Check with your physician to determine if overheating therapy from a sauna or a seaweed bath is all right for you.

# a detox bath is pleasant, easy and stress-free

Holistic healing clinics and spas are famous all over the world for their therapeutic baths. They use mineral clays, aromatherapy oils, seaweeds and enzyme herbs to draw toxins out of the body through the skin, and to put restorative, healing nutrients into the body through the skin.

During a detox program, I recommend a therapy bath at least twice daily to remove toxins coming out on the skin. The procedure for taking an effective healing bath is important. In essence, you soak in an herbal tea, where the skin takes in the healing nutrients instead of the mouth and digestive system.

## There are two good ways to take a therapeutic bath

1. Draw very hot bath water. Put the herbs, seaweeds, or mineral crystals into a large teaball or muslin bath bag. Add mineral salts directly to the water. Steep until water cools and is aromatic. Rub the body with the solids in the muslin bag during the bath.

OR

2. Make a strong tea infusion in a large teapot, strain and add to hot bath water. Soak as long as possible to give the body time to absorb the healing properties.

**Note:** Food grade 35% $H_2O_2$ (hydrogen peroxide) may be used as a detoxifying bath to increase tissue oxygen via the skin. Use 1 ½ cups to a tub of water; or, add ½ cup $H_2O_2$, ½ cup sea salt, and ½ cup baking soda to bath, and soak for ½ hour.

Before a therapeutic bath, dry brush your body all over for 5 minutes with a natural bristle, dry skin brush to remove toxins from the skin and open pores for nutrients.

After a bath, use a mineral salt rub, a traditional spa "finishing" technique to make your skin feel healthy for hours.

# thalassotherapy uses the sea for cleansing and health

Thalassotherapy is another ageless, cleansing, health-restorative technique. Thalassa is the ancient Greek word for sea. The Greeks indeed used the sea for their well-being. I myself have seen 2500 year-old healing sites on the Greek islands of Rhodes and Corfu, and the ancient Greek healing center at Pergamum in what is now Turkey. Even judging by the therapeutic centers still known to us, much of the population of the ancient Greek and Roman world soaked in sea water hot tubs and heated seaweed baths, drank and inhaled sea water for health, got sea water massages, had seaweed facials and body wraps and used sea water pools for hydrotherapy and detoxification. Today, we are learning once again, about the ability of the sea to reduce tension and de-stress our bodies, detoxify the skin and improve circulation, relieve allergies, sinus and chest congestion, and ease arthritis symptoms.

Seaweed baths are Nature's perfect body/psyche balancer. Remember how good you feel after an ocean walk? Seaweeds purify and balance the ocean—they can do the same for your body. A hot seaweed bath is like a wet-steam sauna, only better, because the sea greens balance body chemistry instead of dehydrating it. The electromagnetic action of the seaweed releases excess body fluids from congested cells, and dissolves fatty wastes through the skin, replacing them with depleted minerals, especially potassium and iodine. Iodine boosts thyroid activity, so food fuels are used before they can turn into fatty deposits. Vitamin K in seaweeds boosts adrenal activity, meaning that a seaweed bath can help maintain hormone balance for a more youthful body.

Taking a seaweed bath even once a week stimulates lymphatic drainage and fat burning so you can keep off excess weight, reduce cellulite and rid your body of toxins.

## Here is how to take a hot seaweed bath

If you live near the ocean, gather kelp and seaweeds from the water, (not the shoreline) in clean buckets or trash cans, and carry them home to your tub. If you don't live near the ocean, dried seaweeds are available in most health food stores. Crystal Star (ph. 800-736-6015) packages dried seaweeds, gathered from the coast of Maine, in a made-to-order Hot Seaweed Bath.

Whichever form you choose, run very hot water over the seaweed in a tub, filling it to the point that you will be covered when you recline. The leaves (whether dried or fresh) will turn a variety of rick, deep colors. The water will turn rich brown as the plants release their minerals. Add an aromatherapy bath oil if desired, to help hold the heat in and boost your cleansing program. Let the bath cool enough to get in. As you soak, the gel from the seaweed will transfer onto your skin. This coating increases perspiration to release system toxins, and replaces them with minerals by osmosis. Rub your skin with the seaweed during the bath to stimulate circulation, smooth the body, and remove wastes coming out on the skin surface. When the sea greens have done their work, the gel coating dissolves and floats off the skin, and the seaweeds shrivel—a sign that the bath is over. Each bath varies with the individual, the seaweeds used, and water temperature, but the gel coating release is a natural timekeeper for the bath. Forty-five minutes is usually long enough to balance body pH, encourage liver activity and fat metabolism. Skin tone, color, and circulatory improvement are almost immediately noticeable. After the bath, take a capsule of cayenne and ginger to assimilate the seaweed minerals.

## Don't have time for a bath? Seaweed facials are great tonics for your skin.

The ancient Greeks said that Aphrodite, the goddess of love, rising out of the foaming sea, owed her supple skin, shiny hair, and sparkling eyes to the plants of the sea. In fact, human body makeup is a lot like that of the ocean, so taking in things from the sea can help replace nutrients we may have lost. Seaweed contains huge quantities of minerals that stress and pollution deplete from your skin. The structure of seaweed cells allows your skin to easily absorb and assimilate those minerals.

If your skin has poor tone, a seaweed facial or mask can stimulate lymphatic drainage and dilate capillaries to tone your skin. Seaweed also has mineral salts that help your skin hold its moisture better. When your skin holds moisture well, it plumps up, smoothing out those fine lines and wrinkles. Some seaweeds also have molecules similar to collagen that make the skin more supple and elastic, and add amazing luster. Most people report better skin texture after a seaweed treatment.

## Thalassotherapy seaweed wraps are premier restorative body conditioners

Top European and American spas use seaweed wraps to rapidly cleanse the body of toxins, and to elasticize and tone the skin. As with all sea treatments, the sea herb and mineral solution easily penetrates through

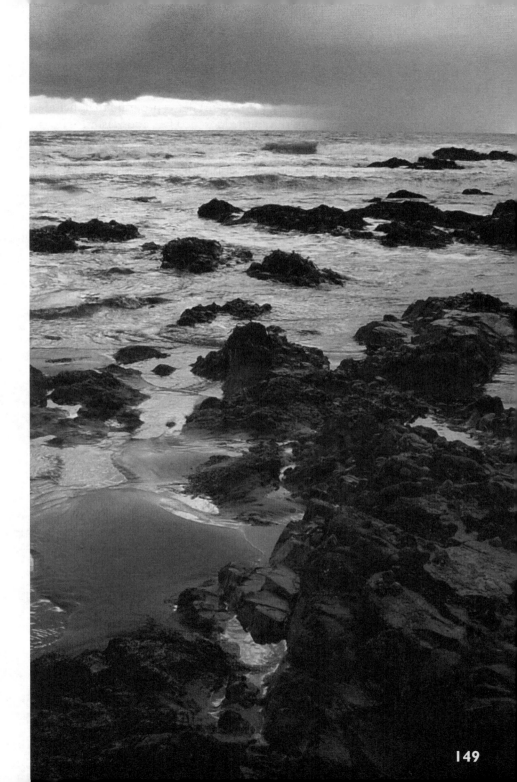

the millions of pores of your skin to break down and shrink unwanted fatty cells and cellulite deposits stored in the fluids between cells. Wraps are most successful when used along with a short detox program that includes 8 glasses of water a day to flush out the loosened fats and wastes.

I have seen almost miraculous benefits from thalassotherapy wraps during my work in the European spas and with sea herbs.

# water therapy helps your cleanse in almost every way

Hot and cold hydrotherapy helps open and stimulate the body's vital healing energies. Alternating hot and cold showers, are effective for improving circulation, relieving throbbing and cramping, toning muscles, relaxing bowel and bladder tightness, and boosting energy. The form of hydrotherapy below is easy and convenient for home use.

Begin with a comfortably hot shower for three minutes. Follow with a sudden change to cold water for 2 minutes. Repeat this cycle three times, ending with cold. Follow with a full or partial massage, or a brisk towel rub and mild stretching exercises for best results.

What are ozone pools? How do they help your body purify? Ozone, or "activated oxygen" ($O^3$) is the fresh, clean scent you smell in the air after a thunderstorm. Ozone is the most powerful natural oxidizer available and one of the fastest, safest and most thorough methods of purification known. Professional spas use ozone pools in their detox treatments today to destroy water and airborne viruses, cysts, bacteria and fungi on contact.

Ozone pool baths are actually the next generation of oxygen baths that you can use in your own home detox plan. They noticeably increase energy and tissue oxygen uptake.

## Take an oxygen bath once a day each day of your cleanse

Start with a food grade 35% hydrogen peroxide. Pour in about 1 cup per bath. Oxygen baths are stimulating rather than relaxing. Most people notice a significant energy increase within 3 days. Other therapeutic benefits include body balance and detoxification, reduction of skin cancers and tumors, clearing of asthma and lung congestion, and arthritis and rheumatism relief.

If you like herbal therapy, certain herbs used in a bath can supply oxygen through the skin. Rosemary is one of the best and most popular; peppermint and mullein are also effective. Just pack a small muslin bath or tea bag with the herb, drop it into the tub or spa, and soak for 15 to 20 minutes. Use the bag as a skin scrub during the bath for skin smoothing and tone.

A baking soda alkalizing bath is a simple but remarkable therapeutic treatment for detoxification. It is especially helpful if you suffer from too little sleep, high stress, too much alcohol, caffeine or nicotine, chronic colds or flu, or over-medication. Baking soda balances an over-acid system leaving you refreshed and invigorated, with extra soft skin.

## Here's how to take a baking soda bath

Fill the bath with enough pleasantly hot water to cover you when you recline. Add 8 oz. baking soda and swirl to dissolve. Soak for 20 to 30 minutes. When you emerge, wrap up in a big thick towel or a blanket and lie down for 15 minutes to help overcome any feelings of weakness or dizziness that might occur from the heat and rapid toxin release. Zia Wesley-Hosford, the author of *Fifty & Fabulous*, recommends this rest time for a face mask, since the hot water will have opened up the pores for maximum benefits.

An arthritis elimination sweating bath can release a surprising amount of toxic material that aggravate your joints. Epsom salts or Dead Sea salts, and herbs with a diaphoretic action, can play a big part in the success of the bath.

## Here's how to take the arthritis bath

Make a tea of elder flowers, peppermint and yarrow. Drink as hot as possible before the bath. Then pour about 3 pounds of Epsom salts or enough Dead Sea salts for 1 bath into very hot bath water. Rub arthritic joints with a stiff brush in the water for 5 to 10 minutes; try to stay in the bath for 15 to 25 minutes. On emerging, do not dry yourself. Wrap up immediately in a clean sheet and go straight to bed, covering yourself with several blankets. The osmotic pressure of the Epsom salt solution absorbed by the sheet will draw off heavy perspiration. Your mattress should be protected with a sheet of plastic. The following morning the sheet will be stained with wastes excreted through your skin—sometimes the color of egg yolk. (This is a strong detox procedure and it happens relatively quickly. Take care if you have a weak heart or high blood pressure.)

Improvement after an arthritic sweat bath experience is notable. Repeat the bath once every two weeks until the sheet is no longer stained, a sign that the body is well cleansed. Drink pure water throughout the procedure to prevent dehydration and loss of body salts.

## A sitz bath puts herbal help where you need it most

A sitz bath is a healing technique for increasing circulation in the pelvic and urethral area It's a good way to relieve anal and vaginal irritations, and improve the pelvic muscle tone of those suffering with incontinence (a fast growing group of people in America). The best sitz baths combine herbs known for their astringent, antiseptic, emollient, and hemostatic properties that will assist the natural healing process. Sitz baths help women recover from hemorrhoids and vaginal infections. They can help men strengthen the prostate/urinary and anal area.

## Here's how to take a sitz bath

**For a cold sitz bath,** use cold water at temperatures ranging from 40° to 85°F. Make a strong, strained tea with your choice of herbs; a good combination includes herbs like goldenseal root, marshmallow root, plantain, juniper berry, saw palmetto berry, slippery elm and witch hazel leaf. Add the tea to 3″ of water in a tub. Soak in the bath for 5 minutes with enough water to reach your navel, once a day for 5 minutes until healed. Use the strained herbs as a compress on the affected area.

OR

**For a hot sitz bath,** start with water about 100° and increase the heat by letting hot water drip continuously into the tub until the temperature reaches about 112°. The water should cover your hips when seated. Place your feet at the faucet end of the tub so that they are soaking in slightly hotter water as the water drips in. Cover your upper body with a towel, and your forehead with a cool, wet washcloth. After 20 or 30 minutes, take a quick, cool rinse in the shower, or splash the body with cool water before drying off to further stimulate circulation. Add Epsom salts, Batherapy bath salts, ginger powder, comfrey or chamomile to the bath water for therapeutic results.

# enemas use water flushing to cleanse your insides

Enemas are an important part of a congestion cleansing detox. They release old, encrusted colon waste, discharge parasites, freshen the G.I. tract and make the cleansing process easier and more thorough. Enemas accelerate any cleanse for optimum results. They are especially helpful during a healing crisis, after a serious illness to speed healing, or to remove drug residues. Migraines and skin problems like psoriasis are relieved with enemas.

Adding herbs to the enema water serves to immediately alkalize the bowel area, control irritation and inflammation, and provide healing action to ulcerated or distended tissue.

## Herbs for specific enemas

Use two cups strong brewed tea to 1 qt. water per enema.

- Garlic helps kill parasites, harmful bacteria, and cleanses mucous congestion. Blend 6 garlic cloves in 2 cups water and strain. For small children, use 1 clove garlic to 1 pint water.

- Catnip is effective for stomach and digestive conditions, and for childhood diseases. Use 2 cups of very strong brewed tea to 1 qt. of water.

- Pau d'arco normalizes body pH, especially against immune deficient diseases like chronic yeast and fungal infections. Use 2 cups of very strong brewed tea to 1 qt. of water.

- Spirulina helps detoxify both blood and bowels. Use 2 tbsp. powder to 1 qt. water.

- Lobelia counteracts food poisoning, especially if vomiting prevents antidote herbs being taken by mouth.

- Aloe vera heals tissues in cases of hemorrhoids, irritable bowel and diverticulitis.

- Lemon juice rapidly neutralizes an acid system, cleanses the colon and bowel.

- Acidophilus relieves gas, yeast infections and candidiasis. Mix 4 oz. powder in 1 qt. water.

- Coffee enemas detoxify the liver, stimulating both liver and gallbladder to remove toxins, open bile ducts, increase peristaltic action, and produce enzyme activity for healthy red blood cell formation and oxygen uptake. Use 1 cup of regular strong brewed coffee to 1 qt. water. Also often effective for migraine headaches.

## How to take a detoxifying, colonic enema

Place warm enema solution in an enema bag. Hang the bag about 18 inches higher than the body. Attach the colon tube, and lubricate its attachment with vaseline or vitamin E oil. Expel a little water to let out air bubbles. Lying on your left side, slowly insert the attachment about 3 inches into the rectum. Never use force. Rotate attachment gently to ease insertion. Remove kinks in the tubing so liquid will flow freely. Massage abdomen, or flex stomach muscles to relieve any cramping. When all solution has entered the colon, slowly remove the tube and remain on the left side for 5 minutes. Then move to a knee-chest position with your body weight on your knees and one hand. Use the other hand to massage the lower left side of the abdomen for several minutes.

Massage loosens old fecal matter. Roll onto your back for 5 minutes; massage up the descending colon, over the transverse colon to the right side and down the ascending colon. Move onto your right side for 5 minutes, to reach each part of the colon. Get up and quickly expel into the toilet. Look for sticky grey-brown mucous, small dark crusty chunks or tough ribbony pieces to be loosened and expelled during an enema. These poisonous looking things are toxins interfering with your normal body functions. An enema removes them. You may have to take several enemas until there is no more evidence of these substances.

Fresh wheatgrass juice enemas stimulate the liver to cleanse. Wheatgrass enema nutrients are absorbed by the hemorrhoidal vein, just inside the anal sphincter, then circulate to the liver where they increase peristaltic action of the colon, and attract waste and old fecal matter like a magnet to be eliminated from the body. Wheatgrass juice tones the colon and is absorbed into the blood, adding oxygen and energy to the body.

- Use pure water for an initial enema rinse of the colon.

- Then use about a cup of water to 4 ounces of fresh wheatgrass juice.

- Hold the juice for ten minutes while massaging colon area. Then, expel.

Herbal implants are concentrated enema solutions for more serious health problems, like colitis, arthritis or prostate inflammation. Prepare for an implant by taking a small enema to clear out the lower bowel. You'll be able to hold the implant longer.

Mix 2 tbsp. herbal powder like spirulina, or wheat grass in l/2 cup water. Lubricate the tip of a syringe with vaseline or vitamin E oil, get down on your hands and knees and insert the nozzle into the rectum. Squeeze the bulb to insert the mixture, but do not release pressure on the bulb before withdrawing, so the mixture stays in the lower bowel. Hold 15 minutes before expelling.

# a colonic irrigation is a "super enema"

I have used both colonics and enemas in detox programs. Benefits are matter of degree but they're dramatically different, both in terms of waste removed and body improvement.

Your colon is over five feet long. If you want to cleanse all of it you need a colonic irrigation. Here's how a colonic works. A colonic irrigation uses special equipment and gravity (or oxygen for more control) to give your colon an internal bath. The person receiving the colonic lies on a special colema-board which is about three feet below the temperature-controlled water flow. A sterilized speculum is gently inserted in the rectum. Under the control of the practitioner, a steady flow of water gently flows from a small water tube. There is no discomfort, no internal pressure, just a steady gentle water flow in and then out of the colon through the evacuation tube, carrying with it impacted feces and mucous. Unlike an enema, a colonic irrigation does not involve the retention of water. As the water flows out of the colon the practitioner gently massages the abdomen to help the colon release its contents, recover its natural shape, tone, and normalize peristaltic wave action. A view tube is available for observation and all colonic matter is contained in the equipment. You do nothing but lie back and relax while the entire colon is cleansed.

A colonic irrigation uses about 40 gallons of water and takes about forty-five minutes. The colonic procedure is not offensive, nor painful. The first things most people feel after a colonic irrigation is a sense of lightness, energy and an improved sense of well-being. Skin condition, digestion and immune response improve. Body odor and bad breath essentially disappear, as does belly distension.

Colonics are best done in the evening so that you can relax and retire for healing rest. For a best results take a green drink before and after the colonic.

## Bentonite clay colonic cleanse

Bentonite clay is a mineral substance with powerful absorption qualities; it can pull out suspended impurities in the body. It helps prevent proliferation of pathogenic organisms and parasites, and sets up an environment for rebuilding healthy tissue. It is effective for lymph congestion, cellulitic fatty tissue, blood cleansing and reducing toxicity from environmental pollutants. It may be used orally, anally, or vaginally. It works like an internal poultice, drawing out toxic materials, then draining and eliminating them through evacuation. Note: Bentonite clay packs are also effective applied topically to varicose veins and arthritic areas.

1. To take bentonite as an enema, mix ½ cup clay to an enema bag of water. Use 5 to 6 bags for each enema set to replace a colonic. Follow normal enema procedure, or the directions with your enema apparatus.
2. Massage across the abdomen while expelling toxic waste into the toilet.

# muscle kinesiology

Muscle kinesiology is a Traditional Chinese Medicine technique being rediscovered in America. The word kinesiology means the study of motion, especially how muscles act to move the body. In the natural health field, kinesiology uses principles from Chinese medicine, acupressure and massage to bring the body into balance and release pain and tension. Applied kinesiology is based on the premise that muscle, glands, and organs are linked by meridians, or energy pathways in the body. Muscle testing is the way most Americans are familiar with applied kinesiology today. Muscle testing is an effective and versatile method for detecting and correcting various energy movements and imbalances in the body.

Muscle testing identifies weak muscles. Weak muscles indicate an energy flow blockage in a body meridian. A kinesiologist uses stress release techniques to unblock the meridians. The muscles are then retested after visualization, massage techniques and movement exercises; if the muscles have regained strength, the restoration of the energy flow of the meridians is confirmed. Kinesiology does not heal, but rather restores balanced energy flow.

You can use personal muscle testing to determine your own individual response to a food or substance. It's a good technique to use before buying a healing remedy, because it lets you estimate the product's effectiveness for your own body before you buy. You will need a partner for the procedure.

## Here's how to use muscle testing

1.  Hold your arm out straight from your side, parallel to the ground. Have a partner place one hand just below your shoulder and one hand on your forearm. Your partner then tries to force your arm down towards your side, while you exert all your strength to hold it level. Unless you are in ill health, you should easily be able to withstand this pressure and keep your arm level.

2.  Then, simply hold the item that you desire to test against your diaphragm (under the breastbone) or thyroid (the point where the collarbone comes together below the neck). The item may be in or out of normal packaging, or in its raw state, like a fresh food.

3.  Holding the item as above, put your arm out straight from your side as before and have your partner try to press it down again. If the test item is beneficial for you, your arm will retain its strength, and your partner will be unable to force it down. If the item is not beneficial, or would worsen your condition, your arm can be easily pushed down by your partner.

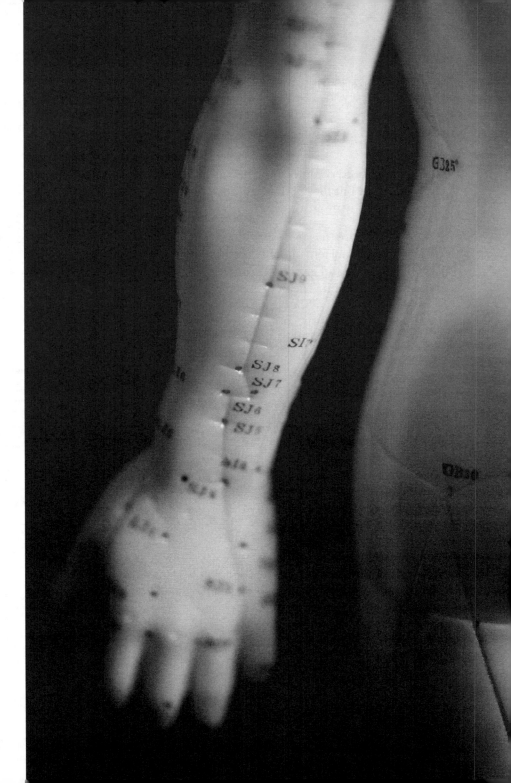

# your skin is a key organ for detoxification

Here are some cleansing methods you can use on your skin to draw out wastes and poisons

## Herbal compresses

Herbal compresses used during a cleanse, draw out waste and waste residues, such as cysts or abscesses, through the skin and release them into the body's elimination channels. Use alternating hot and cold compresses for best results. Apply the herbs to the hot compress, and leave the ice or cold compress plain. I regularly use cayenne, ginger and lobelia effectively for the hot compresses.

### Here are some effective compresses I use

- Add 1 tsp. powdered herbs to a bowl of very hot water. Soak a washcloth and apply until the cloth cools. Then apply a cloth dipped in ice water until it reaches body temperature. Repeat several times daily.
- Green clay compresses are effective toxin-drawing agents for growths. Apply to gauze, placed on the area, cover and leave all day. Change as you would any dressing when you bathe.

## Dry skin brushing

Dry skin brushing helps remove toxins during a detox and opens pores for better assimilation of nutrients. Dry skin brushing removes the top layer of old skin, helping to eliminate uric acid crystals and mucous residues. Dry skin brushing also stimulates circulation, cleanses the lymph system and increases cell renewal. Dry brushing your skin every 24 hours rejuvenates your skin during detoxification. After your detox, dry brushing before a shower once a week will keep your skin beautiful and keep cellulitic build-up down.

Your technique for skin brushing can make all the difference to its success

1. Use a natural bristle brush, not synthetic—it scratches skin surface.
2. Do not wet your skin. It stretches the skin and will not have the same effect.
3. All brush strokes should go towards the heart.
4. Especially brush the bottoms of your feet, nerve endings here affect the whole body.
5. Do circular, counter-clockwise strokes on the abdomen.
6. Brush lighter strokes over and around the breasts. Do not brush nipples.
7. Dry brushing is best when done before you bathe in the mornings. If done before bed, it can cause too much stimulation and may interrupt sleep.
8. Brush the whole body, for best results.
9. Wash your brush every few weeks in water and let it dry.

# massage therapy

Massage therapy has been removing wastes and healing people for thousands of years.

The ancient Romans and Greeks used massage regularly as a healing treatment. Today's massage therapy has joined the alternative medicine techniques of chiropractic and reflexology as a viable health discipline. It's a wonderful detox technique, promoting mucous and fluid drainage from the lungs and increasing peristaltic action in the intestines to promote fecal elimination. I recommend at least one massage treatment during a 3 to 7 day cleanse to stimulate the body's immune response and natural restorative powers.

In the past decade, overwhelming scientific evidence has accumulated in support of massage therapy. Here are some of the research findings:

- Massage therapy is particularly helpful for pain control, stimulating the production of endorphins, the body's natural pain relievers. It is especially effective for back and shoulder pain and spinal/nerve problems.

- Massage therapy is an effective adjunct treatment for cardiovascular disorders, neurological and gynecological problems such as PMS. It is often more helpful than drugs for these problems. Massage actually helps prevent future heart disease.

- Massage therapy helps chronic fatigue syndrome, candida albicans, gastrointestinal conditions, epilepsy and psoriasis.

- Massage therapy helps correct poor posture from spinal curvatures and whiplash.

- Massage therapy helps headaches, temporo-mandibular joint syndrome (TMJ)

- Massage therapy helps respiratory disorders like bronchial asthma, and emphysema.

- Massage therapy promotes recovery from fatigue, muscle spasms and pain after exercise.

- Massage therapy helps break up scar tissue and adhesions.

- Massage therapy effectively treats chronic inflammatory conditions by increasing limbic circulation, especially swelling from fractures or injuries.

- Massage therapy improves blood circulation throughout the entire circulatory system.

## Three types of massage therapy specifically help the body cleansing process

**Swedish massage** uses kneading, stroking, friction, tapping and sometimes body shaking to stimulate and cleanse. These techniques also help cleanse muscle acids, joints, nerves and the endocrine system, by stimulating the body's circulation.

**Deep tissue massage** removes waste in the muscles. Deep tissue therapy uses more direct deep finger pressure across the grain of the muscles to release chronic patterns of tension, and stress accumulation. It also increases circulation to facilitate the movement of waste products out of the muscle tissue. Recent evidence shows that deep tissue massage can break up scar tissue and eliminate it.

**Lymphatic drainage** is a large surface, highly specialized kneading technique, a unique method that uses precise, complex hand movements to encourage the draining of lymph fluids. In comparison, normal massage techniques are much too forceful to allow drainage in the tissues and may hinder transport.

I call the lymphatic system the body's natural antibiotic. When it is flushed and clean, lymph removes body toxins as part of the auto-immune response to disease. Using slow, gentle strokes with a rhythmic pumping action, the massage technician follows the lymph pathways throughout the body to move the flow of lymph and accelerate detoxification.

## There are four primary effects lymphatic massage can have on the body

1. It balances the sympathetic and parasympathetic nervous systems.

2. It activates inhibitory reflex cells which decrease or even eliminate pain sensations.

3. It increases lymph flow for a decongestant effect on connective tissue, stimulates blood capillary flow and increases resorptive capacity of the blood capillaries.

4. It boosts immune response by increasing the lymph flow and stimulating antibodies.

**Note:** As wonderful as massage therapy is, there are some health conditions where massage is not a good idea.

- Don't massage a person with high fever, cancer, tuberculosis or other infections or malignant conditions which might be further spread throughout the body.

- Don't massage the abdomen of a person with high blood pressure or ulcers.

- Don't massage legs with varicose veins, diabetes, phlebitis or blood vessel problems.

- Massage no closer than six inches near bruises, cysts, skin breaks or broken bones.

- Massage people with swollen limbs gently, only above the swelling, towards the heart.

# polarity therapy is a blend of art and science

Today's technology graphically shows that the human body consists of many electromagnetic patterns. We can see that energy both surrounds the body and courses through it in a continual flow of positive and negative charges. Expressed in ancient times as an aura, this magnetic field makes up our physical, mental, and emotional characteristics, directs body systems and maintains energy balance. Popular in holistic spas and detox centers today, a polarity practitioner accesses the magnetic current to release energy blocks.

Polarity Therapy believes that balancing the flow of energy in the body is the underlying foundation of health. Rooted in Ayurveda, polarity therapy uses diet and exercise for cleansing tissues, balancing energy, improving breath and circulation and preventing illness. Polarity therapy is also helpful in treating migraines, low back pain and other stress disorders.

Gentle touch induces a relaxed, meditative state to accelerate energy flow throughout the body, inviting a return to health. There are three types of touch the therapist may use: rajasic is gentle and stimulating, sattvic is a light, balancing touch, tamasic touch goes deeper into the muscles and tissues. Frequently, the touch is so light that one doesn't feel anything at all.

## Magnet therapy works on a balance of negative/ positive magnetic energy

Science has known since the '50s that a magnetic field is critical to normal body function and coordination. (In fact, chronic fatigue syndrome, fibromyalgia and chronic immune deficiency syndrome were first identified as magnetic field deficiency syndromes.)

The positive, acid-producing field, can create conditions like arthritis, mental confusion, fatigue, pain and insomnia- and encourage fat storage. Culprits producing this field are processed foods, caffeine, nicotine, and toxic chemicals in cosmetics, agriculture, auto exhaust, and over-the-counter and prescription drugs.

The negative, alkaline-producing field, increases oxygen, encourages deep sleep, reduces inflammation and fluid retention, relieves pain, and promotes mental acuity. A negative field can act like an antibiotic in helping to destroy bacterial, fungal and viral infections because it lowers body acidity.

In healing, magnets increase blood flow to specific areas of the body, which carries more oxygen to the region (blood is composed of positively and negatively charged particles).

# reflexology works with the body's energy zones through the hands and feet

Reflexology is an ancient natural science based on the belief that each part of the body is interconnected through the nerve system to specific points on the feet and hands. A history of foot massage spans time and place from the Physician's Tomb in Egypt of 2300 B.C. to the Physicians Temple in Nara, Japan of 700 A.D. The ancient Egyptians are believed to have actually developed hand and foot reflexology.

Reflexology is often known as zone therapy, and it's an important part of massage therapy treatment. In reflexology, the nervous system is understood as an electrical system; contact can be made through the feet and hands with each of the electro-mechanical zones in the body to the nerve endings. The nerve endings are called reflex points (referring to the fact that these points are reflexive, like a knee-jerk reaction.) Ten reflexology zone meridians have been extensively mapped connecting all the organs and glands, and culminating in points in the hands and feet. The points are manipulated to open blocked energy pathways. Since the feet serve as reflexes for the entire body, foot reflexology is most often used.

Stress is involved in over 80% of all illness. The first step in healing is relaxation. Reflexology helps the body to heal itself through relaxation. Its goal is to clear the pathways of energy flow throughout the body, to return body balance, and increase immune response. It does this by stimulating the lymphatic system to eliminate wastes adequately, and the blood to circulate easily to poorly functioning areas.

Reflexologists look at the feet as a mini-map of the entire body, with the big toes serving as the head, the balls of the feet representing the shoulders, and the narrowing the waist area. Any illness, injury or tension in the body produces tenderness in the corresponding foot zone. Reflexologists rely on an inchworm-like massage motion of the thumb to produce light or deep pressure on each zone, concentrating on the tender spots, which often feel like little grains of salt under the skin.

For your own individual use, picture your hands and feet as your body's control panels. Get a good reflexology chart—available in health food stores. Then use your fingers or a rounded-end to locate the reflex points. Some points take practice to pinpoint. The best rule for knowing when you have reached the right spot is that it will probably be very tender, denoting crystalline deposits or congestion in the corresponding organ. However, there is often an immediate feeling of relief in the area as waste deposits break up for removal by the body.

Fifteen pounds of applied force on any reflex point can send a surge of energy to the corresponding body area, removing obstructive crystals, restoring circulation, and clearing congestion. The nerve reflex point on the foot for any afflicted area will be tender or sore indicating crystalline deposits brought about by poor capillary circulation of fluids. The amount of soreness on the foot point can also indicate the size of the crystalline deposit, and the amount of time it has been accumulating.

For effective reflexology, press on the reflex point 3 times for 10 seconds each time. The pressure treatment may be used for twenty to thirty minute sessions at a time, about twice a week. Sessions more often than this will not give nature the chance to use the stimulation or do its necessary repair work. Most people notice frequent and easy bowel movements in the first twenty-four hours after reflexology as the body throws off released wastes.

## Documented health benefits of reflexology therapy

- **Reduces PMS.** A study published in 1993 in the journal Obstetrics and Gynecology finds women suffering from premenstrual syndrome experience a 40% reduction in symptoms after using reflexology treatments.

- **Improves asthma.** One case study reports a significant improvement in well being and reduction in asthma symptoms after three months of reflexology therapy.

- **Helps balance blood sugar in cases of type 2 diabetes.** Two different studies (one from China; the other from America) reveal reflexology effectively lowers high blood sugar levels in diabetics.

- **Helps restore some movement and sensation for people paralyzed from spinal cord injuries.** Case studies published in the journal Reflexions find some quadriplegic and paraplegic patients respond to reflexology sessions with movement. Other effects noted: some return of bowel and bladder control; induced sweating below the level of the injury; the sensation of bowel rumbling, improved muscle tone; and a decrease in chronic bladder infections.

## More:

- Medical doctor Julian Whitaker reports in his book, 199 Health Secrets, that just two weeks of reflexology treatment helped remove a ganglion cyst on his hand.

- May help dissolve ovarian cysts. Professional reflexologist Christopher Shirley recounts the story of two women scheduled for surgery to remove ovarian cysts who experienced a mysterious and remarkable disappearance of the cysts (documented by sonograms) after reflexology treatments.

# ear coning for ear cleansing

Ear coning or candling is a comfortable way to clean out excess wax and other accumulations. It's an ancient healing process used by virtually every healing tradition. Chinese Traditional Medicine, Native American and Mayan societies, even the ancient Egyptians all used ear candling to gently remove ear wax, fungus, and yeast from ear canals. Some of these cultures even considered ear coning a spiritual practice that also cleared the mind and senses. Ear candling was believed to detoxify the physical body through the sinus, lymphatic and other systems to realign the flow of cranial fluids.

Ear candles are made from strips of 100% cotton muslin which are dipped into a mixture of wax and herbs with natural antibiotic, decongestant and balancing activity like sage, Swedish bitters, cedar, spearmint, echinacea, goldenseal and rosemary. The waxed muslin is then formed into a tapered cone.

In the coning process, the narrow end of the candle is gently placed at the ear canal, while the opposite end is lit. The spiral design of the cone creates a vacuum which draws the soothing smoke into the ear canal. The smoke goes through the Eustachian tube into the lymphatic system, then by osmosis, it draws accumulations out into the cone. The process is soothing, and takes only about 45 minutes.

Here are the benefits of ear coning:

- helps to stimulate and detoxify the lymphatic system.

- helps remove excessive wax and allows better hearing, usually immediately.

- helps clear "swimmers ear," where ear wax stops water clearing from the ear and allows harmful bacteria to grow and fester.

- relieves pain and pressure from mucous blown into the ear from the Eustachian tube.

- helps clear itching mold caused by candida yeast allergy.

- helps remove parasites growing in the ear

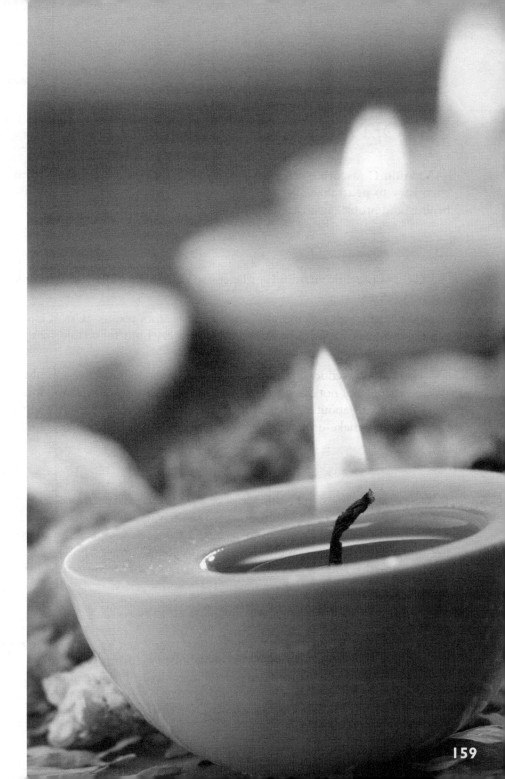

# give your body a detoxifying ascorbic acid flush

Vitamin C (ascorbic acid) accelerates detoxification, changing body chemistry to neutralize allergens, fight infections, promote more rapid healing and protect against illness.

## Here's how

1. Use a non-acidic vitamin C or Ester C powder with bioflavonoids for best results.

2. Take ½ tsp. every 20 minutes until a soupy stool results. (Use ¼ tsp. every hour for a very young child; ½ tsp. every hour for a child six to ten years old.)

3. Then, slightly reduce amount taken so that the bowel produces a mealy, loose stool, but not diarrhea. The body will still continue to cleanse. You will be taking about 8 – 10,000mg of vitamin C daily depending on body weight and make-up. Continue for one to two days for a thorough flush.

## An herbal "vag pac" can detox the vaginal/urethral area

A cleansing herbal combination may be used as a vaginal pack by placing it against the cervix, or as a bolus inserted in the vagina. The pack acts as an internal poultice to draw out toxic wastes from the vagina, rectum or urethral areas. A "vag pac" is effective for cysts, benign tumors, polyps and uterine growths, and cervical dysplasia. It takes 6 weeks to 6 months for complete healing, depending on the problem and severity.

## Here's how to make a pack

**Formula #1:** Mix 1 part each with cocoa butter to form a suppository: squaw vine, marshmallow root, slippery elm, goldenseal root, pau d' arco, comfrey root, mullein, yellow dock root, chickweed, acidophilus powder.

**Formula #2:** Mix 1 part each with cocoa butter to form a suppository: cranesbill powder, goldenseal root, red raspberry leaf, white oak bark, echinacea root, myrrh gum powder.

1. Mix the combined, powdered herbs with warmed cocoa butter to form finger-sized suppositories. Place on waxed paper in the refrigerator to chill and harden slightly.

2. Smear a suppository on the end of a cotton tampon and insert; or insert as is, and use a sanitary napkin to catch drainage. Use suppositories at night and rinse out in the morning with white oak bark tea, or yellow dock root tea to rebalance vaginal pH.

3. Repeat for 6 days. Rest for one week. Resume and repeat.

# chelation therapy cleans out your arteries

Chelation therapy was developed in Germany in the early 1930's and introduced into the United States in 1948 as a method of preventing or reversing heart and artery pathology (hardening of the arteries) from diminished blood circulation. Today chelation is used by medical authorities around the world as a cleansing treatment for heavy metal and radiation toxicity, digitalis intoxication, lead and snake venom poisoning and heart arrhythmias.

A chelating protein called EDTA, a synthetic amino acid, ethylene-diamine-tetracetic acid, is used, because it has the unique property of binding with divalent metals that are clogging arteries. When EDTA is injected, it flushes the cells of ionic minerals, especially calcium, and travels with them out of the body through the kidneys.

Oral chelation refers to specific foods and nutritional supplements that help cleanse the blood vessels of accumulated detritus (waste) and improve blood flow. While experience among chelating physicians indicates that oral chelates take about eight times longer to show health benefits than do IV chelates, oral chelation is successful in improving circulation, reversing heart disease, stroke and sexual impotency due to poor circulation. I use oral chelation as a protective against atherosclerosis and many degenerative diseases.

# detox with the vibe machine

The VIBE machine uses vibrational therapy to recharge the body's cells. A healthy body naturally has a higher frequency. Low frequency is a sign of disease and sickness. The VIBE machine utilizes an electromagnetic field with a high voltage pulse and biophotonic light (a key pathway of cellular communication) to infuse the body with positive energy and eliminate unhealthy frequencies that contribute to disease.

People with cancer, Parkinson's disease, even family pets who are sick can experience health benefits from VIBE. The science emerging behind VIBE is promising, too. Studies on the VIBE machine by Norman Shealy reveal it has stress-relieving and anti-aging activity. The Mayo clinic is planning a double-blind study on VIBE in the near future.

The Stanford girls' swim team broke school records using it. VIBE machines are available at health clinics all across the country. In California alone, there are over 50 practitioners who now include VIBE machine sessions in their daily practice.

## Can a few minutes in front of a VIBE machine really change your life?

The early reports are impressive. Ronda Reinke, a VIBE practitioner I spoke with from Monterey California, says a close friend with Multiple Sclerosis got out of her wheelchair and was walking after just 3 minutes in front of the VIBE machine! Of course, not everyone who uses the VIBE machine has such a dramatic experience, but the technology does have clear promise, especially as an anti-aging therapy and body cleansing protocol.

## EB (Energy Balancing) Foot Bath: a complementary therapy to VIBE

Foot baths have long been used as part of detoxification protocols. Today the EB (Energy Balancing) 305 foot bath is especially popular. It uses a copper coil, which surges positive and negative ions through the bath water. The soles of the feet are highly porous and the bioenergetic ionic exchange of the foot bath increases cellular ATP, enhancing cells' ability to release toxins from the body.

Clients who use the foot bath are shocked when they see how much toxic debris it releases. Heavy metals, yeast overgrowth, lymph congestion, gallbladder and liver stress are evident in materials generated by an EB Detox foot bath. Most people are amazed by how toxic their bodies really are! Combining VIBE sessions with an EB (Energy Balancing) Detox footbath allows the body to discharge even greater toxins with less stress. One of my research associates reports back that she felt a clear long lasting energy lift the day after her VIBE machine session and EB foot bath.

Affordable, non-invasive approaches to detoxification and wellness are urgently needed, and VIBE technology offers a complementary approach to many of the programs in this book.

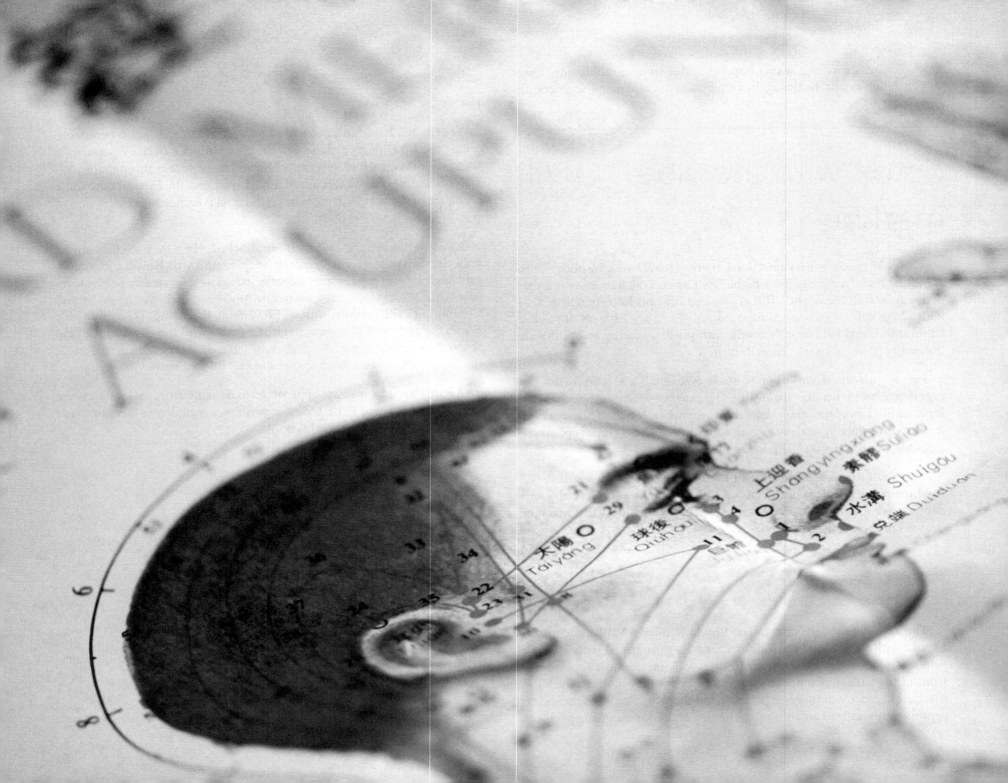

# natural health study guide

# detoxification traditions

## cleansing around the world

**B**ODY CLEANSING HAS BEEN A PART OF HUMAN health care since mankind's ancient times. Cleansing therapies works to keep our species vigorous. The following pages contain a short review of the world's traditional approaches to detoxification.

## Ayurvedic healing

Ayurvedic medicine is the world's oldest recorded healing system, in continuous use for over 6000 years. Originating on the Indian subcontinent in the practices of "Rishis," India's ancient holy men, Ayurvedic practitioners had astounding knowledge of the connections between anatomy, physiology, psychology, the use of herbs, minerals, exercise, even surgery. Their progress in the development of medicine and their success in healing reached around the ancient world, influencing the medical philosophies of the Chinese, Greeks and Romans. During India's colonial period under English rule, Ayurvedic practices were forbidden. Yet the healing knowledge was passed on and preserved. Today, once again, Ayurvedic medicine is a leading edge philosophy in world health care.

Ayurvedic healing is based on body balance for health and longevity, believing that imbalance and disharmony with the rhythms of nature are the foundation of illness.

Detoxification is a cornerstone of Ayurvedic medicine. It is believed that without proper digestion and elimination, toxins build up and disrupt body functions and body balance. There are two main forms of detoxification in Ayurveda. Both can be used in conjunction or alone for restoring health.

**The first is called Shamana,** a palliation therapy involving herbs, oils and therapeutic foods to stimulate digestion, reduce toxins, and return balance and function restoring health.

**The second is Pancha Karma,** a stronger method using massage and sweating therapy, is reserved for imbalances and diseases that are well established.

Ayurvedic practitioners use sign posts from nature to identify imbalances. Man is classified into prototypes or "doshas," based on the five natural elements of air, fire, water, earth and space (ether). The elements are believed to combine in pairs to form the doshas. Each person's emotional and body type is thought to correspond to one of the doshas.

## There are three doshas:

**Vata:** a combination of air and space elements, equated with circulation, the passage of food in the body, breathing and movement.

**Pitta:** a combination of fire and water elements, equated with metabolism and the transformation and assimilation of nutrients.

**Kapha:** a combination of the water and earth elements, equated to body structure like bones, tissue and muscle.

In seeking the cause and cure for an illness, an Ayurvedic healer first determines the dosha that best represents the patient's body and emotional type. While body typing is not absolute, physical attributes like weight, body frame, complexion and behavior provide information for typing. For example: a vata type, governed by air, is generally thin, tall and wiry with prominent bone structure and a dull, darkish complexion. A pitta type, governed by fire, usually has a medium frame and weight with defined musculature and ruddy complexion. A kapha type, governed by water, is often heavy to obese, with large frame and pale complexion.

However, since "dosha" means "that which changes," all the elements are believed to be continually balancing and changing each other. Making it even more complex, each element is also influenced by climates, seasons, stages of life, and one's thoughts and actions. A strong immune system is therefore the key to health in dealing with the constant flux of all the forces.

In Ayurvedic practice, toxins (ama) are deemed one of the main causes of disease, creating imbalances that must be resolved to restore health. When one's dosha is out of balance, digestion, absorption and assimilation are disrupted. This causes the formation of ama or cellular toxins, which clog cell functions and accelerate disease.

In a Pancha Karma detox, a popular spa method, five cleansing methods may be used depending on the type of problem being experienced: 1) therapeutic vomiting, or emetic therapy to purge the stomach and lungs, or the use of expectorant herbs like pepper and ginger; 2) purgation, with herbs like senna and rhubarb; 3) medicated enemas, with herbs like fennel, ginger and licorice in sesame seed oil, flushed into the rectum to be absorbed through the colon and large intestine; 4) blood letting to eliminate toxic blood and stimulate production of new blood; 5) nasal and ear douching to cleanse the head and throat. Gotu kola or licorice oils in drops, cleanse and nourish the brain. Exercise, yoga, breathing techniques and meditation are highly recommended for every detox program.

In a self-administered detox program, Ayurvedic practice begins with a fast of non-sweet vegetable juices—for vata types, 3 to 5 days, for pitta types, 5 to 7 days, and for kapha types, 1 to 2 weeks is recommended. Fruit juices and sweet vegetables juices like carrot juice are not used, since it is thought that sweetness increases waste deposits. Lemon juice mixed with ginger juice is a good choice. Herbal combinations like "Trikuta," (black pepper, long pepper and dry ginger), or a tea of cardamom, cinnamon and ginger increase digestive fire.

Purgatives are included on the first day of the fast, and every three days following, to help clean the digestive system. Digestive bitters like rhubarb, neem, aloe vera and ginger are used. One of my favorite Ayurvedic formulas, "triphala," (a combo of amla, herada, and behera fruits), stimulates digestion gently and gradually and rejuvenates deep tissues. Steams medicated with mint or eucalyptus are used to cleanse the lungs. Diaphoretic herbs are sometimes used to promote sweating.

After the fast, a step 2 cleansing diet is begun, with fruits like lemons, grapefruits and cranberries, vegetables (except heavy roots like potatoes or sweet potatoes), and with grains like barley, or a blend of brown rice and split mung beans called kicharee. Oats, wheat and other beans should be avoided. Vata types should limit the step 2 diet to one or two weeks, pitta types to three weeks, and kapha types to one to two months. The elderly, very young, weak or anorexic people should avoid the step 2 diet.

After the cleansing diet is completed, a maintenance step 3 program, including a well-balanced nourishing diet, proper rest, exercise and tonifying herbs is established. The diet for this stage includes dairy products like ghee (clarified butter), fruits and vegetables, beans, grains, oils like sesame, olive and avocado, and spices like garlic, pepper and curry to promote digestion.

Step 3 maintenance herbs include ashwaganda (Indian ginseng), shatavari (asparagus), amla (high vitamin C berry), gotu kola (a nerve restorative) and triphala (see previous page).

## Traditional Chinese Medicine

Traditional Chinese herbal medicine has a 5,000 year legacy. The first writings about Traditional Chinese Medicine (TCM) date back over 2000 years. The first known herbal materia medica was written during the Han dynasty between 206 B.C. and 5 A.D., and was said to be based on the emperor's personal knowledge of herbalism from nearly 2000 years before. The healing principles of TCM are bound up with the idea of yin and yang, opposing principles that represent both spiritually and physically the daily balance of universal order in Chinese philosophy. Yin and yang are thought to make up all things. Man, too is made up of yin and yang, composing his own balance of opposites for his proper place and function in the universal realm.

Chinese medicine characterizes imbalances in yin and yang as a cause of illness. When disharmony occurs, life energy cannot flow because the balance is upset. TCM assigns yin and yang designations to all body parts, essences and functions depending on their nature. Each designation is connected to an opposite organ or function by energy meridians. Between these flows the life force, or Qi (chee). A TCM practitioner uses this philosophy to find the origin of an illness in order to treat it, rather than treating symptoms of the disease. Identifying the cause of the imbalance allows the TCM practitioner to use herbs and physical stimulation like acupuncture or acupressure to bring the opposites back into balance. Like Ayurveda, Chinese medicine has signposts, designating basic elements like earth, wind, fire and water to body parts, functions, and plants—then assigning qualities of heat and cold, damp and dry to help the practitioner recognize imbalances.

The Chinese belief of interconnectedness makes the TCM healing philosophy seem incredibly complex to the Western mind. Let me try to simplify it for clarity.

Yin and yang are opposites, darkness and light, hot and cold, male and female, yet elements of each are in the other. TCM identifies each vital body organ as yin or yang, between which flows Qi or life force energy. The Qi flows are referred to as meridians and play an important part in maintaining balance in the body. The organs are influenced by the five basic elements— wood, fire, earth, metal and water. The Chinese assign a relationship of the vital organs in the body to the actions of the elements. Thus, the liver and gallbladder are connected to wood; the heart and small intestine are connected to fire; the spleen and stomach are connected to earth; the lung and large intestine are connected to metal; the kidney and bladder are connected to water. Each organ is also related to an emotion; the emotion affects the health of the organ and the organ affects the emotion.

For example, the liver is connected to anger. If a toxic condition exists in the liver it may manifest itself as anger or depression. Through the liver's meridian connection to the gall bladder, the gall bladder is adversely affected. The relationship between the elements is also compromised so that liver/wood that generates heart/fire becomes weak, jeopardizing the heart's ability to function. As imbalances become greater, farther and farther away from the original problem through their interconnection, more body functions suffer.

The health and harmony connections go even further. In TCM, external conditions that cause disease are referred to as the Six Excesses, characterized as weather conditions—wind, cold, summer-heat, dampness, dryness and fire. Imbalances of these may cause immune response to weaken. For example, as spring moves into summer an unusual cold spell may hit; but the body has already geared up for warm conditions, so its resistance to cold is weak, allowing a "spring cold" virus to take hold.

## The TCM practitioner has eight approaches to heal disease

1. perspiration
2. therapeutic emesis
3. purgation
4. neutralization
5. stimulation
6. heat-clearing
7. reduction
8. tonic

For example, to reduce toxicity, a practitioner looks to herbs that take down inflammation and detoxify the blood or liver, reduce and move accumulated phlegm; then to tonic herbs, like ginsengs, for stagnant Qi energy, to nourish and restore balance.

When choosing herbs to treat illness, the TCM practitioner takes into account their "natures" (corresponding to the seasons—cold, hot, warm and cool), their "flavors" (describing the actions—sour, spicy, bitter, sweet and salty), and to their "directions" (movement within the body—rising, descending, floating and sinking), as well as the color and aroma of each herb. Besides their interconnectedness to the five elements and major organs, each herb has an affinity for a specific body organ that it moves and affects. Since the organs are interconnected by meridians, the opposing organ is also affected.

The idea in TCM is to achieve body balance through lifestyle means before an illness occurs—with herbs and food, physical stimulation, aroma and heat therapy, and meditation. For instance, overindulging in a particular food may cause "heat" in the body. A balancing, "cooling" food should be eaten to prevent disease.

Detox treatments provide another example—if toxicity causes heat to occur in the liver, herbs that generate cooling action are used to restore balance. Detoxification is not considered as cleansing, but rather as restoring.

In fact, the success of traditional Chinese medicine is the training its practitioners receive in recognizing symptoms before an illness occurs. Instead, prevention is the primary emphasis.

Western, science-based medicine has lost this personalized skill today, but illness symptoms may be diagnosed from changes in skin color or tone, tongue color or texture, pulse or thirst changes, unusual breath or body odor, behavior changes, etc. Diet, rest, stress, mental and spiritual health, seasons, climate and family history are also seen as major players in one's health. Time, too is a factor. Lifestyle corrections cannot take place without the time to correct lifestyle habits. Traditional Chinese Medicine sees an individual's life health as an ever-changing process of rebalancing. A TCM practitioner does not cure the symptoms to correct the cause of the illness. He is interested in how an illness acts rather than what it is, so

that the origin of imbalance may be traced in order to restore harmony. Unless this process is considered, Chinese healers believe the illness will manifest again.

## The rainforest culture

Rainforest medicine is a system largely based in shamanic tradition; much like Native American medicine, healing is interconnected with spiritual beliefs. Medicine in the rainforest is an herbally based art, not a formal system like Traditional Chinese Medicine or Ayurveda. Although there are vast areas of rainforest around the world, and herbs and beliefs vary widely, rainforest medicinal practices are similar in nature. Healing methods and rituals are still orally passed from shaman to apprentice; herbs are learned by heart. This book focuses on the traditions of the Amazon tribes whose culture extends back to the respected Mayan curandero or healers.

Rainforest healers never have to venture far to collect herbs for their pharmacopia. The rainforest is so rich and diverse in medicinal plants that thousands of herbal remedies lie almost literally within arm's reach. A blur to the average eye, especially to an untrained eye, to the shaman each plant is easily recognizable, as a member of one's family, to the rainforest healer.

Even though the rainforest healing tradition is oral, European explorer's writings tell us that the people of the rainforests were extremely healthy (largely because of their diet of grains, fruits, vegetables and limited meats). The extent of their medicines for the few illnesses the people did have was impressive. The Europeans, who were disease-ridden in comparison, were astonished at the number of remedies available. One of the saddest commentaries of the Spanish conquest was the decimation of huge portions of the rainforest populations despite their extensive pharmacopias. (In the short time their civilizations were being destroyed or absorbed, there was no time to develop resistance or remedies for the new diseases.)

Even though it was less successful, European medicine superseded herbal knowledge, because the Spanish used inquisition tactics to force Christianity upon the rainforest people, and Catholicism conflicted with the spiritual aspects of native healing. Only in remote rainforest areas did the traditional healing practices remain strong. Thankfully, we are beginning to rediscover them today.

Because he is the link between the earthly and spiritual worlds, the shaman, a spiritual healer, is the most powerful medicine man. Disease is seen as stemming from both physical origins and spiritual problems brought by bad spirits that inflict illness. Contact with a bad spirit, or with someone who wishes another harm and uses a person of power to conjure ill will, are believed to poison the body just as any other pathogen or pollutant. Prayers are integral to the healing response against the spiritual or emotional origins of a disease. Fortifying physical rituals are also assigned to the afflicted person to strengthen the power of the medicine. But there are many levels of healers in the rainforest tradition. Other "people of power," like the Mayan curandero, with their vast knowledge of plants, are sought to help with various aspects of a problem. Medicinal plants themselves are considered to possess a spiritual life force beyond their physical existence that may be accessed for healing. Healing spirits are often consulted through an amulet, or "sastun," about which plants to use. The healing spirit of the herbs is acknowledged through ritual or prayer, and thanked for its contribution to the restorative process.

Detoxification is also both a spiritual and a physical process. Today, detoxification is receiving a lot of attention, as even remote rainforest areas are increasingly inundated with the "western" junk food diet. The rainforest culture is being introduced to unnatural food sources and the burden that comes with them. Meanwhile, oral healing traditions are dying as young apprentices no longer want to spend years learning the thousands of herbs and their uses. Allopathic medicine is an easier option and it "comes with the territory" in the cities to which the rainforest people are migrating. With the demise of the old herbal ways goes the recognition of thousands of plants and their thousands of uses gathered over thousands of years.

Modern rainforest curanderos recognize that present day foods "are ruining people's diets, and that junk or "cuchinada" (pig food) is at the root of most patients' ailments, and getting worse. Foods full of chemicals and preservatives have made a people who had almost no instance of civilization diseases, more vulnerable to high blood pressure, heart disease, arthritis, diabetes, and cancer.

We can only hope that we learn from the Spanish conquest of centuries ago, that ancient wisdom will prevail. Unfortunately, we know the "chemical food equals disease" scenario all too well. It has happened over the last 50 years in China, Japan and Southeast Asia, where western food products have brought more disease to more people than all the wars fought there.

Detoxification and cleansing methods are largely plant based. Herbs are used for both their physical healing properties and for their purifying power. The herbs chosen are tailored to the individual and condition being treated. For example, to cleanse the body of "modern food disease," Balsam bark tea is used to detoxify the kidney and the liver.

## Here is a small sampling of detox remedies currently in use

**Purgative herbs to correct digestive problems** abound throughout the rainforest tradition. Chewing gum is a favorite method of delivery.

**A yearly parasite cleanse** is commonly followed in almost every rainforest healing system, sometimes with oje (ficus insipida).

**Liver cleansing is common,** with teas like aguacate (persea gratissima), assacurana (erythrina glauca) or the bark of the Brazil nut tree (bertholletia excelsa). Trumpet tree may be combined with papaya as a liver or kidney tonic during a cleanse.

**Stinking toe (senna grandis), and China root** (smilax lanceolata) are used to rid the blood and tissues of toxins and to help the body recover from toxicity resulting in fatigue and anemia.

**Sangre de grado:** A Rainforest home remedy for insect bites including those from: wasps, hornets, fire ants, bees, mosquitoes, even jellyfish. As little as a single drop can diminish pain from bites and sting by blocking nerve activity. In Peru, the herb is used as a vaginal bath to ease childbirth). New scientific research suggests Sangre de Grado is one of the most potent herbal antivirals available. It is currently undergoing FDA Phase 2 and Phase 3 clinical trials for viral respiratory infections (used orally) and for herpes (topically). Sangre de grado also shows great promise for reducing AIDS-related diarrhea.

**Blood purifying rituals use gumbolimbo** (bursera simaruba), jack-ass bitters (neurolaena lobata), or purslane (portulaca oleracea), to flush the kidneys, and to fight infections. The fresh juice from jack-ass bitters is used on the skin to heal sores and fungal infections.

**Heat therapy herbal steam baths,** are a respected detox practice in the rainforest to sweat out toxins. Green stick (eupatorium morifolium) leaves are used as a healing steam for skin conditions, flus and fevers. Steamed herbs like trumpet tree (cecropia peltata) or pheasant tail (anthurium schlechtendalii) are applied for relief from arthritic conditions and sprains.

**Massage and palpation** are widely used during cleansing. A skilled therapist can even move a misplaced organ to its correct setting through massage therapy. I have witnessed this phenomenon myself during a session with a Guatemalan healer.

## The Native American tradition

Native American religious and philosophical beliefs centered, as with all early human civilizations, on the concept that mankind was an integral part of the cosmic balance of all living things. Balance meant universal harmony and health; disruption of the balance meant illness, drought, famine, death. Respect for all life was very important—permission was even asked of plants before picking them. Indians believe that what is needed is provided. Taking too much, or more than one needed, was considered to deplete the Earth, disrupt the balance, and create bad energy.

Health in the Native American view signifies harmony and balance between the human and the supernatural world, a natural human condition given to each individual at birth. Disease was, and is today, believed to be caused by spiritual disharmony.

Native American healing practices are often similar to rainforest medicine traditions. Healing ideas are related to spiritual beliefs. Native Americans also include bad spirits as pathogens inducing illness. As with the rainforest cultures, modern circumstances have made it difficult for Native American healing practices to flourish. Unlike rainforest cultures, Native Americans divide diseases into white man categories and Indian categories, believing that their cleansing and healing methods work only for their own people and their own health conditions. Diseases they deem as originating from the white man and the white American way of life are treated by allopathic medicine.

Still, although it's not well-publicized, Native American medicine is experiencing a renaissance, especially in healing through body purification. Healing methods once again reflect the philosophy that everything is all one

with both mind and spirit stimulating the healing process and cleansing actions. Purity of mind and soul are once again considered the way to good health. Purification rituals as always address all of life. Body detoxification for instance, clears out both bad influences and spirits as well as toxins. In the well-known sweat lodges, both spiritual cleansing and body cleansing take place. While the high heat helps the body kill bacteria and viruses, sweating helps the skin release toxins. Aromatherapy from the burning of cleansing herbs like cedar and sage stimulates body functions, and prayers carry the purifying herbal smoke to the creator.

Sweat lodges were first famous as cleansing places for purification prior to religious rituals, hunting, or war. It was felt that men's and women's cleansing needs were different, and they had separate sweat lodges. As social norms changed, the purpose of the sweat lodge changed to cleaning out impurities and toxins for physical as well as spiritual health. The act of sweating became the ritual instead of a precursor. Men and women used the same lodge.

Herbs were the primary cleanser and healers used in the sweat lodges. Body parts were often wrapped with an herb, then held over hot coals to allow the herb and heat combination to act upon the disease. Sage was the favorite herb in the sweat lodge, both as a sacred plant to drive out bad spirits, and as a body cleansing herb. It was spread on the floor of the lodge, made into cleansing poultices and rubbed on the body, and burned in spaces thought to be contaminated by communicable diseases. I myself have participated in a Native sweatlodge and Medicine Wheel ceremony on a tour I led to the Southwest USA. My experience was both powerful and transformation, never to be forgotten.

Smudging—slowly burning bundles of fresh sage, sweetgrass, cedar or other herbs that draw in good influences, is a Native American cleansing ritual popular everywhere today. The herbal smoke is gathered in the hands, inhaled, rubbed on the body, then carried throughout a house or other space to cleanse it. Chanting or prayers are spoken or sung along with the smudging.

An interesting form of cleansing, practiced throughout Native American healing, is shamanic extraction—the cleansing of a foreign object (like a rock, stick or bone piece) left by a bad spirit or supernatural force. The objects are felt to be the cause of major illnesses, and must be found and removed to heal the afflicted person. Extraction takes place after a shaman journeys into the soul of the ill person either through trance or in dreams, and sees the disease. Then through a process of sucking, either with the mouth directly on the spot of the illness, or by using a hollow stick, or laying on of hands, or a sacred feather to sweep it away, the offending object is removed and destroyed. Herbs are sometimes applied to aid the extraction process. While to white Americans, this type of spiritual cleansing may seem to be based on the powers of suggestion alone, to the Native American it is as real and effective as a massage for stiff muscles.

Native Americans considered medicinal herbs as primary healing foods to restore body balance in order to restore normal health. The spring body cleanse popular in America today has its roots in Native American cleanses that celebrate the spirit of new growth and the rhythm of life with spring herbal elixirs. Slowly, the powerful effective healing ways of our Native American culture are becoming known and available to everyone who wishes to seek them out and incorporate them into an alternative medicinal approach for good health.

## European detox techniques

Since the early middle ages, the power of the Catholic Church and its controlling influence has been extreme in Europe. Through the Church, Christian beliefs connected illness to evil, and often dealt with it through exorcisms. The idea that an illness could be the result of a natural antigen was considered blasphemy. As a result, medicines and detoxification treatments for illness were slower than in other healing traditions.

The first inklings about the physical nature of illness did not develop until well into the Renaissance when man began to understand Nature as science. Thus, assigning meaning to the mystery of disease took a scientific rather than a spiritual turn.

Still, detoxification techniques had long been known. The Roman penchant for cleansing baths had been established throughout Europe. Many of the best spa locations today have been in use since Roman times. The hot springs connected to health in Scandinavian countries led to discoveries about the benefits of mineral waters, mud baths, and overheating therapy as body cleansers.

During medieval times, hot, sulphurous-smelling water boiling from the hot springs was thought to come from the devil. Yet, at the same time, there was the search for the Fountain of Youth, (an offshoot of the quest for the Holy Grail), where waters bubbled forth from the earth that could reverse the aging process or offer immortality. Eventually this idea lead to the development of therapeutic spas where special treatments were aimed at detoxifying, rejuvenating organs and overall health.

Over the last 200 years spas have developed more precise treatments. A German clergyman, Sebastian Kneipp who believed that mind, body, and spirit were all integral to health, refined many of the spa techniques used today. His therapies focused on the cause of illness, enhancing the body's natural defenses and establishing patterns for disease prevention. Kniepp suffered from tuberculosis declared incurable by allopathic medicine, yet he treated himself successfully using hot and cold hydrotherapy to improve his circulation and stimulate his immune system.

Today, spas treat psychosomatic exhaustion, recuperation from illness or postoperative conditions (with follow-up rehabilitation treatment), and support treatments for cardiovascular diseases, rheumatic disorders, metabolic imbalances, digestive tract afflictions, respiratory diseases, neurological illness, male and female hormone disturbances, childhood diseases, allergies and hypersensitive reactions.

Their programs incorporate herbal remedies, hot and cold hydrotherapy, massage, aromatherapy, special cleansing diets and exercise. Mineral mud baths and ionized hydro-treatments are popular. Herbal packs and wraps are especially used for detoxifying and cleansing effects and for long-term immune stimulation.

In fact, today, in some European countries, a "spa tune-up" is considered preventive health care, part of the general health care program. In German and Austrian Kur spas (derived from the Latin cura meaning care), where I worked in the early sixties there were specific spas for specific ailments, even spas to detoxify specific body parts, like the liver.

Nutrition is a focus at the spas. I worked in the spa kitchens part of my time there, and knew well the saying that "If the father of a disease is unknown, its mother will always be false nutrition." Customized therapeutic nutrition counseling, juice fasting and vegetarian diets are provided to guests for diet balance and correction based on individual needs.

Bodywork as part of the cleansing process ranges from massage therapies to tailored exercise programs like yoga, stretching and hydro-exercises to improve circulation, oxygen uptake, structural support and psychological well being. Hiking, walking, and cross-country skiing in the winter months, are encouraged.

Emotional harmony is treated as the glue binding the detoxification therapies together. Relaxation techniques, like yoga, breathing exercises, creativity exercises, autogenic training and psychological counseling are used to focus and unburden the mind so the soul and body can harmonize.

Many European spas are located in mountain settings where the clear air, aromatherapy from plants and springs, and the serenity offered by abundant trees promote better rest. (Strict noise restriction laws halt auto traffic near the spas in the afternoons and at night to improve sleep.)

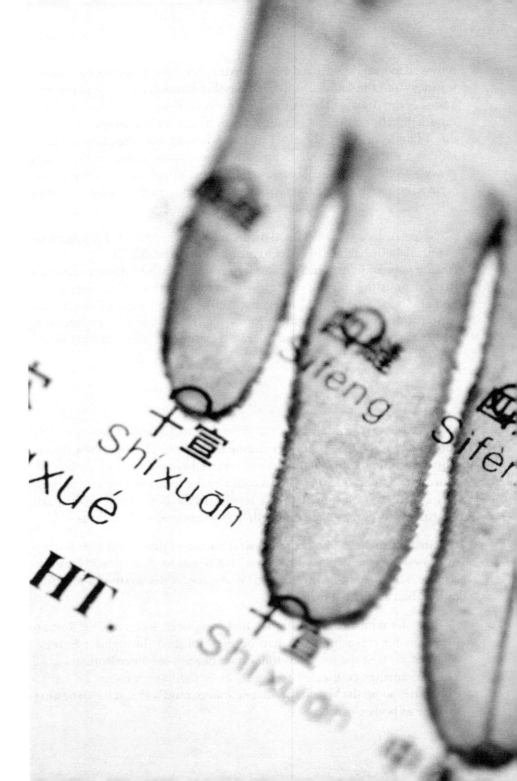

# quick detox glossary

Detoxification and body cleansing rituals have been around for so many millennia that they have developed a language and terminology all their own. Many methods and techniques come to us from ancient times. This short chapter is an easy glossary of alternative medicine and herbal therapy with examples for detoxification.

## Absorbents

Herbs used to produce absorption of diseased tissues. Examples of absorbents include mullein and slippery elm.

## Adaptogens

Herbs that help normalize body chemistry and resistance to stress. Examples of adaptogens include Siberian eleuthero, panax ginseng, jiaogulan, astragalus and rhodiola.

## Alkalizing enzyme cleanse

A good "spring cleaning" technique for liver, digestive and elimination system support. Balances and increases enzyme and systol/diastole activity, alkalizing an over-acid system. Used in spas in enzyme body wraps through herbal-infused gels applied to the skin for easy absorption. Examples of alkalizing, enzyme-stimulating herbs are aloe vera, ginger, bladderwrack, spearmint and alfalfa.

## Alteratives

Tonifying herbs that restore proper body function and vitality by normalizing blood composition. Alteratives improve metabolism, increasing the body's ability to eliminate waste through the kidneys, liver, lungs or skin. Examples of alterative herbs include echinacea, burdock, garlic, red clover, sarsaparilla, goldenseal, turmeric and yellow dock.

## Amino acids

Cysteine, methionine, tyrosine and taurine support internal cleansing. Cysteine converts to glutathione, one of the most powerful natural detoxifiers of heavy metals, radiation, chemicals and drugs. Glutathione is found in asparagus, broccoli, parsley and spinach.

## Antacids

Herbs which correct acidic conditions in the stomach, blood and bowels. Examples of antacids include comfrey, flax seed, hops, fig, aloe vera, mullein, raspberry and slippery elm.

## Anthelmintics

Herbs that help destroy or expel intestinal worms and parasites from the digestive system. (see also Vermifuge) Examples of anthelmintics include wormwood, pumpkin seed, tansy, aloe vera, rue, thyme, black walnut hulls and garlic.

## Anti-arthritics

Herbs used to relieve and heal arthritic-type conditions. Examples of anti-arthritic herbs include yucca, devil's claw, black cohosh, burdock, cayenne, St. John's wort, chaparral, dandelion, Irish moss, sarsaparilla, scullcap, wintergreen and yellow dock.

## Anti-bilious

Herbs that help neutralize and remove excess bile, and overcome jaundice conditions. Examples of antibilious herbs include barberry, dandelion root, goldenseal, wild yam and gentian.

## Antibiotics (anti-bacterial)

Herbs that kill and arrest the growth of harmful micro-organisms (see Anti-microbials). Examples of antibiotic herbs include goldenseal root, echinacea, myrrh, olive leaf, oregano, eucalyptus, St. John's wort, lomatium and garlic.

## Anti-catarrhal

Herbs that help remove excess mucous and congestion, particularly from sinus, bronchial and chest areas. Examples of anti-catarrhal herbs include boneset, echinacea root, garlic, goldenseal, cayenne, elecampane, marshmallow, mullein, sage and yarrow.

## Anti-emetic

Herbs that relieve nausea and vomiting, and upset stomach. Examples of anti-emetic herbs include ginger root, cayenne, cloves, Oregon grape, peppermint and spearmint, fennel, lemon balm, wild yam, alfalfa and dill.

## Anti-fungal

Herbs that destroy or prevent the growth of fungal infections. Examples of anti-fungal herbs include black walnut hulls, tea tree oil, licorice, propolis, maitake mushroom, wormwood and garlic.

## Anti-hydropics

Herbs that eliminate excess body fluids or dropsy. Examples of anti-hydropic herbs include anise, asparagus, barberry, black cohosh, burdock seeds and root, carrot, celery, chaparral, dandelion, fennel, flaxseed, mullein and rosemary.

## Anti-inflammatory

Herbs that help reduce and overcome inflammation both externally and internally. Examples of anti-inflammatory herbs include calendula, goldenseal, chamomile, devil's claw root, St. John's wort, feverfew, turmeric and white willow.

## Anti-lithics

Herbs that help remove and prevent the formation of sediment, gravel and stones in the urinary/urethral area. Examples of anti-lithic herbs include gravel root, hydrangea, stone root, cornsilk, buchu, tribulus, uva ursi and parsley root.

## Anti-microbials

Herbs that help the body to destroy or resist pathogenic micro-organisms. Examples of anti-microbials include myrrh, garlic, echinacea, calendula, elecampane, goldenseal and astragalus.

## Anti-neoplastics

Hrbs that combat tumorous growth. Examples of anti-neoplastics include calendula, red clover, burdock, dandelion, cleavers, green tea, maitake, shiitake, and tremella mushrooms, mistletoe, guaiacum and echinacea.

## Anti-oxidants

Agents that unite with oxygen, protecting the cells and body constituents like enzymes from being destroyed or altered by oxidation. Although oxygen is vital to our body functions, the presence of either too much or too little oxygen creates toxic by-products called free radicals. These highly reactive substances can damage cell structures so badly that immunity is impaired and DNA codes are altered, resulting in degenerative disease and premature aging. Specifically, free radical attacks are the forerunners of heart attacks, cancer, and opportunistic diseases such as HIV infection or candidiasis. Anti-oxidants "quench" free radicals and render them harmless. Antioxidants are selective, acting against undesirable oxygen reactions but not against desirable oxygen activity. A poor diet, inadequate exercise, illness and emotional stress result in a reduction of the body's system antioxidants. (See also Free Radicals.) Examples of antioxidants that are important in detoxification include the herbs ginkgo biloba, white pine, sea vegetables, astragalus, turmeric, and reishi mushrooms; enzyme stimulators—CoQ10, glutathione peroxidase and SOD; minerals—germanium and selenium; amino acids—cysteine, methionine and glutathione; and vitamins—beta-carotene, vitamins C and E.

## Anti-carcinogens

Substances that prevent or delay tumor formation and development. Examples of anticarcinogens include panax ginseng, ashwagandha, shiitake mushroom, garlic, echinacea, goldenseal, licorice, black cohosh, wild yam, sarsaparilla, maitake mushroom and cruciferous vegetables.

## Anti-parasitics

Like viruses, parasites have adapted and become stronger in order to survive, developing defenses against the drugs designed to kill them. In fact, most drugs commonly used to treat parasites not only lose effectiveness against new parasitic strains, but also cause a number of unpleasant side effects in the host. Herbal remedies have been successfully used for centuries as living medicines against parasites, with little or no side effects. Antiparasitic herbs include black walnut hulls, garlic, quassia, cloves, pumpkin seed, gentian root, wormwood, butternut bark, fennel seed, cascara, mugwort, slippery elm and false unicorn.

## Anti-phlogistics

Herbs that reduce inflammation or swelling (see Anti-inflammatories). Examples of anti-phlogistic herbs include arnica (external), balm of Gilead, bayberry, black cohosh (nerves), blue cohosh (uterus), burdock root (external), cayenne, comfrey and licorice.

## Anti-pyretics

Herbs that help reduce fevers. (See Febrifuge.)

## Anti-septics

Herbs that combat and neutralize pathogenic bacteria, and prevent infection. (See Anti-microbials and Antibiotics.)

## Anti-spasmodics

Muscle relaxant herbs that relieve cramping and spasms in a wide variety of uses, from hiatal hernias to PMS cramps, to lower back pain. Examples of anti-spasmodic herbs include cramp bark, black haw, kava kava, lady's slipper, motherwort, lobelia, scullcap, wild yam, chamomile and valerian.

## Anti-syphilitics

Herbs that help overcome venereal disease. Examples of anti-syphilitics include sarsaparilla, black walnut, black pepper, burdock, lobelia, white oak bark, goldenseal and myrrh.

## Anti-tussive

Herbs to prevent and relieve coughing. Examples of anti-tussive herbs include licorice, horehound, comfrey, mullein, plantain, coltsfoot, wild cherry bark and valerian.

## Anti-venomous

Antidote herbs against poisons. Examples of anti-venomous herbs include plantain (powerful), black cohosh, fennel, garlic, juniper berry, lobelia, marigold, olive oil, parsley, slippery elm and wormwood.

## Anti-virals

Herbs that combat and neutralize viruses. Examples of anti-virals include echinacea, St. John's wort, shiitake mushroom, lomatium dissectum, myrrh, goldenseal, astragalus and propolis.

## Aperients

Herbs with mild, gentle laxative activity. Examples of aperients include rhubarb root, flax seed, barberry, butternut root, rose hips and cleavers.

## Aphrodisiacs

Herbs that help impotency problems and strengthen sexual desire and vitality. Examples of aphrodisiacs include yohimbe, gotu kola, kola nut, all the ginsengs, damiana, saw palmetto, maca, horny goat weed, muira pauma (potency wood) and dong quai.

## Aromatics

Herbs with strong, pleasant odors, that stimulate digestion and well-being through both carminative activity and smell. Examples of aromatics include anise seed, basil, bay leaf, peppermint, fennel, cinnamon, dill, rosemary, ginger, cloves, chamomile and coriander.

## Astringents

Herbs that tighten tissue, reducing irritation, secretions and discharges (including heavy menstrual flow). Examples of astringent herbs include bayberry, St. John's wort, red raspberry, lady's mantle, and white oak bark.

## Balsamics

Herbs that soothe and heal skin inflammation. Examples of balsamics include avocado leaves, balm of Gilead buds, clary sage, ox-eye daisy petals, poplar buds and spikenard.

## Bentonite

A natural clay used for internal cleansing and externally as a poultice.

## Bitters

Herbs with a bitter taste that stimulate the digestive system, producing healthful counteractive juices and bile secretions. Examples of bitters herbs include gentian, angelica, wormwood, chamomile, barberry, goldenseal, dandelion and Oregon grape.

## Blood cleansing

Ridding the blood, liver, kidneys and lymph glands of toxins while normalizing blood chemistry. Examples of blood cleansers include echinacea, red clover, sarsaparilla and goldenseal.

## Calmatives

Herbs that calm stress and nervous tension. Examples of calmatives include peppermint, chamomile, scullcap, catnip, rosemary, hops and Siberian ginseng.

## Cardiotonics

Herbs that strengthen and tonify heart and circulatory activity. Examples of cardiotonic herbs include hawthorn, arjuna, cayenne, motherwort and Siberian ginseng.

## Carminatives

Herbs that normalize digestive system peristalsis to relieve gas. Examples of carminatives include anise seed, catnip, cayenne, licorice, peppermint, ginger root, cinnamon, caraway, ginger and thyme.

## Cathartics

Herbs that stimulate bowel purging (see Purgative). Examples of cathartic herbs include cascara, senna, butternut bark, barberry, aloe vera, buckthorn, rhubarb, and bentonite.

## Cell proliferants

Herbs that promote rapid new cell growth. Examples of cell proliferants include aloe, comfrey, chlorella, spirulina, barley grass, horsetail, evening primrose, sea vegetables and ginsengs.

## Charcoal, activated

A natural agent that relieves gas and diarrhea—an antidote for many poisons. An antacid, depurative and carminative that neutralizes and absorbs toxins allowing the kidneys to work more efficiently. Neutralizes acids and relieves flatulence in the stomach and intestinal tract. Helps normalize dysentery, diarrhea and constipation. Effective as a poultice for malodorous ulcers and wounds. An antidote for almost all poisons. Note: For cases of severe poisoning, call the Poison Control Center 1-800-222-1222.

## Chelation therapy

A safe intravenous therapy that increases blood flow and decreases excess plaque deposits in arteries and organs. EDTA, (ethylenediamine tetra-acetic acid), used in chelation therapy, removes toxic, clogging minerals from the circulatory system, particularly those that impair membrane function and contribute to free radical damage. EDTA puts these minerals into solution where they can be excreted by the kidneys. Oral chelation products are more affordable, accessible choice, and also help remove heavy metals and toxins that damage the cardiovascular system. Consider Metabolic Response Modifiers CardioChelate.

## Cholagogue

Herbs that stimulate bile secretion from the gallbladder, engendering natural laxative activity and digestive improvement. Examples of cholagogues include artichoke, barberry bark, wild yam, dandelion rt., Oregon grape, calendula, golden seal, garlic and gentian root.

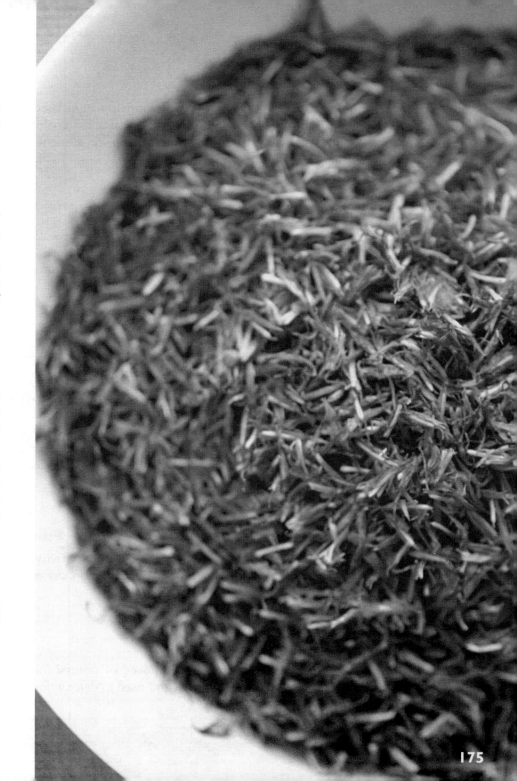

## Clay, white, purified

Absorbs and antidotes toxins to normalize intestinal inflammation. Used in formulas to relieve diarrhea and soothe the intestinal tract. Externally used as part of a poultice to disperse healing properties for skin ailments like eczema, boils, tumors and rashes.

## Colonic

A gentle, warm water cleansing of the colon. The procedure lasts approximately 45 minutes. A small nozzle or hose is inserted into the anus, allowing the water to flow in under gentle pressure and dislodge toxic wastes which are flushed out the rectum.

## Colloidal silver

A universal antibiotic natural substance, pure metallic ionic silver is held in suspension by the minute electrical charge of each particle. Colloidal silver is tasteless, non-addictive and non-toxic. Many forms of bacteria, viruses and fungi utilize a specific enzyme for their metabolism. Colloidal silver acts as a catalyst to disable the enzyme. In fact, it proves toxic to most species of fungi, bacteria, parasites, even many viruses. Even more important, harmful organisms do not develop an immunity to silver as they do to chemical antibiotics.

## Cordials

Tonic herbs that warm the stomach and stimulate cardiac activity. Examples of cordials include ginger, ginsengs, cardamon, cinnamon, cloves and coriander.

## Dead Sea Salts

Obtained from the Dead Sea in Israel—composed of potassium, chlorine, sodium, calcium and magnesium salts, and used in detoxifying baths.

## Demulcents

Soothing, coating mucilaginous herbs that protect irritated and inflamed tissue. Examples of demulcent herbs include comfrey, marshmallow, milk thistle, slippery elm, flax seed, parsley root, Irish moss, licorice, aloe vera and mullein.

## Depurant

Blood purifying herbs that stimulate elimination of toxins. Examples of depurants include garlic, goldenseal, chaparral, "Essiac" formula, chlorella, buckthorn, barley grass, cranberry and sea plants.

## Diaphoretics

Skin cleansing herbs that induce sweating, releasing body toxins through perspiration. Examples of diaphoretic herbs include cayenne, elder, garlic, ginger, chamomile, boneset, angelica, bayberry, prickly ash, yarrow, spikenard and buchu.

## Digestants

Enzyme-containing herbs that promote digestion and nutrient assimilation. Examples of digestant herbs include ginseng, chlorella, barley grass, spirulina, yellow dock, sea vegetables, ginger, basil, peppermint, papaya and garlic.

## Discutients

Herbs that dissolve and remove tumors or abnormal growths. Effective in poultices and fomentations or taken internally as teas. Examples of discutients include aloe vera, ginseng, pau d' arco, wheat grass, medicinal mushrooms, calendula, echinacea and sea plants. (See anti-neoplastics)

## Diuretics

Herbs that stimulate kidney/bladder activity, and increase the flow of urine. Examples of diuretics include uva ursi, cleavers, dandelion leaf, parsley, celery seed, buchu, couchgrass, juniper, yarrow, corn silk and gravel root.

## Electuary

A sweet paste, food or drink used to mask bitter or medicine-tasting herbs so they may be taken by children. Examples of electuaries include peanut butter, fruit juice, honey/butter pastes, bread or cream cheese.

## Emetic

Herbs that in high doses cause vomiting to rid the body of toxic substances or excess mucous congestion. Examples of emetic herbs include lobelia, elder flowers, boneset and ipecacuanha (Ayurveda).

## Emmenagogues

Herbs that stimulate and normalize menstrual flow. Examples of emmenagogues include pennyroyal, blue cohosh, dong quai, blessed thistle, motherwort, lovage, angelica and tansy.

## Emollient

Externally applied, soothing herbs that smooth and soften the skin and reduce inflammatory skin conditions. Examples of emollient herbs include slippery elm, marshmallow, plantain, comfrey, Irish moss, tremella mushroom, chickweed, borage, mullein and aloe vera.

## Essiac

An herbal tea formula of the Ojibway Indians, made famous by Rene Caisse for cleansing the body of cancer cells, has been rediscovered today. The name "Essiac" is actually an anagram of her last name "Caisse." The formula consists of sheep sorrel, burdock root, turkey rhubarb and slippery elm bark.

## Expectorants

Herbs that help remove mucous congestion from the chest and respiratory system. Examples of expectorant herbs include licorice root, horehound, pleurisy root, coltsfoot, comfrey, anise seed, marshmallow, eucalyptus, wild cherry and thyme.

## Free radicals

Unstable fragments of molecules produced from oxygen and fats in cell membranes when high energy chemical oxidation reactions in the body get out of control. Atoms and molecules consist of protons, neutrons and electrons, which normally come in pairs. Electron pairs form chemical bonds which hold all molecules together. A free radical contains an unpaired electron. In this unbalanced state, the free radical is stimulated to combine with other molecules, and in combination is capable of destroying an enzyme, a protein, or a complete cell. The destruction causes chain reactions that release thousands more free radicals and stimulate aging skin pigment, damage protein structures, and impair fat metabolizing enzymes. While the body normally produces some free radicals in its ordinary metabolic breakdown of organic compounds (like those released to fight bacteria during immune response), it also produces the necessary substances (like antioxidant enzymes) to deactivate them.

**Free radical formation can be caused by:**

- Infections from viruses, bacteria, or parasites.
- Trauma from surgery, injury, inflammation, burns and wounds.
- Smoking or passive exposure to cigarette smoke.
- Excessive alcohol and/or addictive drug intake.
- Exposure to toxic chemicals, like pesticide residues and household chemicals.
- Exposure to radiation, including excessive UV rays from sunlight.
- Cytotoxic drugs, such as the anticancer drug Adriamycin.
- Oxidant drugs that steal electrons, such as acetaminophen (Tylenol).
- Consumption of nitrites, nitrates and other food additives.

- A diet low in antioxidant foods; partially-hydrogenated fats in many snack and junk foods.
- Chronic degenerative disease like cancer, heart disease or arthritis.

## Hemostatic

Herbs that help stop bleeding (see Styptic). Examples of hemostatics include shepherd's purse, comfrey, lady's mantle, turmeric, plantain, witch hazel, cayenne, buckthorn and cranesbill.

## Hemoglobin builder

A compound that aids absorption of iron and other minerals for red blood cell production. Examples of hemoglobin building herbs are beet root, chlorella, alfalfa, dandelion, Siberian ginseng, yellow dock root, parsley root, nettles, burdock root, dulse, capsicum.

## Heavy metal poisoning

Long term exposure to metals like lead, mercury, cadmium, arsenic, nickel and aluminum affects cell growth, behavior and immune response. Examples of herbs that help remove heavy metals are bugleweed, bladderwrack, sea buckthorn (radiation), licorice root, astragalus, kelp and all sea vegetables.

## Hepatics

Herbs that support and stimulate the liver, gall bladder and spleen to increase bile flow. Examples of hepatics include barberry, Oregon grape, beet root, burdock, red sage, dandelion, goldenseal, hyssop, wild yam, fennel and cleavers.

## Herbal wraps

Spas use herbal wraps as restorative body-conditioning techniques. Wraps are also body cleansing methods that may be used to elasticize, tone, alkalize and release body wastes quickly. For best results, use in conjunction with a short cleansing program, and 6 to 8 glasses of water a day to flush out loosened fats and toxins. Alkalizing enzyme wraps replace and balance minerals, enhance metabolism and alkalize the body.

## Juice fasting

A raw vegetable and fruit juice cleanse for 24 hours to 7 days for detoxification. Fruit juices promote cleansing; vegetable juices help build and regenerate.

## Kidney flush

Ridding the kidneys of metabolic wastes such as ammonia and urea, allowing them to operate more efficiently. A purifying, kidney cleansing drink should have balancing potassium and other minerals, and naturally-occurring amino acids for protein synthesis. Examples of kidney flushing herbs are juniper, dandelion leaf, uva ursi, cleavers, cranberry extract.

## Lactobacillus

Beneficial bacteria, including L. acidophilus, L. bifidus, L. caucassus, and L. bulgaricus, that synthesize nutrients in the intestinal tract, counteract pathogenic microorganisms and maintain a healthy intestinal environment. Lactobacillus organisms are fragile flora readily destroyed by harmful chemicals and drugs, particularly chlorine and antibiotics. A single, long course of antibiotics can destroy most bowel flora, leading to an overgrowth of yeasty pathogens like candida albicans, which are resistant to antibiotics. Eating antibiotic-laced meats and dairy products leads to a decline of Lactobacillus organisms in the body. Skin disorders, chronic candidiasis, irritable bowel syndrome, intestinal disorders, hepatitis, lupus and heart disease are all associated with a Lactobacillus deficiency. Top food sources include yogurt, kefir, miso, tempeh and cold-cooked or "raw" sauerkraut.

## Laxatives

Herbs that promote evacuation of the bowels. Examples of laxative herbs include cascara, senna, aloe vera, Oregon grape, rhubarb rt., butternut bark, buckthorn and barberry.

## Lithotropics

Herbs that dissolve and discharge urinary and gall bladder stones and gravel. Examples of lithotropics include barberry, gravel root, buchu, cascara, chaparral, cornsilk, dandelion, horsetail, juniper berry and parsley.

## Liver flush

A liver flush releases wastes from the liver and surrounding organs, tones liver tissue and stimulates protein synthesis to increase production of new liver cells to replace damaged ones. Examples of liver flushing herbs include dandelion and yellow dock roots, burdock, watercress, pau d'arco, hyssop, parsley, Oregon grape, red sage, licorice, milk thistle seed.

## Lymphatics

Herbs that stimulate and cleanse the lymph system. Examples of lymphatics include black walnut, garlic, chaparral, dandelion, echinacea root, red root, sea vegetables, Oregon grape and yellow dock.

## Lymphatic massage

A gentle, whole-body massage aimed at stimulating the lymphatic system to carry away excessive fluid in the loose connective tissue.

## Mucilaginous

Herbs with high mucilage content that have soothing, demulcent action. Examples of mucilaginous herbs include comfrey, slippery elm, Irish moss, Iceland moss, flax seed, psyllium, aloe vera and marshmallow root.

## Mucous cleanse

Releases excess mucous from the lungs, respiratory and digestive system allowing other body functions to operate more efficiently.

## Nervines

Herbs that tone, relax and strengthen the nervous system. Examples of nervines include lady's slipper, passionflowers, mistletoe, chamomile, oatstraw, lobelia, cramp bark, wood betony, hops, valerian and scullcap.

## Nutritional Yeast

An excellent source of protein, B vitamins, amino acids and minerals. Chromium-rich nutritional yeast significantly improves blood sugar metabolism, and substantially reduces serum cholesterol, raising HDL's. Helps speed wound healing by increasing production of collagen. Antioxidant properties allow the tissues to take in more oxygen for healing. B vitamin and mineral content improve skin texture and heal blemishes. (I use it in a cleansing facial mask.) Nutritional yeast is not the same as Candida albicans yeast. It is one of the best immune-enhancing supplements available.

## Nutritives

Food supplement plants, rich in minerals, that nourish and promote growth. Examples of nutritive herbs include chlorella, spirulina, barley grass, ginseng, wheat grass, sea vegetables, suma and astragalus.

## Parasiticides

Herbs that kill and remove parasites from the skin. Examples of parasiticide herbs include black walnut, wormwood, cinnamon and cajuput oils, chaparral, garlic, echinacea, rue, thyme, gentian and wood betony.

## Pectoral

Herbs that helps heal and strengthen the lung and respiratory system. Examples of pectorals include comfrey, coltsfoot, goldenseal, elecampane, mullein, licorice, marshmallow, pleurisy root and hyssop.

## pH

The scale used to measure acidity and alkalinity. H is hydrogen, or the "H" ion concentration of a solution. "p" stands for the power factor of the H ion. pH of a solution is measured on a scale of 14. A neutral solution, neither acidic nor alkaline, such as water, has a pH of 7. Acid is less than 7; alkaline is more than 7.

## Pycnogenol

A concentrated, highly active bioflavonoid extract from pine bark. A powerful antioxidant, 50 times stronger than vitamin E, 20 times stronger than vitamin C. Helps the body resist inflammation, and blood vessel and skin damage caused by free radicals. Strengthens arteries and improves circulation. Reduces capillary fragility, develops skin smoothness and elasticity. Stimulates collagen-rich connective tissue against atherosclerosis and for joint flexibility in arthritis. Helps diabetic retinopathy, varicose veins and hemorrhoids. One of the few dietary antioxidants that easily crosses the blood-brain barrier to protect brain cells and aid memory.

## Phytochemicals

Natural constituents in plants that have specific pharmacologic action. Also known as nutraceuticals, pharmafoods and phytonutrients, the best way for your body to utilize phytochemicals is to ingest the plant source in its whole form. Here are some phytochemicals that are of important interest to a cleansing balancing diet;

Anti-carcinogen phytochemicals prevent or delay tumor formation. Some herbs and foods with known anticarcinogens include ginseng, soy foods, garlic, echinacea, goldenseal, licorice root, black cohosh, wild yam, maitake mushroom and cruciferous vegetables.

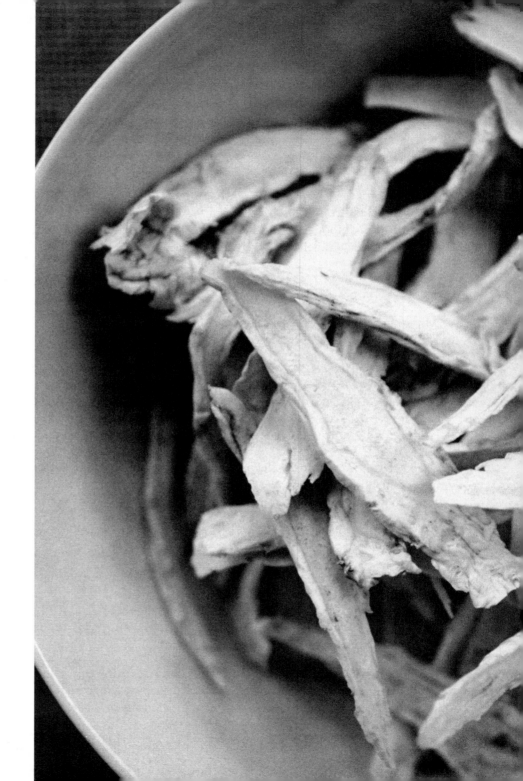

Phytohormones contain substances with hormonal actions. Plant hormone chemicals are quite similar to human hormones and are capable of binding to human hormone receptor sites. Unlike synthetic hormones, plant hormones show little or no adverse side effects. Some food plants and herbs that have phytohormone activity include soy foods, licorice root, wild yam, sarsaparilla root, dong quai, damiana and black cohosh.

**Phytoestrogens are plant estrogens remarkably similar to human estrogens.** Important in inhibiting hormone-driven cancers, phytoestrogens bind to human estrogen receptor sites without the negative side effects of synthetic estrogens. Recent studies show phytoestrogens are essentially hormone balancers, inhibiting proliferation of both estrogen-receptor positive and negative breast tumor cells. Some plants with phytoestrogenic activity include dong quai, panax ginseng, licorice, fennel, alfalfa and red clover.

**Phytoprogesterones are plant hormones** similar to human progesterone. They normally contain diosgenin, a chemical precursor to progesterone. Progesterone participates in almost every physiological process, biochemically providing material out of which other steroid hormones (cortisone, testosterone, estrogen and salt-regulating aldosterone) can be made. A precursor to estrogen, its tremendous increase during pregnancy serves to stabilizes hormone adjustment and growth of mother and child. When progesterone is deficient, there tends to be hypoglycemia, often combined with obesity. Some diosgenin sources are sarsaparilla, licorice root and wild yam.

**Phyto-testosterone, or plant testosterone,** is a similar substance to the androgen or male hormones found in both men and women. Testosterone determines sex drive in both sexes. Testosterone is essential for normal sexual behavior and the occurrence of male erections. Ginseng is an herb known to affect production of human testosterone.

## Probiotics

Beneficial microorganisms, including Lactobacillus, Bifidobacteria, and Streptococcus termophilus, that compete with disease-causing microorganisms in the gastrointestinal tract. Probiotics are responsible for the manufacture of B vitamins like biotin, niacin, folic acid and pyridoxine (B6), improving digestion, combating vaginal yeast infections, killing harmful bacteria by normalizing acid/alkaline balance and depriving harmful bacteria of nutrients they need.

## Purgatives

Herbs that promote watery evacuation of the bowels (see Laxative).

## Rubefacient

Herbs that increase circulation and stimulate dilation of the capillaries. Examples of rubefacient herbs include cayenne, ginger, horseradish, mustard, nettles, rosemary, peppermint oil, cloves, black pepper and garlic.

## Sauna heat therapy

A sauna is a way to use heat cleansing principles. A 20 to 30-minute sauna not only induces a healing, cleansing fever, but also causes profuse therapeutic sweating. The skin, in effect, acts as a "third kidney" to eliminate body wastes through perspiration. Native Americans used sweat lodges on much the same principle. Health benefits of a dry sauna include dramatic increase in the cleansing capacity of the skin, increased metabolism, a jump start for a weight loss program (especially for sugar cravers), gland and organ stimulation, enhanced immune response, and inhibition of virus replication. **Note:** Although cleansing heat is a natural means of biological healing, supervision from a practitioner is recommended.

## Sedatives

Herbs that calm the nerves and reduce stress and tension. Examples of sedatives are valerian, scullcap, hops, black cohosh, black haw and passionflowers.

## Stimulants

Herbs that accelerate, enliven and vitalize body functions. Examples of stimulant herbs include bayberry, cayenne, ginger root, horseradish, cardamom, peppermint, wild yam and ginsengs of all kinds.

## Stomachics

Agents that stimulate and strengthen the stomach, improving digestion and appetite. Examples of stomachics include peppermint, wild yam, catnip, fennel and goldenseal.

## Styptics

Herbs to reduce and stop external bleeding (see Hemostatics and Astringents). Examples of styptics include plantain, St. John's wort, witch hazel, yarrow, bayberry bark, cranesbill, white oak bark and cayenne.

## Sudorifics

Herbs that stimulate and increase perspiration. (see Diaphoretic)

## Tonics

Herbs that strengthen and tone specific organs and body parts. Examples of tonic herbs include ginsengs, hawthorn, black cohosh, dandelion, garlic, gotu kola, licorice rt. and damiana.

## Toxins

Toxic or poisonous compounds produced by microorganisms, that promote disease. Examples of toxins include heavy metals, environmental and chemical pollutants, chemical laced foods, tobacco smoke, drugs of all kinds, pesticides and food additives.

## Triphala

A detoxifying compound of three herbal fruits terminalia chebula, terminalia bellerica and emblica officinalis. Triphala has both laxative and tonic properties that regulate elimination, cleanse the digestive tract and colon, and revitalize the blood and liver. It is a specific for regulating bowel activity, constipation, diarrhea, biliousness, dyspepsia, and for headaches.

Triphala regulates menstrual activity, helps weight control through cleansing, and is an effective eyewash to relieve redness and soreness.

## Vasodilators

Herbs that relax and expand blood vessels. Examples of vasodilators include ephedra, hawthorn, ginkgo biloba, feverfew and Siberian ginseng.

## Vermifuge

Herbs that help expel and/or destroy intestinal parasites (see Anthelmintics). Examples of vermifuge herbs include thyme, black walnut hulls, chaparral, garlic, barberry, psyllium husks, tea tree oil, tansy and wormwood.

**T**HIS MATERIA MEDICA IS A SHORT, QUICK-LOOK catalogue of notable herbs for detoxification and cleansing. While many of the herbs have a wide range of therapeutic activity, the elements discussed in this listing are those that specifically relate to their cleansing activity.

## materia medica of detoxification herbs

## Alfalfa *(Medicago sativa)*

**FAMILY:** Leguminoseae

**MEDICINAL PARTS:** leaves, flowering tops and seeds.

**DOSAGE:** tea: 6 oz. 3x daily; tincture: 5 – 10 drops 3x daily; extract: ½ to 1 tsp. 3x daily; capsules: 2 caps 3 – 4 times daily with meals.

**NUTRITION PROFILE:** a highly nutritive herb, rich in vitamin C (can even counteract scurvy), carotenes, vitamin K, amino acids, octacosonal and a full spectrum of minerals and trace minerals; an excellent source of fiber and chlorophyll with a balance of elements almost identical to human hemoglobin. One of the world's richest mineral foods, pulling up earth sources from root depths as great as 130 feet!

**CLEANSING PROPERTIES & DETOX ACTIVITY:** Alfalfa binds and neutralizes a wide range of carcinogenic agents in the colon, and is a proven nutritive for colon cancer protection… As a green superfood, alfalfa helps neutralize allergens, overcome anemia and jaundice, and balance over-acidity. It is used therapeutically for arthritis, bursitis and gout, stimulating removal of inorganic mineral deposits from the blood. As a blood clotting agent, it counteracts internal bleeding from ulcers. It is an estrogen precursor for menopause. Alfalfa is beneficial for indigestion, in reducing blood sugar levels, in lowering cholesterol and in the prevention of tooth decay. It is a healer for a wide range of intestinal and skin disorders, liver problems, breath and body odor, even morning sickness.

**SAFETY PRECAUTIONS:** none in common use

**SYNERGY WITH OTHER HERBS:** With pau d' arco and mineral-rich herbs like carrot root to help detoxify, rebuild and restore foundation body strength. With dandelion for better digestion and to detoxify the liver. With yucca to help relieve pain and inflammation of arthritis.

## Aloe Vera *(Aloe barbadensis, Aloe vera)*

**FAMILY:** Liliaceae

**MEDICINAL PARTS:** bottom leaves yield the most gel with the most healing potential.

**DOSAGE:** external: cover affected area 3x a day; internal: 1 tsp. of juice 3x daily as a cathartic. Effective in ridding children of roundworms by injection: 10 grains to 3 oz. of water.

**NUTRITION PROFILE:** Aloe has medicinal amounts of protein for healing, almost 18% dietary fiber, up to 5% of 22 amino acids and all B complex vitamins. Aloe contains active enzymes for enzyme therapy. Skin-building nutrients include vitamin E, selenium and silicon.

**CLEANSING PROPERTIES & DETOX ACTIVITY:** Aloe juice penetrates injured tissue, relieving pain through anti-inflammatory activity; dilates capillaries to increase blood supply to an injured area. Aloe is a colon, bowel and digestive cleanser. Both aloe vera gel and juice are beneficial for gastrointestinal complaints, like diverticulitis, peptic, gastric or duodenal ulcers, Crohn's disease and ulcerative colitis. Aloe treats liver symptoms like jaundice and cirrhosis. (Tests on liver cirrhosis show that after six months of aloe treatment normal liver enzymes are achieved.) Aloe also contains a substance which inhibits liver cancer. Because of its blood cleansing qualities, drug detoxing patients treated with aloe have fewer complications than those given regular therapy. Synergistic with vitamin C in treating arthritis, aloe helps prevent or slow tissue breakdown and reduce inflammation.

**SAFETY PRECAUTIONS:** Large doses of aloe are purgative; large doses can cause rectal piles. Don't take internally during pregnancy or nursing (it will purge the suckling child).

**SYNERGY WITH OTHER HERBS:** A tea of aloe, fennel, catnip and St. John's wort cleanses the liver and reduces stomach cramping. As a poultice: with comfrey (50:50). With ginger as a liver tonic.

## Astragalus (Astragalus membranaceous) (Huang chi)

**FAMILY:** Leguminosae

**MEDICINAL PARTS:** root

**DOSAGE:** for health maintenance: 2 capsules 3x daily at mealtime; for recovery from illness: 4 capsules 4x daily.

**NUTRITION PROFILE:** high in flavonoids, amino acids and trace minerals including selenium. Rich in key nutrients like folic acid, calcium, iron and potassium. Immuno-active polysaccharides are responsible for its amazing immune-defense power.

**CLEANSING PROPERTIES & DETOX ACTIVITY:** Astragalus is a toning diuretic in kidney inflammation formulas. It nourishes exhausted adrenals to combat fatigue. It is a strong antiviral agent, producing extra interferon in the body. Promotes the regeneration of bronchi cells after a viral infection. Astragalus stimulates immune system white blood cell activity to help destroy invading microorganisms. Damaged immune system cells taken from cancer patients have been restored to full function in tests with Astragalus extract. Astragalus also increases the number of stem cells in bone marrow and lymphatic tissue to stimulate their development into immune cells. Astragalus is especially useful in the rebuilding and maintaining stages of a cleanse to increase disease resistance against repeated infections.

**SAFETY PRECAUTIONS:** Do not take if you have an acute disease, high fever or severe inflammation.

**SYNERGY WITH OTHER HERBS:** For anemia: a tea with equal parts astragalus and angelica, 2 cups daily. For cold and numbness: a tea with 2 parts astragalus bark and 1 part cinnamon bark, 1 cup twice a day. In combination with ligustrum to boost the immune system.

## Barberry (Berberis vulgaris)

**FAMILY:** Berberidaceae

**MEDICINAL PARTS:** bark of stem and root, and berries.

**DOSAGE:** Barberry is a "bitters" herb, take in small doses. Capsules: 2, 3x a day; tincture: ½ to 1 tsp.; tea: 2 – 3 tbsp. 3x a day; extract: 10 – 20 drops every 3 – 4 hours (extract has the widest range of effects).

**NUTRITION PROFILE:** rich in vitamin C and fiber, the root has about 6.6% protein. Has measureable B vitamins, and the minerals calcium, chromium, cobalt, magnesium, potassium, selenium and silicon.

**CLEANSING PROPERTIES & DETOX ACTIVITY:** Barberry's bitters compounds improve digestion, stimulate bile production, dilate blood vessels and have a mild laxative effect for cleansing. Anti-microbial against a wide range of organisms, including candida albicans yeast, and several intestinal parasites. Diarrhea is a common symptom of candidiasis—barberry has remarkable anti-diarrhea activity even in severe cases.

Barberry's astringent compounds tighten and shrink inflamed tissues. In the upper digestive organs, (liver, stomach and duodenum), barberry's bitters break up and remove morbid matter from the intestinal tract, while helping bile to flow more freely through a stagnant liver and gallbladder, important for liver problems. Barberry helps clean out bronchial mucous clogs, and is a recuperative tonic for bronchitis and the early stages of tuberculosis. Barberry dilates the blood vessels, so it's good for high blood pressure. It is a specific for diseases like cholera and its side effects like scabs, itch, tetters, and ringworm.

**SAFETY PRECAUTIONS:** Use only root and berries—small doses for best effects. (Leaves and seeds contain methylcysticine a poisonous purgative in large doses.) Do not take if there is digestive weakness. Avoid use as a single herb during pregnancy. A high dose may slow down the heart muscle and respiratory system, constricting the bronchial tubes. Discontinue if the tincture causes nosebleeds or dizziness.

**SYNERGY WITH OTHER HERBS:** With turmeric to regulate liver function. With cayenne, golden seal and lobelia is a specific for jaundice and hepatitis. Equal parts with wild yam root helps eliminate gas. With goldenseal, burdock, yellow dock, fringe tree and wild cherry as a body cleanser.

## Barley Grass (Hordeum vulgare)

**FAMILY:** Gramineae

**MEDICINAL PARTS:** stem and juice

**DOSAGE:** 2 – 3 capsules 3x daily, or one to two tsp. daily. For recovery: 6 – 8 capsules daily. For weight loss: take before meals with an 8 oz. glass of water.

**NUTRITION PROFILE:** Barley has a broad spectrum of concentrated vitamins, minerals, enzymes, proteins, chlorophyllins and antioxidants. Considered a "superfood," and an exceptional source of protein and essential amino acids, barley has eleven times the calcium of cow's milk, five times the iron of spinach, and seven times the vitamin C and bioflavonoids as orange juice. One of its most important contributions is to the vegetarian diet with 80mcg of vitamin B12 per hundred grams of powdered juice. Barley also contains glucan, the same fiber found in oat bran to reduce cholesterol levels. Barley (along with alfalfa) is one of the few foods that contains enough nutrition to sustain life from birth to old age.

**CLEANSING PROPERTIES & DETOX ACTIVITY:** Barley, rich in chlorophyll, normalizes metabolism and neutralizes heavy metals like mercury in the body that precipitate disease. Its small molecular proteins are absorbed directly through the cell membranes to purify and rebuild blood, and promote anti-aging. A compound in barley grass, 2-0-GIV, has antioxidant properties similar to vitamin E, that cleanse the cell membranes. Mega antioxidant enzymes in barley (including SOD, super-oxide dismutase) stop free radical attacks, destroy nitro-compounds, (environmental pollutants which build up in the body) and stimulate healing. Barley eliminates fecal matter and toxins in the colon.

A green drink with barley is a tonic, regenerating drink—a chlorophyll-containing aid to the digestive system, an ideal anti-inflammatory food for healing stomach and duodenal ulcers and hemorrhoids. It's a specific for blood sugar balance, particularly in cases of hypoglycemia and diabetes. Barley grass acts directly on DNA to repair cellular damage, and boosts the cells' ability to fight diseases like cancer.

**SAFETY PRECAUTIONS:** None in common use.

**SYNERGY WITH OTHER HERBS:** with spirulina, bee pollen and alfalfa to restore strength after exhaustion or illness. With vitamin c and sea vegetables, to neutralize and cleanse the body of heavy metals.

## Bee Pollen

**MEDICINAL PARTS:** High quality, unsprayed, dried granules.

**DOSAGE:** Pollen granules, 2 tsp. daily; capsules: 1 to 2 daily for longterm maintenance. Use only unsprayed pollen for therapeutic applications.

Short term, a therapeutic amount of bee pollen is about three times the preventive amount.

**NUTRITION PROFILE:** A highly bio-active, complete food, bee pollen is completely balanced for all 105 of the known nutritional ingredients. No other food contains as many enzymes… an estimated 5000, with 22 amino acids, 27 minerals and all known vitamins, in fact every nutrient needed to maintain life. Bee pollen has 35% protein, about half of which is in the form of free amino acids (excellent for healing). It contains 5 to 7 times more amino acids than beef, eggs or cheese of equal weight. Bee Pollen is rich in chromium, vitamin A, B-complex vitamins (especially B12) and vitamins C, D and E. It has one of the highest food amounts of rutin, for tissue strength. Bee pollen is a low-calorie food with 15% lecithin that helps burn away body fat. It is also 40 to 80 percent free-form glutamic acid, which can cross the blood/brain barrier, accounting for its ability to curb cravings for alcohol and increase powers of concentration.

**CLEANSING PROPERTIES & DETOX ACTIVITY:** Bee pollen enhances a feeling of youthful vitality and provides energy. It is valuable for weight control because it helps correct metabolic chemical imbalance.

Well-documented evidence shows pollen counteracts the effects of severe toxins like radiation and environmental chemicals. More importantly, bee pollen antioxidants are clinically proven to strengthen immune response. Recent clinical tests on women with inoperable uterine cancer, show that pollen significantly reduces the side effects of both radium and cobalt-60 radiotherapy at a level of 2 tbsp. a day. Red and white blood cell counts and serum protein levels both increase. The women reported notably better health, with stronger immune responses than those who did not take pollen. Pollen is regularly used in Russia to improve the immune status of patients with M.S. Pollen effectively helps chronic diarrhea and constipation, rheumatism with heart complications, kidney and liver disease, anemia (increases amount of hemoglobin), intestinal infection, fatigue, circulatory disorders, depression, colitis and prostatitis.

Bee pollen's main use is as a tree pollen and spore antidote during allergy season for control and neutralization of seasonal allergy symptoms. It relieves respiratory problems like bronchitis and sinusitis.

**SAFETY PRECAUTIONS:** Pesticides used on the plants where bees gather pollen affect an extremely small number of people. Discontinue if itching, dizziness or difficulty swallowing occurs. Start with small doses.

**SYNERGY WITH OTHER HERBS:** With panax ginseng, Siberian ginseng and "green superfoods" such as chlorella, alfalfa and spirulina; and with CoQ10 for immune enhancement.

## Beets *(Beta vulgaris)*

**FAMILY:** Chenopodiaceae

**MEDICINAL PARTS:** leaves and root

**DOSAGE:** Four capsules 3x daily with water at mealtime.

**NUTRITION PROFILE:** Beets owe their medicinal benefits to the active ingredient betaine, a substance that helps vitalize the blood. Betaine is an essential hepatotropic, a lipotropic amino acid similar to methionine. Betaine acts on the methylation cycle of liver cells and the conversion of triglycerides for fat transport. It is a good source of vitamin A, specifically indicated for fatty degeneration of the liver.

**CLEANSING PROPERTIES & DETOX ACTIVITY:** Beet juice is a blood detoxifying, blood builder that cleanses eliminative, digestive and lymphatic systems, then enlivens with rich minerals and natural sugars. Beet juice is an anti-inflammatory, scouring medicinal, especially effective for the kidneys, making beet juice a good choice for a cancer program. Beet juice also aids liver and spleen function to cleanse toxic waste. It can help restore organs damaged from alcohol abuse.

**SAFETY PRECAUTIONS:** none in common use.

**SYNERGY WITH OTHER HERBS:** A tea with vinegar heals itching, cleanses dandruff and dry scabs, and relieves running sores and ulcers.

## Bilberry *(Vaccinium myrtillus)*

**FAMILY:** Ericaceae

**MEDICINAL PARTS:** fruit and leaves

**DOSAGE:** For diarrhea, boil 3 tbsp. for 10 minutes in ½ liter of water. Extract: 15 drops 2x daily; capsules: 180 mg. per day for preventive purposes, 300 mg per day for therapeutic purposes.

**NUTRITION PROFILE:** Bilberry is rich in vitamin C, bioflavonoids, manganese, phosphorus, iron and zinc. The fruit has as much as 13% protein and 31% EFAs. Bilberries contain important medicinal compounds called anthocyanosides, bioflavonoids that provide a wide range of benefits.

**CLEANSING PROPERTIES & DETOX ACTIVITY:** Bilberry extract is well documented for reducing and reversing damage caused by blood vessel deterioration or inflammation. It supports, strengthens and protects collagen structures, inhibits bacteria growth, and produces anti-carcinogenic benefits. It clears toxins and restrains infection. Its anthocyanodins are active free radical scavengers to boost immunity. Anthocyanodins also have cardiac protective, anti-aging activity for impressive effects on the circulatory system. Regular use of bilberry reduces hardening of the arteries by preventing oxidative damage, thus limiting calcium plaque deposits, and maintaining flexible blood vessels. Research shows impressive effects on circulation, restoring normal blood flow in patients ranging from 18 to 75 years old.

Bilberry promotes kidney cleansing and urination, to help prevent urinary tract infections. Bilberries help heal inflammation of the intestinal mucosa that accompanies chronic constipation. Flavonoids increase mucous secretion that protects the stomach lining. Also used to treat intestinal parasites, diarrhea and vaginal disharge.

Externally, bilberry extract ointment helps dermatitis, eczema, dandruff, burns and inflammations, and speeds recovery from grazes, bruises and swelling. Bilberry helps promote a clearer fresher complexion due to its astringent effect, lessening the marks of cellulite, strengthening collagen structures.

**SAFETY PRECAUTIONS:** Bilberry leaf contains hydroquinone; if used for diabetes or bladder infections, it should not be taken continuously. Use for 3 weeks, then take a break for a week.

**SYNERGY WITH OTHER HERBS:** An energizing tea: equal parts of bilberry, thyme and strawberry leaves.

## Black Walnut (*Juglans nigra*)

**FAMILY:** Juglandaceae

**MEDICINAL PARTS:** fruit, leaves and bark, green nut, rind, hulls and root.

**DOSAGE:** leaves are used for skin conditions as a tea or 1 – 3 capsules, two times daily; hull extract: 10 – 30 drops three times a day.

**NUTRITION PROFILE:** Black walnuts are rich in oil and high in food energy, with almost as much protein as sirloin steak! The nut is rich in linolenic, linoleic and oleic fatty acids, (important for nerves, brain and cartilage), juglone (believed to have antifungal properties), in vitamin B15, and manganese. The hulls are especially high in tannins, vitamins A, B, C and E and organic iodine, useful in anti-parasite cleansing.

**CLEANSING PROPERTIES & DETOX ACTIVITY:** Black walnut hulls are useful in cleansing programs for the organs, lungs, kidneys and brain. The bark helps chronic constipation (a cleansing purgative), and liver congestion. The bark and leaves are astringent, antiseptic cleansers useful as a douche for leucorrhea, as a vermifuge for amoebic dysentery and as a mouthwash for mouth sores or sore tonsils. One study finds that several constituents of black walnut even have anti-cancer activity. Black walnut oxygenates the blood to rid the body of excessive toxins and fatty material, and is especially effective in expelling parasites. The extract of the hulls is good internally and externally for skin diseases, eczema, genital herpes, psoriasis and skin parasites. Chinese medics use black walnut to kill tapeworm with excellent success.

**SAFETY PRECAUTIONS:** Avoid during pregnancy.

**SYNERGY WITH OTHER HERBS:** For giardia (amoebic dysentery): equal parts: black walnut, goldenseal root, mugwort or wormwood, chaparral and licorice root. For cold sores: equal parts with licorice root.

## Boneset (*Eupatorium perfoliatum*)

**FAMILY:** Compositae

**MEDICINAL PARTS:** tops and leaves

**DOSAGE:** tea: 3 oz. three times daily. Drink 4 to 5 cups while in bed to encourage sweating; capsules: ½ to 1 gram; extract: ½ to 1 tsp. three times daily; tincture: 10 to 40 drops three times daily; 2 tbsp. tincture added to hot water can be used for sweating to break fevers.

**NUTRITION PROFILE:** Boneset contains vitamin C, calcium, some PABA, magnesium and potassium.

**CLEANSING PROPERTIES & DETOX ACTIVITY:** Boneset is closely related to gravel root and has similar cleansing constituents. As a hot tea, boneset is widely used and practically unequalled in its effectiveness as a reliable diaphoretic, providing slow, gentle perspiration to clear flu and cold infections. As a cold tea, it works as a soothing tonic on the stomach, liver, bowels and uterus, relaxing the muscular structures, and clearing areas of waste buildup and congestion. Liver detoxification helps clear the skin, bilious fevers, and other inflammation (like that associated with arthritis and rheumatism.)

**SAFETY PRECAUTIONS:** Overdose may result in flu-like symptoms.

**SYNERGY WITH OTHER HERBS:** To treat flu, combine with yarrow, elder flowers, cayenne or ginger. Use with ginger and anise for coughs for children. Use as a fomentation with hops for tumors.

## Borage (*Borage officinalis*)

**FAMILY:** Boraginceae

**MEDICINAL PARTS:** the whole plant and the oil

**DOSAGE:** extract: 2 – 10 ml three times a day; powder: 12 to 20 grains; tea: 2 teaspoons dry herb steeped 10 – 15 minutes, three times daily; oil: 500mg daily.

**NUTRITION PROFILE:** the most potent natural, currently known source of GLA (22% gamma-linolenic acid) which shows promise in the treatment of alcholism and diabetes, Contains vitamin C, and large amount of salts of potassium and calcium salts. The fresh juice has almost 30 percent potassium. The stems and leaves supply rich saline mucilage, responsible for the invigorating properties of borage.

**CLEANSING PROPERTIES & DETOX ACTIVITY:** Borage purifies the blood by promoting kidney activity. It is anti-inflammatory against pleurisy and pneumonia. It may be used as a tonic for exhausted adrenals as a restorative agent for the adrenal cortex, especially after cortisone or steroid drugs. It is a remedy for jaundice and ringworm. Borage is used for heart and lung congestion. Its demulcent properties make it effective against ulcers, both internal and external. The leaf tea can be a poultice for external inflammations.

**SAFETY PRECAUTIONS:** Pyrrolizide alkaloids are present in very small amounts. Though used by traditional people around the world for thousands of years, borage is not the type of nutritive tonic herb to take regularly over a period of months. It is more of an occasional acute remedy for fevers and might be considered safe to use as a sole agent for no more than three to seven days maximum.

**SYNERGY WITH OTHER HERBS:** With marshmallow or mullein as an expectorant.

## Buchu (Barosma betulina)

**FAMILY:** Rutaceae

**MEDICINAL PARTS:** leaves

**DOSAGE:** 2 cups tea daily; 20 drops three times a day; three 200mg capsules three times a day.

**NUTRITION PROFILE:** The essential oil has antiseptic properties and is highly bacteriocidal.

**CLEANSING PROPERTIES & DETOX ACTIVITY:** Buchu is effective for chronic cystitis, irritation of the urethra, first stage diabetes, urine retention, nephritis and cystitis. It is highly regarded for cleansing the kidney and urinary tract, increasing the quantity of urinic fluids and solids, acting at the same time as a tonic, astringent and disinfectant. Its volatile oil is excreted virtually unchanged by the kidneys, rendering the urine itself antiseptic.

**SAFETY PRECAUTIONS:** too strong a diuretic to use during pregnancy. Don't use during acute inflammatory conditions or serious kidney infections. Large doses produce mouth burning, nausea, severe diarrhea, heart palpitations and sweating. Breaks of several days are advisable every two weeks.

**SYNERGY WITH OTHER HERBS:** With uva ursi for water retention. For urinary tract infections: with juniper berry and gentle, antiseptic and anti-inflammatory herbs, like cornsilk or marshmallow. With yarrow, uva ursi or couchgrass for cystitis.

## Buckthorn (Rhamnus cathartica)

**FAMILY:** Rhamnaceae

**MEDICINAL PARTS:** the branch and young tree bark

**DOSAGE:** Fluid extract: 15 drops per dose; decoction in teaspoon doses; syrup: 1 – 2 tablespoons daily for a purgative effect.

**NUTRITION PROFILE:** contains anthraquinones and bitters for better digestion and elimination.

**CLEANSING PROPERTIES & DETOX ACTIVITY:** A gentle laxative for chronic constipation—does not cause cramping, is not habit forming, relieves hemorrhoids. Buckthorn is a blood cleansing tonic remedy for gallstones, hardening of the liver and spleen, lead poisoning, clearing toxic blood, gout and rheumatism. Taken hot, diaphoretic properties cause perspiration and help lower fevers.

**SAFETY PRECAUTIONS:** Bark must cure for at least one year prior to use or it acts as an irritant on the gastrointestinal tract, causing griping pains and nausea. Contraindicated for pregnancy.

**SYNERGY WITH OTHER HERBS:** For persistent constipation, combine with senna, peppermint and caraway seed, or with chamomile and fennel as a tea.

## Bugleweed (Lycopus virginicus)

**FAMILY:** Labiatae

**MEDICINAL PARTS:** the whole fresh flowering herb

**DOSAGE:** infusion: three times a day; tincture: take 1 – 2 ml three times a day.

**NUTRITION PROFILE:** flavone glycosides, volatile oil, tannins

**CLEANSING PROPERTIES & DETOX ACTIVITY:** Treats Graves' disease (an overactive thyroid condition with tightness of breathing and nervous heart palpitations), where a thyroid-stimulating antibody is found in the blood. The antibody binds to and is inhibited by bugleweed extract. Very useful for relieving widespread pain regardless of location. It is a mild gastric tonic and a remedy for painful indigestion. As a sedative cough reliever, it eases irritating coughs. Bugleweed's cardiotonic properties aid a weak heart, especially where there is build-up of fluid retention.

**SAFETY PRECAUTIONS:** Use with caution during pregnancy.

**SYNERGY WITH OTHER HERBS:** With dong quai, honeysuckle and licorice root for abscess swelling and pain. With nervines like skullcap or valerian as a natural sedative. With motherwort for the high thyroid condition Grave's disease. With kelp, bladderwrack, vitamin C, astragalus, Irish moss, licorice rt., parsley and prickly ash it helps neutralize and release hazardous chemicals from the blood.

## Bupleurum (Bupleurum falcatum) (Chai hu)

**FAMILY:** Umbelliferae

**MEDICINAL PARTS:** root

**DOSAGE:** 3 – 10 grams daily.

**NUTRITION PROFILE:** Sakiosaponins found in bupleurum are capable of inhibiting measles, herpes simplex virus. Rich in flavonoids.

**CLEANSING PROPERTIES & DETOX ACTIVITY:** An ideal herb in a detoxification program, bupleurum is a prime liver detoxifier, toner and strengthener. Its antibiotic abilities inhibit micro-organisms like influenza and polio. A tonic immune-enhancer with the ability to stimulate T, B, and phagocyte immune cells. Stabilizes the central nervous system with an antispasmodic quality, especially effective for menstrual cramping. Clears and reduces blood cholesterol levels.

**SAFETY PRECAUTIONS:** May cause nausea or vomiting in large doses.

**SYNERGY WITH OTHER HERBS:** With bee pollen, white pine bk., elecampane, scullcap, royal jelly, ephedra, acerola cherry, and ginger rt. to maintain harmony during high risk seasons. Used with ginseng and gotu kola to promote strong nerves, energy and raise vitality.

## Burdock (Arctium lappa)

**FAMILY:** Compositae

**MEDICINAL PARTS:** root, herb and seeds

**DOSAGE:** tea: 1 cup 3x daily; tincture: 30 to 60 drops 3x daily; extract: ½ to 1 tsp. 4x daily; capsules: 6 – 10 daily.

**NUTRITION PROFILE:** abundant in iron and insulin for the blood. High in chromium, magnesium, manganese, silicon and thiamine. Also high in dietary fiber, phosphorus, potassium, vitamin A and zinc.

**CLEANSING PROPERTIES & DETOX ACTIVITY:** Burdock is one of the herb world's best blood purifiers. It helps arthritis, rheumatism and sciatica inflammations, reducing swelling around joints and ridding the body of calcification deposits. It helps cleanse the blood of toxins during a weight loss regimen. Burdock is useful for arthritis, rheumatism, gout, asthma and sciatica. It has volatile oils which make it a good diaphoretic which clears the kidneys of excess wastes and uric acid by increasing the flow of urine. Aids the pituitary gland in releasing an ample supply of protein to help adjust hormone balance. Burdock alleviates ulcerated, glandular and white tumors.

Documented effects include treatment of venereal eruptions (particularly gonorrhea) and skin conditions, such as ringworm and eczema. Homeopaths prescribe the tincture of fresh root for acne, since most poor skin conditions result from blood toxicity. Herbal formulas for weight loss include burdock to help cleanse the body of toxins. Burdock markedly enhances liver, gallbladder and bile functions. It helps cleanse the body of toxins and wastes that accumulate during illness.

**SAFETY PRECAUTIONS:** none in common use.

**SYNERGY WITH OTHER HERBS:** For detoxifying the liver from addictions: equal parts turmeric, barberry, gotu kola and burdock. With calendula, oregon grape, gumweed, cleavers, black haw for herpes. With sheep sorrel, slippery elm and turkey rhubarb in the cancer-fighting "Essiac" formula.

## Butternut (Juglans cinerea)

**FAMILY:** Juglandaceae

**MEDICINAL PARTS:** inner bark of young stems and roots, leaves and nut

**DOSAGE:** decoction: 1 – 2 teaspoons 3x daily; tincture: up to 5ml a day for skin ailments, liver health or slow digestion; infusion: 1 oz. bark in 1 cup of water.

**NUTRITION PROFILE:** contains juglandic acid, juglandin and juglone and tannins.

**CLEANSING PROPERTIES & DETOX ACTIVITY:** Used for constipation, sluggish digestion, as a liver cleanser and stimulant, and for skin diseases and fevers. Especially helps skin ailments resulting from incomplete cleansing of the body via the bowels. It has been used as a vermifuge and is recommended for syphilis and old ulcers. The expressed oil of the fruit removes tapeworms.

**SAFETY PRECAUTIONS:** As a purgative, it should not be used on fragile persons.

**SYNERGY WITH OTHER HERBS:** To combat infections, fevers and colds, some part of the treatment should be laxative to help the body rid itself of bacteria-laden wastes. With barberry, rhubarb, psyllium husk, fennel seed, licorice, ginger, Irish moss and capsicum for evacuation of the bowels.

## Capsicum (*Capsicum annuum, Capsicum frutescens*)

**FAMILY:** Solanaceae

**MEDICINAL PARTS:** fruit and seeds

**DOSAGE:** One to 2 capsules with meals or ¼ tsp. extract 3x daily. Apply powder externally to stop bleeding.

**NUTRITION PROFILE:** Capsaicin, a main constituent of capsicum is rich in carotenoid, iron and zinc. High in Vitamins A, B complex, and C; lower in calcium, potassium and magnesium, to allow the stimulant effects to work at maximum potential.

**CLEANSING PROPERTIES & DETOX ACTIVITY:** Capsicum is a catalyst in the blood purification process, stimulating the vital organs to greater activity, promoting cardiovascular activity, lowering blood pressure. Capsicum is popular today as an ointment for relief of arthritis pain, rheumatism, neuralgia, sprains and bruises, for skin ailments like shingles, even gangrene. It increases circulation, and is used as a stimulant for people with sluggish metabolisms. Recent studies point to capsicum's fat burning qualities with proven thermogenesis enhancement; it slows fat absorption from the small intestine. Stimulates circulation in the stomach and intestines to improve digestion. It acts directly as a diaphoretic, stimulating excretion of wastes in sweat. Also effective for fatigue, infections, tumors, and healing stomach ulcers.

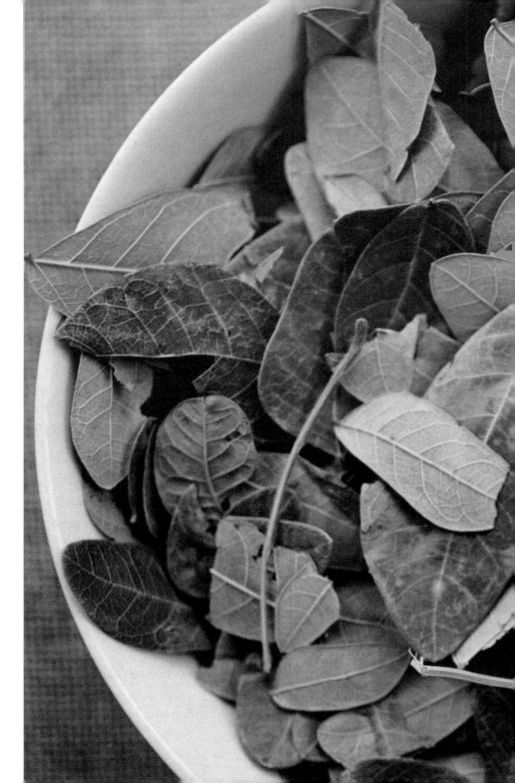

**SAFETY PRECAUTIONS:** Keep away from the eyes.

**SYNERGY WITH OTHER HERBS:** With herbs like ginger and garlic protects against colds and flu.

## Cascara Bark *(Rhamnus purshiana)*

**FAMILY:** Rhamnaceae

**MEDICINAL PARTS:** aged, dry bark. The bark must be aged for at least one year prior to use.

**DOSAGE:** dried powdered bark: 2 – 4 tsp. at bedtime; extract: 2 – 5 ml at bedtime.

**NUTRITION PROFILE:** high in calcium, cobalt, and vitamin A.

**CLEANSING PROPERTIES & DETOX ACTIVITY:** Cascara is a cleansing laxative for stagnant conditions and general toxicity, and non-habit forming for chronic constipation. A bitters tonic that stimulates digestive secretions for the liver, gallbladder, stomach and pancreas. It is a proven remedy for colitis, ridding the body of gallstones, indigestion, intestinal mucous congestion, gout, hemorrhoids, and liver disorders, especially an enlarged liver. A specific for chronic constipation and flatulence from gas. Useful for hemorrhoids because of poor, flaccid bowel structure or constipation. There is evidence of anti-tumor activity.

**SAFETY PRECAUTIONS:** Pregnant and nursing mothers should avoid— transfers in milk. Large doses of the bark may cause inflammation; habitual use can result in diarrhea.

**SYNERGY WITH OTHER HERBS:** With dandelion, licorice, celery seed, cayenne and wild yam for liver disorders. With butternut bark, rhubarb, ginger, licorice rt., Irish moss and cayenne as a laxative. With red clover, chaparral, licorice rt., Oregon grape, stillingia, burdock, sarsaparilla, prickly ash, buckthorn and kelp for detoxification and toning. With butternut, barberry, rhubarb, psyllium husk, fennel seed, licorice, ginger, Irish moss and capsicum for evacuation of the bowels by normal peristalsis.

## Chaparral *(Larrea tridentata)*

**FAMILY:** Zygophyllaceae

**MEDICINAL PARTS:** leaves and stems

**DOSAGE:** tea ½ oz. infused in a pint of water; tincture: 10 – 30 drops, 3 times daily.

**NUTRITION PROFILE:** Famous for its primary constituent NDGA, a significant antioxidant, antitumor and anticancer element. Its amino acid content is rich: arginine, tryptophane, phenylalanine, glycine, glutamic acid, aspartic acid, cystine and tyrosine. Also contains carotenes, vitamin C, potassium, calcium, magnesium, iron, chlorine, natural salts, and sulfur.

**CLEANSING PROPERTIES & DETOX ACTIVITY:** Chaparral's blood purifying, antioxidant value is legendary. Effective blood purifying uses include kidney infections, respiratory infections, allergies, auto-immune diseases and several types of cancers. It often works for difficult toxic blood conditions when other herbs are ineffective. Chaparral is a specific analgesic to relieve arthritis and rheumatic pain. It is a system toner to rebuild tissue strength. It is one of the best herbal antibiotics, effective internally and externally against bacteria, viruses and parasites. It is used for colds and flu, TB, diarrhea, urinary tract infections, venereal disease, leukemia, acne, eczema, some STD's and tetanus. It is effective externally as a poultice for sores and bruises. I have seen it used successfully in reduced dosage for dogs with certain cancers.

**SAFETY PRECAUTIONS:** Because of its potency and swift action, chaparral must be used with care and direction. NDGA in concentrated and overlong use can affect liver health leading to jaundice and possibly hepatitis. Longterm heavy dosages should be avoided to prevent possible formation of kidney lesions.

**SYNERGY WITH OTHER HERBS:** With echinacea, goldenseal, garlic and usnea to heighten its antibiotic, detox properties.

## Chlorella

**MEDICINAL PARTS:** Entire plant

**DOSAGE:** average nutritional level: 15 tablets per day; poor nutritional levels: 30 tablets per day; very poor nutritional level: 45 tablets per day. Children under 15 should take the number of tablets daily that corresponds to their age in years.

**NUTRITION PROFILE:** Chlorella is 60% protein, rich in minerals and contains 12% chlorophyll, the largest amount of any plant on Earth. The richest food source of vitamin B12, higher than liver or sea vegetables, with a protein yield greater than soy beans, corn or beef. Phytoplankton like chlorella are the most potent source of beta carotene in the world with all B vitamins, vitamin C and E, an abundance of the antioxidant superoxide dismutase (SOD), and many trace minerals high enough to be supplementary amounts. Phytoplankton are the only foods, other than mother's milk, with GLA, an essential fatty acid and precursor to the body's master hormones (GLA deficiency contributes to obesity, heart disease and PMS).

**CLEANSING PROPERTIES & DETOX ACTIVITY:** The cell wall material of chlorella has a particular effect on intestinal and bowel health, detoxifying the colon, stimulating peristaltic activity, and promoting the growth of beneficial bacteria. Chlorella is effective in eliminating heavy metals, such as lead, mercury, copper and cadmium. Antitumor research shows it is an important source of beta carotene in healing. It strengthens the liver, the body's major detoxifying organ, so that it can free the system of infective agents that destroy immune defenses. It reduces arthritis stiffness, lowers blood pressure, and relieves gastritis and ulcers. Its rich nutritional content has made it effective in weight loss programs, both for cleansing ability, and in maintaining muscle tone during lower food intake. Chlorella also enhances tissue growth and repair (beneficial to hypoglycemic and diabetic people), accelerates healing, protects against radiation, prevents degenerative diseases and promotes longer life. It improves the complexion and aids in skin disorders such as eczema, recurrent cold sores, warts, atopic dermatitis and acne.

But its most important benefits come from a unique molecular composition called Controlled Growth Factor, that provides a noticeable increase in stamina and immune health when eaten on a regular basis.

**SAFETY PRECAUTIONS:** none in common use.

**SYNERGY WITH OTHER HERBS:**

1. an herbal revitalizer: American ginseng and chlorella.

2. in a whole green drink with chlorophyllins, trace minerals and full spectrum amino acids: barley and alfalfa sprouts, bee pollen, acerola fruit, Siberian eleuthero, sarsaparilla rt., dandelion, quinoa and oat sprouts and chlorell.

## Cleavers (Galium aparine)

**FAMILY:** Rubiaceae

**MEDICINAL PARTS:** aerial portions

**DOSAGE:** 3 – 9 grams of tea infusion.

**NUTRITION PROFILE:** contains chlorophyll, saponins (to prevent red blood cell destruction), tannins (useful as astringents), citric acid, coumarins, trace minerals, glycosides and a mild laxative, asperuloside.

**CLEANSING PROPERTIES & DETOX ACTIVITY:** Cleavers is a blood cleansing diuretic with mild laxative activity. Used to dissolve kidney stones and sediment. It eliminates excess fluid, both as a diaphoretic and as a diuretic. It counteracts inflammations, urinary infections, hepatitis and venereal disease. It is an astringent herb for the treatment of psoriasis and various skin diseases. A lymphatic cleanser for swollen or enlarged lymph glands, including prostate disorders, glandular fever and tonsillitis. Also for ailments where toxic conditions and skin problems exist as well as urinary ailments like cystitis and stones.

**SAFETY PRECAUTIONS:** Care should be taken if diabetes exists.

**SYNERGY WITH OTHER HERBS:** With juniper berry, uva ursi, goldenseal and marshmallow as a diuretic and sediment dissolver. To prevent itching, scaling and skin discomfort, use with burdock rt., dandelion rt., echinacea purpurea rt., St. John's wort herb, yellow dock rt., nettle's herb, kelp and tumeric. To gently relieve and relax, use with parsley, cornsilk, uva ursi, dandelion, juniper berry, ginger, marshmallow rt. and kelp.

## Comfrey Root (Symphytum officinalis)

**FAMILY:** Boraginaceae

**MEDICINAL PARTS:** root and leaves

**DOSAGE:** 3 – 9 grams, 10 – 30 drops tincture, 1 tsp. extract 3x daily, 30 – 60 grains powder 3x daily, no more than two weeks at a time.

**NUTRITION PROFILE:** A main constituent, allantoin, works like calcium stimulating cell production for healing connective tissue, bone and collagen. High in sodium, calcium, cobalt, iron, manganese, potassium and vitamins A and B2. One of the few plants that can produce vitamin B12 from the cobalt in the soil.

**CLEANSING PROPERTIES & DETOX ACTIVITY:** Comfrey leaves and root cleanse the upper respiratory system—effective for asthma, bronchitis, colds, tuberculosis and pleurisy. Helps stop lung hemorrhage accompanying severe inflammation of coughing. The richest source of mucilage, soothing and stimulating mucous membranes, it is also an expectorant, removing toxic material from the lungs. Comfrey is a blood cleansing tonic that treats cystitis, colitis, bladder and prostate infections. It works both internally and externally to promote healing of sores, bones, muscles and tissues. It works well for anemia, arthritis and rheumatism, and for boils, bruises, burns, diarrhea, eczema and other skin infections.

**SAFETY PRECAUTIONS:** Although used for thousands of years safely and effectively, recent investigation shows comfrey contains hepatotoxic pyrrolizidine alkaloids (PA's), such as echimidine. Whether this is from environmental toxins or is naturally present in the plant, but neutralized by other plant substances, has not been determined. Until a safe source can be guaranteed, comfrey should not be used during pregnancy and nursing or for children. I recommend using an organically grown source for a short limited time, or using comfrey externally until more information on these alkaloids is known. Not for use when on dietary potassium restrictions.

**SYNERGY WITH OTHER HERBS:** With goldenseal, slippery elm and aloe vera as a laxative to detoxify and heal inflamed tissues in the digestive system. With peppermint, marshmallow, slippery elm, pau d'arco, ginger, aloe vera, wild yam and lobelia as a gentle bowel cleanser when there is irritable bowel disease.

## Cornsilk (Zea mays)

**FAMILY:** Gramineae

**MEDICINAL PARTS:** silk hair surrounding ears of corn.

**DOSAGE:** tincture: 5 to 20 drops 3x daily; extract: ½ tsp. 3x daily; infusion: ½ cup as needed; powder: 1 to 5 caps 3x daily.

**NUTRITION PROFILE:** Very high in silicon, high in iron, significant in zinc, magnesium, Vitamin B1, chromium, cobalt, phosphorus and potassium.

**CLEANSING PROPERTIES & DETOX ACTIVITY:** Cornsilk is effective for cleansing when there is inflammation of the urethra, bladder, prostate or kidneys. Helps conditions such as cystitis, urinary stones and painful urination, prostatitis, edema from hypertension, and inflamed kidneys. Helps lower high blood pressure and high cholesterol, and clear arteriosclerosis.

**SAFETY PRECAUTIONS:** None in common use.

**SYNERGY WITH OTHER HERBS:** To relieve fluid retention, with uva ursi, juniper bry., parsley, dandelion lf., plantain, marshmallow rt., ginger and cleavers. Or with juniper bry., uva ursi, dandelion, marshmallow rt., goldenseal rt., ginger, parsley and honey.

## Cranberry (Vaccinium macrocarpon)

**FAMILY:** Ericaceae

**MEDICINAL PARTS:** berries

**PREPARATION FORMS:** juice, powder and douche.

**DOSAGE:** 16 oz. per day of juice.

**NUTRITION PROFILE:** high in phosphorus, potassium, and calcium; contains significant amounts of iron, magnesium, manganese, sodium and B-complex vitamins.

**HERBAL HEALING ACTIONS:** Antibacterial compounds in cranberries inhibit urinary infecting bacteria from adhering to tract walls so that they are flushed from the system. It is a good source of bioflavonoids and vitamin C for tissue tone. Has anti-cancer, blood purifying and immuno-stimulant effects.

**CLEANSING PROPERTIES & DETOX ACTIVITY:** A specific for cystitis and other urinary tract infections because it helps neutralize acids and dissolve sediment. New research shows excellent results in clearing kidney stones. Now used successfully in the prevention of asthma attacks, dilating bronchial passages during an attack. A good antidote for reducing ammonia urinary odors in the elderly. A natural benzoyl peroxide which is a preventative of acne. It prevents the acne-causing bacteria from penetrating the skin so breakouts are less frequent and less severe.

**SAFETY PRECAUTIONS:** none in common use

**SYNERGY WITH OTHER HERBS:** In a balancing, cleansing combination rich in bioflavonoids with pau d'arco, cranberry, rose hips, burdock, damiana, echinacea rt., myrrh, lemon balm, cinnamon, hibiscus.

## Dandelion (Taraxacum officinalis)

**FAMILY:** Compositae

**MEDICINAL PARTS:** The root, roasted or raw, and the leaves

**DOSAGE:** tincture: 10 – 15 drops 3x daily; capsules: 1 – 2 capsules with each meal; tea: 1 cup in the morning and the evening for 4 – 6 weeks.

**NUTRITION PROFILE:** Dandelion is very high in Vitamin A, with balanced mineral content.

**CLEANSING PROPERTIES & DETOX ACTIVITY:** Because of its high potassium level, dandelion is an excellent diuretic choice over pharmaceutical diuretics. It can even maintain potassium in the body often leached by over-ambitious pharmaceutical formulas. It is a blood purifying herb that soothes the digestive tract while absorbing toxins, inhibiting unfriendly bacteria, and allowing friendly fauna to thrive. It scours the liver and kidneys, softens deposits, encourages urination and removes intestinal congestion. As a bitters tonic, dandelion helps the liver and gall bladder produce bile for better assimilation.

Dandelion is beneficial for a wide variety of ailments including arthritis, rheumatism, gout, skin eruptions, eczema, herpes, acne, abscesses, ulcers, bladder irritation, kidney infections and stones, jaundice, hepatitis, anemia, edema, high blood pressure, tumors, constipation, and heartburn.

**SAFETY PRECAUTIONS:** Large amounts may cause heartburn.

**SYNERGY WITH OTHER HERBS:** Use with red clover, licorice rt., chaparral, burdock, pau d'arco, echinacea rt., ascorbate vitamin C, goldenseal rt., garlic, kelp, alfalfa, poria mushroom, American ginseng, sarsaparilla, astragalus, yellow dock, butternut, milk thistle seed, ginger, prickly ash

and buckthorn bk. for a strong detoxification formula. With watercress, yellow dock, pau d'arco, hyssop, parsley, Oregon grape rt., red sage, licorice rt., milk thistle seed and hibiscus for a liver flush. Use with bancha lf., kukicha and chicory as a cleansing coffee substitute.

## Echinacea (Echinacea angustifolia and purpurea)

**FAMILY:** Compositae

**MEDICINAL PARTS:** root and whole plant

**DOSAGE:** 10 – 50 drops of extract or tincture; 2 to 3 capsules every two hours for acute conditions—three times a day for chronic conditions.

**NUTRITION PROFILE:** high in cobalt, silicon and zinc, chromium, iron, manganese, selenium and in vitamins C, B-3 and riboflavin.

**CLEANSING PROPERTIES & DETOX ACTIVITY:** Echinacea is indicated whenever reinforcement for resistance is needed and to stimulate body defense mechanisms—for the onset of colds, flus and other respiratory infections, or for any acute inflammatory condition, like mumps, measles, scarlet fever, rheumatic fevers, urinary infections, venereal infections, food borne infections, bites, stings, Also used for skin conditions: acne, eczema, psoriasis; for congested lymph gland diseases, like chicken pox, ulcers, goiter, strep throat, even cancer and tumors.

**SAFETY PRECAUTIONS:** none known in common use

**SYNERGY WITH OTHER HERBS:** With ginsengs, goldenseal and other tonifying herbs for rebuilding and restoring health. With red clover, licorice root, chaparral, burdock root for blood purifying.

## Eleuthero, Siberian (Siberian Ginseng, Wujiashen) (Eleutherococcus senticosus)

**MEDICINAL PARTS:** root

**DOSAGE:** Take 2 capsules dried herb 2 – 3 times daily; or take 1 dropperful of tincture two to three times daily.

**NUTRITION PROFILE:** Assists carbohydrate metabolism to normalize blood sugar levels in diabetics. Effective in lowering blood pressure and cholesterol. A highly complex herb—contains ginsenoids, polysaccharides, triterpenoids, saponins, lignans, sterols, B complex vitamins, vitamins A, D and E, selenium, amino acids, minerals and enzymes. Its glycosides provide antioxidant influence and overall resistance to chemical factors. Its generous amount of germanium preserves oxygen and stimulates immunity.

**CLEANSING PROPERTIES & DETOX ACTIVITY:** Siberian eleuthero exhibits many of the rejuvenative, adaptogen properties of panax ginseng in terms of energy and endurance and raising sexual potency. It is an all-body tonic and an energizer which combats depression and fatigue, and helps the body rebuild system strength after mental or physical exhaustion. It should be a prime part of any immune rebuilding herbal combination to increase body resistance to disease, especially heart disease. In fact, Siberian eleuthero promotes an enormous increase in the number of immune cells (particularly natural killer cells) to support the immune system against infections of all types. It is an excellent nutritive tonic for both the adrenal and circulatory systems, helping the body withstand heat, cold, infection and radiation.

**SAFETY PRECAUTIONS:** Not recommended for persons with hypertension. Avoid caffeine while using. Some people may experience insomnia when consuming large doses.

**SYNERGY WITH OTHER HERBS:** With kava kava, kirin ginseng, American ginseng, prince ginseng, dong quai, fo-ti rt., suma, kola nut and gotu kola for mental inner energy. With American ginseng, Chinese kirin ginseng, prince ginseng, fo-ti rt., suma, gotu kola, wild oat tops and sarsaparilla for active physical energy.

## Fennel Seed (Foeniculum vulgare)

**FAMILY:** Umbelliferae

**MEDICINAL PARTS:** seeds

**DOSAGE:** Infusion: 6 oz. 3x daily; fluid extract: 5 to 60 drops 3x daily.

**NUTRITION PROFILE:** Fennel seeds are high in calcium, magnesium, phosphorus, selenium, sodium and vitamin B1, and contain significant amounts of iron, manganese, potassium, zinc, and vitamins B2 and B3.

**CLEANSING PROPERTIES & DETOX ACTIVITY:** In a cleansing compound, fennel is helpful for indigestion, abdominal cramping, urinary incontinence and bladder irritation, urinary stones, nausea and PMS. As an expectorant, it relieves coughs, hoarsness, loss of voice, bronchial asthma. For nausea and vomiting; for inflammation of the eyes and floaters in the vision; and externally for healing snake bites.

**SAFETY PRECAUTIONS:** Because they have a stimulating effect on the uterus, fennel seeds are contraindicated during pregnancy. Fennel oil may cause pulmonary edema, respiratory problems and seizures.

**SYNERGY WITH OTHER HERBS:** With rhubarb root for digestive disorders. To calm and soothe coughs: with wild cherry bk., slippery elm bk. and licorice rt. For digestion in kids: with peppermint, chamomile, papaya, ginger and orange peel.

## Fenugreek (Foenum graceum)

**FAMILY:** Leguminosae

**MEDICINAL PARTS:** seeds

**DOSAGE:** tincture: 1 – 2ml 3x daily; powder: 1 – 2 tsp. daily or 1 – 2 capsules with meals.

**NUTRITION PROFILE:** The seed is 30% galactomannan-like mucilage with lecithin, making an excellent choice for a poultice; 20% protein and high in fiber, making the seed a good choice for a cleansing fiber.

**CLEANSING PROPERTIES & DETOX ACTIVITY:** Fenugreek helps reduce total and LDL (bad) cholesterol without altering levels of HDL (good) cholesterol, makings it helpful in preventing atherosclerosis. It reduces blood glucose, plasma glucagon, and somatostatin levels including sugar-induced hyperglycemia allowing less insulin doses in diabetics. Fenugreek can reduce the amount of calcium oxalate deposited in the kidneys. It helps relieve excess mucous and respiratory congestion and lower blood pressure.

**SAFETY PRECAUTIONS:** Large doses may result in hypoglycemia.

**SYNERGY WITH OTHER HERBS:** To help breakdown toxic buildup, use with gotu kola, garlic, red sage, black cohosh, lecithin, goldenseal rt., quassia wood, bilberry, poria mushroom, fennel sd., milk thistle sd., tumeric, kola nut and kelp. For a cleansing combination, use with flax sd., gotu kola, fennel sd., parsley, uva ursi, senna, bancha, burdock rt., gymnema sylvestre, red clover, lemon peel, hisbiscus and bladderwrack. With cranberry juice ext., echinacea ang. rt., coriander, wild yam rt., dandelion, marshmallow, juniper bry., uva ursi and kava kava for a tissue toning formula. For respiratory ailments, use with marshmallow, mullein, ma huang, rosemary, ginkgo biloba, passionflowers, wild cherry bk., angelica, lobelia, cinnamon.

## Fo-Ti-Tieng Root (Polygonum multiflorum) (See Ho-Shou-Wu)

## Garlic (Allium sativum)

**FAMILY:** Liliaceae

**MEDICINAL PARTS:** bulb

**DOSAGE:** One clove 3x daily; Garlic oil capsules: 3 a day or 3 capsules 3x daily when infection occurs.

**NUTRITION PROFILE:** Loaded in fiber, garlic is high in calcium, iron, magnesium, phosphorus, potassium, vitamin A and C, and B-complex vitamins. It contains 33 sulphur compounds. Garlic's primary benefit comes from its rich antioxidant compounds (at least 15 different), including germanium, chromium, selenium, zinc, vitamins A and C and 17 amino acids.

**CLEANSING PROPERTIES & DETOX ACTIVITY:** Garlic's list of cleansing and detox benefits is wide ranging. It is a blood purifying tonic that helps restore good body chemistry against pollutants and allergens. Garlic is a part of almost every kind of detoxification compound, especially those involving digestive waste elimination. It is a specific for removing candida albicans yeast overgrowth. It is effective for almost every type of respiratory congestion problem, from colds, coughs and flu to chronic bronchitis and asthma. Recent tests show that garlic has anti-cancer (especially stomach cancer) and antitumor effects. Garlic is good as an enema for detoxification and to expel worms as a liver stimulant for bile production and as part of a compound to re-establish friendly, beneficial flora in the digestive tract. It is effective as part of a compound for arthritis and rheumatism.

**SAFETY PRECAUTIONS:** stomach irritating if taken raw; not for use in

medicinal doses during pregnancy.

**SYNERGY WITH OTHER HERBS:** With echinacea angustifolia, siberian ginseng, rosehips, goldenseal rt., hawthorn, guggul, pau d' arco, astragalus, elecampane, peppermint for herbal defense in high risk seasons.

## Ginger Root (Zingiber officinalis)

**FAMILY:** Zingiberraceae

**MEDICINAL PARTS:** root

**DOSAGE:** tea: 2 oz. 3x daily; tincture: 15 to 30 drops 3x daily; extract: 5 – 20 drops 3x daily; caps: 2 to 4 3x daily.

**NUTRITION PROFILE:** Ginger is very high in aluminum, manganese and silicon; contains high amounts of magnesium and potassium, and vitamins C, B2 and B3. Contains a wealth of amino acids.

**CLEANSING PROPERTIES & DETOX ACTIVITY:** Use ginger for colds and flu, fever, bacterial and viral infections, bronchitis, tonsilitis, laryngitis, stomach upset, ulcers, flatulence and bloating, motion and morning sickness, food poisoning, and PMS congestion. Promotes toxin cleansing through the skin by opening pores and stimulating perspiration. Helps cleanse the bowels and kidneys, and stimulates digestion. It is effective for nausea, gas, heartburn, flatulence, diarrhea and dizziness.

**SYNERGY WITH OTHER HERBS:** With capsicum, wormwood and gentian for indigestion and heartburn. With mullein, pleurisy rt, marshmallow, rose hips, ephedra, licorice, calendula, boneset, peppermint and fennel seed to clear mucous congestion.

## Ginkgo Biloba (Bai guo) (Ginkgo biloba)

**FAMILY:** Coniferales

**MEDICINAL PARTS:** leaves

**DOSAGE:** 1 tablet 3x daily.

**NUTRITION PROFILE:** The leaves contain flavone glycosides, bioflavones, sitosterol and anthocyanin.

**CLEANSING PROPERTIES & DETOX ACTIVITY:** Stimulates circulation and supplies oxygen to the brain, specifically to brain-damaged areas.

Ginkgo protects and nourishes brain cells, enhances mental alertness and defends against disorders that cause senility or Alzheimer's. It increases circulation in people with hardening of the arteries, helping to return elasticity to cholesterol-hardened blood vessels. Provides specific cardiac protection against stroke and atherosclerosis. Because Ginkgo inhibits PAF (platelet activating factor), it can prevent blood clotting in congestive heart disease, asthma, skin problems and hearing problems. Ginkgo boosts acetylcholine levels—thus the ability to better transmit body electrical impulses.

**SAFETY PRECAUTIONS:** In extremely large, high doses, ginkgo may cause irritability, restlessness and diarrhea. The fruit pulp and raw seed are toxic. Direct contact with the pulp may cause contact dermatitis. Swallowing the seeds may cause stomach ache, nausea, diarrhea, convulsions, difficulty in breathing and shock. Not recommended for pregnant or lactating women. Do not use ginkgo if taking anticoagulants.

**SYNERGY WITH OTHER HERBS:** It is a specific in anti-aging and regenerative compounds. For relief of respiratory and circulatory conditions, use with mullein, wild cherry bk., pleurisy rt., plantain. and horehound. For asthma, use with marshmallow rt., fenugreek sd., mullein, ma huang and rosemary. For mental clarity, use with gotu kola and panax ginseng.

## Ginseng (Ren-shen) *(Panax ginseng)*
## American Ginseng *(Panax quinquefolium)*

**FAMILY:** Araliaceae

**MEDICINAL PARTS:** root, dried or fresh

**DOSAGE:** about 500 mg daily or ½ tsp. powdered root 3x a day. Ginseng benefits are cumulative in the body. Taking ginseng as a tonic for several months to a year is more effective than short term doses.

**NUTRITION PROFILE:** Ginseng has measurable amounts of germanium for tissue healing. Ginseng's saponins retard plaque formation on the aorta to help prevent stroke. Ginseng's polysaccharides protect against alcohol induced ulcers and increase the protective cells in the gastrointestinal lining.

**CLEANSING PROPERTIES & DETOX ACTIVITY:** Ginseng is a strong tonic

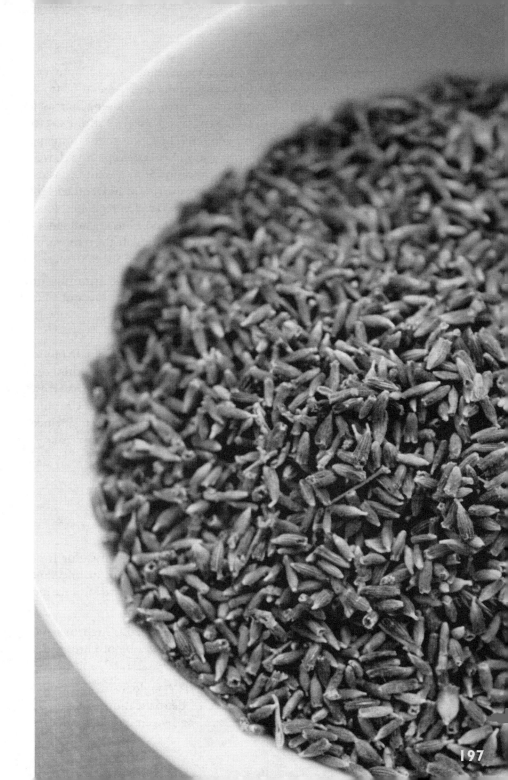

for boosting energy and rejuvenation during detoxing. As an adaptogen, ginseng provides energy to all body systems, promotes regeneration from stress and fatigue, and rebuilds foundation strength. Ginseng increases the body's ability to fight disease. Ginseng is an effective stimulant to the central nervous system, but in a gentler, calmer way than stimulant drugs like caffeine and nicotine, so it also improves sleep and relieves pain. Ginseng can improve memory, concentration, alertness, visual motor control and reaction time. It reduces the risk of heart attacks by thinning the blood, suppresses arrythmias, and helps regulate blood pressure by regulating cholesterol levels in the blood. Ginseng influences carbohydrate metabolism and has the ability to stimulate the removal of sugar from the blood, preventing hypoglycemic blood sugar swings.

**SAFETY PRECAUTIONS:** In large amounts, may cause insomnia or high blood pressure. Avoid while consuming caffeine. Do not take during pregnancy or during acute diseases, high fever or severe inflammation.

**SYNERGY WITH OTHER HERBS:** Use with licorice rt. to regulate blood sugar swings. Use with prince ginseng, kirin ginseng, suma, echinacea angustifolia and purpurea rt., pau d' arco, astragalus, St, John's wort, ashwagandha and aralia to energize and restore body defenses. Use with bee pollen, Siberian ginseng rt., gotu kola, fo ti rt., kirin ginseng, prince ginseng., suma, aralia rt., alfalfa, dong quai to revitalize the system.

## Goldenseal (Hydrastis canadensis)

**FAMILY:** Ranunculacaea

**MEDICINAL PARTS:** root

**DOSAGE:** capsules: 2 to 4 caps 3x daily; tincture: small doses for liver restoration; medium doses for astringent, decongestant, disinfectant and anti-inflammatory actions; large doses for laxative and stimulating actions.

**NUTRITION PROFILE:** Very high in cobalt and silicon; high in iron, magnesium, zinc and vitamin C; significant amounts of chromium, phosphorus, potassium, selenium, and vitamins A, B1, B2, and B3.

**CLEANSING PROPERTIES & DETOX ACTIVITY:** Goldenseal is a broad spectrum medicinal with a wide range of detoxification benefits. Its properties include effective blood cleansing by removing circulatory congestion to restore veins and enliven the blood. It stimulates blood supply to the spleen, increasing spleen activity to release immune potentiators. It is a bitter tonic with laxative, bowel regulating effects against constipation, diarrhea and hemorrhoids. It helps resolve infectious tumors of the breast, uterus, stomach and skin. It is effective in cleansing and healing formulas for cystitis, gonorrhea, candida albicans, eye inflammations, head and sinus congestion, bronchitis, gallstones, gastric ulcers and chronic gastritis, fevers, flu and tonsillitis.

**SAFETY PRECAUTIONS:** Not for use during pregnancy—a uterine stimulant; not for use with high blood pressure. Extended use can weaken good intestinal flora.

**SYNERGY WITH OTHER HERBS:** With echinacea, garlic and antibiotic herbs for immune stimulation. With chaste-tree berry for PMS. With licorice rt., chaparral, burdock, pau d' arco, echinacea, ascorbate vit. C, goldenseal rt., garlic, kelp, alfalfa, dandelion, poria mushroom, American ginseng, sarsaparilla, astragalus, yellow dock, butternut, milk thistle seed, ginger, prickly ash and buckthorn bark in a detox formula.

## Gravel Root (Eupatorium purpureum)

**FAMILY:** Compositae

**MEDICINAL PARTS:** root

**DOSAGE:** tincture: ½ to 1 tsp. 3x daily; or 10 – 30 drops 3x daily; infusion: 1 oz. root to 1pt. water.

**NUTRITION PROFILE:** A flavonoid-rich, high tannin herb with strong bitters principles for digestion.

**CLEANSING PROPERTIES & DETOX ACTIVITY:** Gravel root is a diuretic for the urinary and reproductive systems that also reduces inflammation and fever, with disinfecting action. It clears excess uric acid, and strengthens the tissues against urinary incontinence. Especially effective for urinary infections, stones and irritation, excess uric acid, urinary incontinence, edema, gout, rheumatism and arthritis.

**SAFETY PRECAUTIONS:** none in common use

**SYNERGY WITH OTHER HERBS:** To aid in elimination of sediment, use with dandelion rt., parsley rt., hydrangea rt., wild yam rt., marshamallow rt., licorice rt., lecithin, lemon balm herb, ginger rt., and milk thistle sd. Use with devil's claw rt., red clover blsm., Oregon grape rt., ginkgo biloba, licorice rt., horsetail, slippery elm, elm bk., prickly ash bk., ginger rt., flax sd. for a soothing and relaxing formula.

## Green Tea (*Thea sinensis*)

**MEDICINAL PARTS:** leaves (unfermented), leaf buds.

**DOSAGE:** 1 cup green tea daily or 1 capsule (5 – 15 mg) daily.

**NUTRITION PROFILE:** rich in flavonoids with antioxidant and anti-allergen activity; contains potent polyphenols like catechins, that act as antioxidants, yet do not interfere with iron or protein absorption.

**CLEANSING PROPERTIES & DETOX ACTIVITY:** Traditionally a good fasting tea, providing energy support and clearer thinking during cleansing. Combats free radical damage to protect against degenerative disease. Boosts enzyme production in the body. Green tea is fully enzyme-active for weight loss and cleansing. Green tea is a vasodilator and smooth muscle relaxant in cases of bronchial asthma. Highly valued as a cancer preventive. Recent research in Japan shows that several cups of green tea on a regular daily basis are effective in reducing lung cancer death rates, even in men who smoked two packs of cigarettes a day. Other studies in Tokyo indicate the same success with stomach and liver cancers. It shows definite evidence of tumor and skin cancer prevention in animals, even when exposed to ultraviolet radiation.

Green tea is equally valuable as a heart protector, especially against atherosclerosis. Prevents LDL cholesterol development and PAF (platelet aggregation factor), blood stickiness. Green tea has antibiotic qualities, amazingly even combatting antibiotic-resistant microorganisms. It can lower iron levels in the body, having a direct anti-viral effect on abnormal types of hepatitis viruses.

**SAFETY PRECAUTIONS:** none in common use.

**SYNERGY WITH OTHER HERBS:** With burdock rt., gotu kola herb, kukicha twig, fo ti rt., hawthorn bry., cinnamon bk., and hisbiscus flowers for a cleansing, energizing antioxidant tea.

## Hawthorn (*Cratageus oxyacantha*)

**FAMILY:** Rosaceae

**MEDICINAL PARTS:** berries, flowers and leaves

**DOSAGE:** Cumulative effects over a lengthy period for best effects. Tincture: 15 – 30 drops 3x daily; extract: 10 – 15 drops 3x daily; infusion: 1 cup 3x daily.

**NUTRITION PROFILE:** high in chromium and selenium and contains significant amounts of calcium, cobalt, magnesium, phosphorus, potassium, sodium and vitamins A and C with bioflavonoids.

**CLEANSING PROPERTIES & DETOX ACTIVITY:** Hawthorn is a specific for a wide range of circulatory conditions: congestive heart failure, angina, arrhythmias, arteriosclerosis, high blood pressure, difficult breathing, hypertension and insomnia from cardio-pulmonary problems. It relieves edema and fluid congestion, and promotes hormone balance. It acts quickly as well as longterm, to offer a feeling of well-being.

**SAFETY PRECAUTIONS:** None in common use

**SYNERGY WITH OTHER HERBS:** Use with red clover, pau d'arco, nettles, sage, alfalfa, horsetail herb, milk thistle seed, gotu kola, echinacea, blue malva, yerba santa and lemon grass for a blood cleansing and purifying tea. Use with spirulina, bee pollen, rose hips, barley grass, Siberian ginseng, alfalfa, sarsaparilla, raspberry, kelp, parsley, carrots, golden seal, mullein to rebuild the body.

## Ho-Shou-Wu, Fo-Ti-Tieng Root (*Polygonium multiflorum*)

**FAMILY:** Polygonaceae

**MEDICINAL PART:** root.

**DOSAGE:** capsules: 2 capsules with meals 2x daily.

**NUTRITION PROFILE:** A source of beta-carotene, calcium, carbohydrates, chromium, fiber, iron, lecithin, potassium, selenium, vitamin C, thiamin and zinc. Also contains leucoanthrocyanidins (LAC), a bioflavnoid-like compound, which have anti-inflammatory, cardiotonic, hypotensive and vasodilating action. Currently being studied for one of its compounds, LAC, effective in reducing inflammatory conditions such as ulcers and arthritis.

**CLEANSING PROPERTIES & DETOX ACTIVITY:** Ho-shou-wu rejuvenates, restores energy, increases fertility. For the elderly, it helps maintain strength and vigor. Strengthens and tonifies the liver, kidneys and blood. A good choice for diabetes because of blood glucose lowering activity. Lowers blood cholesterol levels and inhibits atherosclerosis by decreasing blood coagulation. Reduces hypertension and coronary disease. It moistens the intestines and unblocks bowel movements.

**SAFETY PRECAUTIONS:** Use caution in cases of spleen deficiency, phlegm and diarrhea. Do not use while taking or using onion, chives or garlic.

**SYNERGY WITH OTHER HERBS:** Use with bancha lf., burdock, gotu kola, kukicha twig, hawthorn bry., cinnamon, orange peel for a cleansing, energizing tea with antioxidants. For calm energy, use with St. John's wort, kava kava, American ginseng rt., ashwagandha, gotu kola, scullcap, Siberian eleuthero rt., rosemary, wood betony and ginger. To boost vigor, use with American ginseng rt., Chinese ginseng rt., Siberian eleuthero, suma, gotu kola, prince ginseng rt., dong quai, sarsaparilla and ginkgo biloba.

## Horseradish (Cochlearia armoracia or Armoracia rusticana)

**FAMILY:** Cruciferae

**MEDICINAL PARTS:** root

**DOSAGE:** grated root: 2 – 4 grams; tincture: 1 to 1 ½ teaspoons or 6 – 12 drops.

**NUTRITION PROFILE:** high in potassium and vitamin C, with significant amounts of calcium, iron, phosphorus, potassium, sulphur, protease, selenium and vitamin B.

**CLEANSING PROPERTIES & DETOX ACTIVITY:** A cold and flu herb that warms the body, relieves sinus ache, and releases excess mucous. Particularly good for asthma. An herb to relieve urinary infections and stones. Helps rheumatism, gout, colitis, asthma, chronic bronchitis, sore throat and coughing, intestinal parasites, skin ulcers and acne.

**SAFETY PRECAUTIONS:** Very strong. Don't use if there is acute inflammation, during pregnancy or thyroid imbalance. Overdose can irritate the kidneys or gastric mucosa. Discontinue if diarrhea or nightsweats occur.

**SYNERGY WITH OTHER HERBS:** Use with honey and apple cider vinegar for rheumatism. Use with mustard seed for water retention. Use with water and honey for a sore throat gargle.

## Horsetail (Equisetum arvense)

**FAMILY:** Equisetaceae

**MEDICINAL PARTS:** above ground portions

**DOSAGE:** Extract: 30 drops 3x daily.

**NUTRITION PROFILE:** very high in chromium, iron and silicon; high in calcium, magnesium, manganese, potassium and vitamin A; significant amounts of cobalt, phosphorus, selenium, and vitamins C, B2 and B3.

**CLEANSING PROPERTIES & DETOX ACTIVITY:** Horsetail herb is useful as a diuretic and tonic for a "spring cleaning" detox. It nourishes and strengthens the kidneys, lungs, bones and connective tissue. Recent tests show that it helps build strong blood. It is anti-inflammatory, restraining infection and clearing toxins through antiseptic activity. It promotes urination, scours the kidneys and softens sediment deposits. It is rich in silica which benefits the skin, hair and nails by assisting tissue and collagen repair.

**SAFETY PRECAUTIONS:** Caution during pregnancy. Horsetail breaks down B vitamins; take with nutritional yeast for B vitamins.

**SYNERGY WITH OTHER HERBS:** Use with nettles or sage or Irish moss for chronic lung conditions; use with parsley or cornsilk for bladder conditions. Use with dandelion for connective tissue ailments.

## Lemon Balm (Melissa officinalis)

**FAMILY:** Labiatae

**MEDICINAL PARTS:** leaf

**DOSAGE:** tincture: 5 – 10 drops; essential oil 1 – 2 drops in water; infusion: 1 – 2 cups daily. Its gentle properties and mild bitters provide a pleasant flavor for children who find it difficult to consume strong bitter herbs.

**NUTRITION PROFILE:** Lemon balm citronella terpene has sedative-like effects. High in antispasmodic and antibacterial volatile oil that acts on the digestive tract and central nervous system. Polyphenols and tannin give lemon balm its anti-viral properties and are, perhaps, responsible for its success and effectiveness in inhibiting the herpes simplex virus and mumps.

**CLEANSING PROPERTIES & DETOX ACTIVITY:** Lemon balm restores the nervous system and has relaxing tonic action upon the heart (especially palpitations) and circulatory system. It helps calm coughing spasms and asthma spells and expels phlegm. It resolves fever and expels phlegm, disperses heat and helps to break down tumors. Lemon balm is a good choice for insomnia, tension headaches and depression. It is an effective compress for herpes and cold sores; a good wash for eye inflammations.

**SAFETY PRECAUTIONS:** none in common use.

**SYNERGY WITH OTHER HERBS:** With elecampane and sage as a restorative from depression and exhaustion. With senna, fennel seed, ginger, papaya, hibiscus, peppermint, parsley and calendula for a laxative.

## Licorice Root (*Glycyrrhiza glabra*)

**FAMILY:** Papilionaceae

**MEDICINAL PARTS:** root

**DOSAGE:** Extract: 1 – 1.5 tsp. 3x daily.

**NUTRITION PROFILE:** very high in magnesium, silicon and sodium; high in chromium, cobalt, iron and vitamin B3; significant amounts of calcium, manganese, potassium and vitamins C and B1.

**CLEANSING PROPERTIES & DETOX ACTIVITY:** Both antibacterial and antiviral, licorice is effective against many infections, including hepatitis, herpes, dermatitis, eczema and most respiratory infections. It cleanses the blood of toxic pollutants, making it effective for allergies, asthma, candida albicans and arthritis. It restores exhausted adrenals, making it a good choice for fatigue and weakness, including serious adrenal conditions, such as Addison's disease. It is a specific for sore throat, laryngitis and vocal strain.

Licorice is a good remedy for flu, colds and all lung problems; it is a good expectorant for coughs and bronchial congestion. Its action is complex in normalizing vital blood salt concentrations to stimulate and sustain proper adrenal function. Licorice enhances blood purity by protecting the body's blood detoxification plant: the liver.

**SAFETY PRECAUTIONS:** Not when high blood pressure is a problem.

**SYNERGY WITH OTHER HERBS:** Use with mullein, pleurisy, marshmallow, rose hips, ephedra, calendula, boneset, ginger, peppermint and fennel seed for a tea to clear mucous congestion. Use in a capsule with sarsaparilla, bladderwrack, Irish moss, uva ursi, rose hips, ginger, capsicum for an adrenal activator.

## Lobelia (*Lobelia inflata*)

**FAMILY:** Lobeliaceae

**MEDICINAL PARTS:** The whole plant

**DOSAGE:** capsules 2 – 4; tincture: 5 – 15 drops.

**NUTRITION PROFILE:** high in manganese and vitamins A and C; significant amounts of calcium, iron, magnesium, phosphorus, potassium and vitamins B1 and B3.

**CLEANSING PROPERTIES & DETOX ACTIVITY:** Lobelia is a specific for bronchial asthma, both to calm spasms and open passages, and as an emetic to throw out mucous obstruction. Lobelia extract may be used as an emergency measure to revive a person who has overdosed on a narcotic or is in convulsions from epilepsy. It cleanses in cases of blood poisoning, both food and heavy metal. Lobelia antidotes poison though emesis. It works for several childhood diseases including colds, fevers, chicken pox, mumps, measles, scarlet fever, croup and allergies. It helps clear both lung and lymphatic congestion. It is a specific in formulas to relieve the pain and swelling of insect bites and stings, and poison ivy or oak.

**SAFETY PRECAUTIONS:** There is a long standing debate over whether lobelia is poisonous or not—allopathic doctors and FDA say yes; alternative medicine says no. Use small amounts or it will cause vomiting.

**SYNERGY WITH OTHER HERBS:** Use with capsicum, grindelia and ephedra for asthma. Use with peppermint/ peppermint oil, comfrey, marshmallow, slippery elm, pau d'arco, ginger, aloe vera powder and wild yam for gentle cleansing of the bowel for irritable bowel, colitis inflammation or diverticular disease.

## Ma Huang (Ephedra sinica)

**FAMILY:** Ephedraceae

**MEDICINAL PARTS:** aerial parts

**DOSAGE:** 2 to 6 grams in tea daily; 2 – 4 capsules daily.

**NUTRITION PROFILE:** ephedrine, alkaloids and pseudo-ephedrine are responsible for bronchial dilating effects and central nervous stimulation.

**CLEANSING PROPERTIES & DETOX ACTIVITY:** Ephedra is a long lasting CNS stimulant that calms the mind as it stimulates the body. Excellent for mental energy during a long test or meditation. Helps relieve congestive conditions almost immediately from allergies and bronchitis and sinusitis. Beneficial in balancing combinations for circulatory stimulation, strengthening and restoring the body's vitality. Ma huang is thermogenic and can raise metabolism, making it a primary herb in weight loss programs. It is extremely effective without being overly strong in its actions, but only when properly utilized.

**SAFETY PRECAUTIONS:** For best results, use in combination with other herbs. Not for those suffering from hypertension, not for long-term use, and not for people who are using MAO inhibitors for depression. Should also be avoided in severe cases of glaucoma and coronary thrombosis. A cardiac stimulant that should be used with caution by anyone with high blood pressure. Other precautions may include heart palpitations, nervousness, insomnia, headaches and dizziness.

**SYNERGY WITH OTHER HERBS:** Use with marshmallow rt., bee pollen, goldenseal rt., white pine bk., burdock, juniper bry., parsley, acerola cherry, mullein, rosemary, lobelia and capsicum as a breathing formula. An asthmatic aid, use with marshmallow rt., fenugreek sd., mullelin lf., rosemary lf., ginkgo biloba, passionflowers, wild cherry bk., angelica, lobelia and cinnamon. For a cleansing combination, use with licorice rt., mullein, pleurisy rt., rose hips, marshmallow, boneset, calendula, ginger, fennel sd., peppermint and stevia.

## Marshmallow (Althea officionalis)

**FAMILY:** Malvaceae

**COMMON NAMES:** mallards, mauls, schloss tea, mortification root, mallowwild.

**MEDICINAL PARTS:** leaves, roots and flowers

**DOSAGE:** tincture: 30 – 60 drops 3x daily; extract: 1 – 2 tsp. 3x daily; capsules: 2 to 4 daily.

**NUTRITION PROFILE:** very high in iron, magnesium and selenium; high in chromium, sodium and vitamin C; significant amounts of calcium, cobalt, manganese, potassium, silicon and vitamin B3.

**CLEANSING PROPERTIES & DETOX ACTIVITY:** Marshmallow is used to reduce inflammation for arthritis, respiratory infections including allergies and asthma, urinary tract infections, kidney stones and venereal diseases. It is effective for diarrhea, hemorrhoids and ulcers. It is a soothing to insect bites and for any skin sore or inflammation. Marshmallow's mucilaginous properties help bind and eliminate toxins regulating bowel activity and increasing colonic flora to allow the body to cleanse itself. It soothes and heals the mucous membranes to lubricate the lungs, intestines and kidneys.

**SAFETY PRECAUTIONS:** none in common use.

**SYNERGY WITH OTHER HERBS:** With spearmint for urinary ailments. With mullein, pleurisy, rose hips, ephedra, licorice, calendula, boneset, ginger, peppermint and fennel seed as an expectorant tea. With peppermint/peppermint oil, comfrey, slippery elm, pau d'arco, ginger, aloe vera powder, wild yam and lobelia for a mild, gentle cleansing of the bowel.

# medicinal mushrooms

## Kombucha *(Fungus japonicus)*

**MEDICINAL PARTS:** fungus cap

**DOSAGE:** Use as a tea only as directed.

**NUTRITION PROFILE:** An enzyme-rich, immune boosting detoxification agent effective in cleansing the liver, eliminating toxic deposits and promoting optimal digestion and absorption.

**CLEANSING PROPERTIES & DETOX ACTIVITY:** Kombucha is especially effective as a blood and liver cleanser. As a detoxifier, kombucha is considered a good source of Glucuronic Acid, a substance that can interact with body toxins, make them easier to excrete, and prevent them from being absorbed by the intestines.

**SAFETY PRECAUTIONS:** Avoid using kombucha if you drink large amounts of alcohol; it may cause adverse effects, such as jaundice, dizziness, nausea, even liver damage. Use commercial preparations instead of home-brewed kombucha. There is high risk of contamination with dangerous pathogens if the mold is not managed correctly. Persons with HIV are not recommended for kombucha treatment.

**SYNERGY WITH OTHER HERBS:** Use alone, or with green tea and echinacea for immune strengthening.

## Maitake Mushroom *(Grifola frondosa)*

**MEDICINAL PARTS:** fungus cap

**DOSAGE:** As a preventative: 2 – 3 caplets per day. For hypertension: 6 caplets daily then 2 – 4 caplets per day to maintain lowered blood pressure. For immune suppression: 4 – 10 caplets per day. For diabetics: 10 caplets per day, then 3 – 6 caplets once blood sugar balanced. For tumors: 4 – 10 caplets daily.

**NUTRITION PROFILE:** contains amino acids, enzymes, lectins, triglycerides, EFAs, vitamins, nucleotides, amino acids. Taking maitake is more effective than taking reishi or shiitake; its polysaccharide, beta-glucan, is more readily absorbed than other mushroom immune-stimulating polysaccharides.

**CLEANSING PROPERTIES & DETOX ACTIVITY:** Maitake is a specific in formulas to combat cancers (especially leukemias, prostate cancer, fibroid and breast cancers, ovarian and uterine cancers). Many healers use it as an alternative or adjunct approach to chemotherapy drugs. Maitake have strong immuno-stimulating properties for diseases like chronic fatigue syndrome and rheumatoid arthritis. They inhibit replication of HIV by increasing T-cell counts. In one test, maitake inhibited tumor growth 86% after 31 days. Four of ten animals showed complete tumor resolution. Another study reports maitake activates various immune effector cells (macrophages, natural killer cells, T-cells) to attack tumor cells, including lymphokines and interleukin.

**SAFETY PRECAUTIONS:** None in common use.

**SYNERGY WITH OTHER HERBS:** Use with echinacea in an immune boosting compound. Use with reishi and shiitake for a medicinal mushroom superfood. Use as a specific in a weight control formula with thermogenic herbs like garcinia, sida cordifolia and ephedra.

## Reishi Mushroom *(Ganoderma lucidum)* (Ling zhi)

**MEDICINAL PARTS:** fungus cap

**DOSAGE:** tincture: 10ml 3x day; tablets: 1g. tablets 3x day.

**NUTRITION PROFILE:** contains protein, lipids, minerals, fiber, carbohydrates, high levels of germanium, and ergosterol, a provitamin which converts into vitamin D with the presence of sunlight.

**CLEANSING PROPERTIES & DETOX ACTIVITY:** Promotes longevity and health. Increases vitality and immunity during a cleansing program. Has special effectiveness against wasting syndrome, and degenerative diseases like cancer and AIDS. Stimulates T-cell activity and inhibits the replication of the HIV virus and demonstrates anti-tumor activity. In 1977, an extract of reishi (PSK) was approved in Japan as a treatment for cancer. (After five years, 62 percent of PSK treated cancer patients were disease-free, compared with 35 percent treated with surgery alone.) Helps reduce the side effects of chemotherapy for cancer. In several Chinese hospitals, a reishi formula tested on 2,000 cases of chronic bronchitis, one of the hardest-to-handle allergic reactions, is proven effective in up to 91% of cases. After several months of treatment with reishi, patients showed an increase in their immunoglobulin A (Ig A), the major immune system defender in the respiratory tract. Reishi is also a powerful antioxidant, used therapeutically for a wide range of serious conditions like hepatitis and Chronic Fatigue Syndrome. Detoxifies and regenerates the liver. Lowers cholesterol and triglycerides. Reduces coronary symptoms and high blood pressure. Calms the nervous system and relieves insomnia. Helps strengthen recovery from longterm illness. Excellent even for children.

**SAFETY PRECAUTIONS:** Use only when needed, not continuously. Do not use during pregnancy. Do not mix with aspirin. Take with food. If overused, reishi may cause diarrhea and skin rash.

**SYNERGY WITH OTHER HERBS:** Works well with ginseng or chlorella to rebuild the system after illness.

## Shiitake Mushroom (Lentinus edodes) (Hsiang-ku)

**MEDICINAL PARTS:** fungus cap

**DOSAGE:** 1 – 2 capsules a day before breakfast. The dried or fresh mushroom may be added to soups.

**NUTRITION PROFILE:** contains LEM, vitamins, minerals, amino acids, polysaccharides and abundant in nutrients such as potassium, phosphorus, silicium, magnesium, calcium, sulphur.

**CLEANSING PROPERTIES & DETOX ACTIVITY:** Shiitake mushrooms are a tonic mushroom useful for maintaining immune defenses after a cleanse. Shiitakes have precise activity on immune response: they stimulate the immune system powerhouses, the macrophages and NK (natural killer) cells to act more quickly and aggressively against invading pathogens; they combat existing infections; and they increase antibody production and interferon for greater disease resistance. Shiitakes are now used all over the world to fight cancer, Candida infections and environmental allergies.

**SAFETY PRECAUTIONS:** None in common use

**SYNERGY WITH OTHER HERBS:** Use with chlorella as a superfood immune booster for anti-cancer activity. In miso soup and brown rice for strengthening immunity.

## Milk Thistle (Silybum marianum)

**FAMILY:** Compositae

**MEDICINAL PARTS:** seed and herb

**DOSAGE:** tincture or extract: 20 drops 3 – 4x daily.

**NUTRITION PROFILE:** Very high in chromium, iron, manganese, phosphorus and selenium; high in magnesium and zinc; contains significant amounts of calcium, cobalt, potassium and vitamin A.

**CLEANSING PROPERTIES & DETOX ACTIVITY:** Milk thistle is a specific for all liver, spleen and gallbladder conditions including jaundice, hepatitis (chronic and viral), liver cirrhosis and fatty liver. It is also effective for asthma and allergy attacks. Extensive clinical trials substantiate the ability of milk thistle to reverse the symptoms of liver disorders, like hepatitis and cirrhosis, and to stimulate liver cells to replace tissue that which has been damaged or destroyed by disease.

**SAFETY PRECAUTIONS:** None in common use.

**SYNERGY WITH OTHER HERBS:** Use with beet, Oregon grape, dandelion, wild yam, yellow dock, licorice, ginkgo biloba, barberry bark, gotu cola, ginger, wild cherry bark for liver cleansing and support.

## Mullein (Verbascum thapsus)

**FAMILY:** Scrophulariaceae

**MEDICINAL PARTS:** flowers and leaves

**DOSAGE:** tincture: 30 – 60 drops, often; oil: 2 – 3 drops 3x daily.

**NUTRITION PROFILE:** Very high in iron; high in calcium, chromium, cobalt, magnesium, manganese, phosphorus, silicon and in vitamins A, C and B3; contains significant amounts of potassium.

**CLEANSING PROPERTIES & DETOX ACTIVITY:** Mullein is an anti-spasmodic and astringent herb, a specific for all types of respiratory problems asthma, bronchitis, swollen glands, whooping and hacking coughs, sinus congestion and hay fever. Mullein is particularly good in treating damaged lung tissue in emphysema. It is a main ingredient for ear infections, especially for children, and is also effective for other childhood diseases—mumps, fevers, toothaches, diarrhea and constipation. Topically, the oil is used for bruises, skin ailments, warts and swellings.

**SAFETY PRECAUTIONS:** none in common use.

**SYNERGY WITH OTHER HERBS:** With horehound, lobelia and coltsfoot for use against bronchitis. With pleurisy, marshmallow, rose hips, ephedra, licorice, calendula, boneset, ginger, peppermint and fennel seed for a tea to clear mucous congestion.

## Nettles (Urtica dioica)

**FAMILY:** Urticaceae

**MEDICINAL PARTS:** leaves

**DOSAGE:** tincture: 5 – 15 drops as needed; juice: 1 tsp. as needed, infusion: as needed.

**NUTRITION PROFILE:** Nettles is very high in calcium, chlorophyll and magnesium; high in chromium, cobalt, iron, phosphorous, potassium, zinc, and in vitamins A, C, and B1. Contains significant amounts of manganese, selenium, silicon and vitamins B2 and B3 and vitamin K.

**CLEANSING PROPERTIES & DETOX ACTIVITY:** Nettles is useful for arthritis, sciatic pain, and all types of respiratory conditions, including asthma, chronic bronchitis, hacking coughs and excess mucous. Nettles has a draining action, clearing mucous through expectoration. It has a role against cancer and tumors. Its diuretic qualities make it helpful for cardiac edema. Used in cleansing formulas for hives, hepatitis, kidney stones, kidney and bladder infections, diarrhea and constipation. Its tonic qualities make it a favorite for fatigue, anemia and thyroid conditions. Its chlorophyll and mineral content make it a good choice for digestive problems such as gastric acidity and allergies.

**SAFETY PRECAUTIONS:** none in common use.

**SYNERGY WITH OTHER HERBS:** With marigold, burdock and figwort for an ointment for skin conditions. With beets, alfalfa, dandelion, Siberian eleuthero, yellow dock, parsley, burdock, dulse, bilberry and capsicum as a hemoglobin builder. With alfalfa, Irish moss, yellow dock, watercress, parsley, borage seed, dulse and barley grass for an effective mineral formula.

## Oregon Grape (Mahonia aquifolium)

**FAMILY:** Berberidaceae

**MEDICINAL PARTS:** root bark

**DOSAGE:** tincture: 10 – 30 drops 3x daily; fluid extract: ½ tsp. 3x daily; capsules: 2 to 4 3x daily.

**NUTRITION PROFILE:** Contains measureable calcium, chromium, iron, cobalt, magnesium, phosphorus, potassium, selenium, silicon and vitamins B1, B2 and B3.

**CLEANSING PROPERTIES & DETOX ACTIVITY:** Oregon grape is effective liver support against jaundice and lymphatic congestion, enhancing the flow of bile through the liver and gallbladder to purify the blood. It may be used for all liver diseases including hepatitis and gallstones. Its blood cleansing properties are strong against arthritis, acne, herpes, psoriasis, eczema, syphilis, vaginitis, bronchitis, anemia and even some cancers. Also used for skin diseases, bronchial congestion, arthritis, cancers and tumors.

**SAFETY PRECAUTIONS:** Not when pregnant or when hyperthyroid. Overdosing can cause fatal poisoning.

**SYNERGY WITH OTHER HERBS:** Use with dandelion root for a tea for hepatitis and jaundice. Use with dandelion, watercress, yellow dock, pau d'arco, hyssop, red sage, licorice, milk thistle seed and hibiscus for a liver flush tea. Use with beet, milk thistle seed, dandelion, wild yam, yellow dock, licorice, ginkgo biloba, barberry bark, gotu kola, ginger, wild cherry bark, for a liver cleansing and support formula.

## Parsley (Petroselinum crispum)

**FAMILY:** Umbelliferae

**MEDICINAL PARTS:** leaf and root

**DOSAGE:** tincture: 20 – 40 drops 3x daily, fluid extract: ½ to ¾ tsp. 3x daily; capsules: 2 – 4, 3x daily.

**NUTRITION PROFILE:** Parsley is rich in chlorophyll, potassium, and vitamin A, making it a strengthening diuretic to relieve fluid congestion. It is a specific for liver, kidney and bladder problems. It is a nutritive digestive aid that stimulates secretion of stomach acids. It enhances the immune system, acts as a tonic on the blood and is a chlorophyll source to clean up toxic blood.

**CLEANSING PROPERTIES & DETOX ACTIVITY:** Useful for all kidney and bladder problems, including kidney and gall stones, bladder infections and bloating, jaundice, hepatitis and anemia. Helps indigestion, gas, flatulence and ulcers. Effective in formulas for arthritis, PMS, asthma, hay fever and swollen glands.

**SAFETY PRECAUTIONS:** Not during pregnancy in high doses.

**SYNERGY WITH OTHER HERBS:** Use with kelp, dulse, barley grass, spirulina, dandelion, watercress, alfalfa to revitalize metabolic activity. Use with beets, alfalfa, dandelion, Siberian eleuthero, yellow dock, nettles, burdock, dulse, bilberry and capsicum for a hemoglobin builder. Use with dandelion, watercress, yellow dock, pau d'arco, hyssop, Oregon grape, red sage, licorice, milk thistle seed and hibiscus for a liver flush tea.

## Pau d' Arco Bark (Tabebuia impetiginosa)

**FAMILY:** Bignoniaceae

**MEDICINAL PARTS:** inner bark

**DOSAGE:** 2 – 5 capsules 3x daily.

**NUTRITION PROFILE:** Rich in quinones, mainly lapachol. In fact, pau d' arco contains 18 different quinones including naphthoquinones and anthraquinones which are rarely found together in a plant. High in iron, iodine and the bioflavonoid quercetin. A good source of natural COQ10. Pau d'arco gets most of its chemical and mineral substances from the soil in which the tree grows and not the bark itself.

**CLEANSING PROPERTIES & DETOX ACTIVITY:** A primary blood cleanser and immune stimulant, especially purifying blood toxicity against dermatitis and psoriasis. Anticancer against leukemia. Anti-viral qualities boost the immune system against viruses such as HPV, flu, herpes and hepatitis, and, amazingly, against AIDS. Effective against warts, diabetes, ulcers, rheumatism and liver disease.

**SAFETY PRECAUTIONS:** May produce nausea and loose bowels; anti-coagulant blood effects in high doses.

**SYNERGY WITH OTHER HERBS:** Use with dandelion, gentian, myrrh, goldenseal rt., witch hazel, lomatium, grapefruit sd., propolis, vitamin D gel to provide relief for itchy skin conditions. Use for serious cleansing, with red clover, licorice rt., burdock, ascorbate vitamin C, sarsparilla, alfalfa, kelp, echinacea rt., garlic, butternut, panax ginseng, goldenseal rt., astragalus, poria mushroom, yellow dock, buckthorn bk, prickly ash, dandelion, and milk thistle sd.

## Peppermint (Mentha piperita)

**FAMILY:** Labiatae

**MEDICINAL PARTS:** leaf and oil

**DOSAGE:** tincture: 20 – 40 drops 3x daily; oil: 5 – 10 drops 3x daily; tea: 1 cup 3x daily.

**NUTRITION PROFILE:** Peppermint is very high in magnesium, phosphorus and in vitamins A, B1 and B2; high in calcium, iron, potassium, sodium and in vitamin B3, and contains significant amounts of manganese, selenium and vitamin C.

**CLEANSING PROPERTIES & DETOX ACTIVITY:** Peppermint is an effective body cleanser and toner. It reduces inflammations and expels phlegm to benefit the skin and lungs. Peppermint is a good enzyme therapy herb to stimulate the liver and gall bladder, promote the flow of bile, cleanse the colon and improve digestion. Peppermint is a good choice for the onset of colds, flu, cough and fever, bronchitis and asthma.

**SAFETY PRECAUTIONS:** Don't use while breast feeding (reduces the flow of milk); use sparingly with very young children; oil may cause contact dermatitis on the skin. Keep oil away from eyes.

**SYNERGY WITH OTHER HERBS:** Use with comfrey, marshmallow, slippery elm, pau d'arco, ginger, aloe vera, wild yam and lobelia for a mild gentle cleanser for the bowel when there is irritable bowel soreness, colitis, or diverticular disease. Use with senna, fennel seed, ginger, papaya, hibiscus, lemon balm, parsley and calendula for a simple herbal laxative. Use with mullein, pleurisy rt., marshmallow, rose hips, ephedra, licorice, calendula, boneset, ginger and fennel for an herbal expectorant tea.

## Plantain *(Plantago lanceolata)*

**FAMILY:** Plantaginaceae

**MEDICINAL PARTS:** leaves

**DOSAGE:** juice: 2 tsp. 3x daily; tincture: 2 – 60 drops 3 – 4x daily; extract: ½ to 1 tsp. 3 – 4x daily.

**NUTRITION PROFILE:** contains vitamins A, C, K, B2, B3; also calcium, iron, zinc and tyrosine.

**CLEANSING PROPERTIES & DETOX ACTIVITY:** A cleanser in cases of chronic diarrhea, dysentery, leucorrhea, kidney and bladder infections and inflammations, lymphatic infections, edema, lung and throat inflammations and infections, bronchitis, allergic asthma, hayfever, rhinitis, venereal infections, wounds, burns, boils, abscesses, bug bites and stings, snakebites, rashes, poison oak, blood poisoning, skin infections, dry skin, ulcers, eye, mouth and ear inflammations and hemorrhoids.

**SAFETY PRECAUTIONS:** None in common use.

**SYNERGY WITH OTHER HERBS:** Use for respiratory aid with mullein, wild cherry bk., horehound, ginkgo biloba, slippery elm bk., marshmallow rt., chickweed, licorice rt., kelp, acerola cherry, cinnamon, ma huang and capsicum.

## Psyllium Husk *(Plantago psyllium)*

**FAMILY:** Plantaginaceae

**MEDICINAL PARTS:** The seed husk

**DOSAGE:** powder: 1 – 2 tsp. in warm water or juice 3x daily.

**NUTRITION PROFILE:** husk contains measureable calcium, iron, phosphorus and vitamin A.

**CLEANSING PROPERTIES & DETOX ACTIVITY:** Widely used as a laxative for chronic constipation and detoxifying the bowels and colon. Helpful for inflammatory diverticulitis and colitis, and is a lubricant for ulcerous intestinal tract tissue, for dysentery, gastritis, hemorrhoids and ulcers. Psyllium also decreases LDL cholesterol.

**SAFETY PRECAUTIONS:** May cause allergic response in a small number of people.

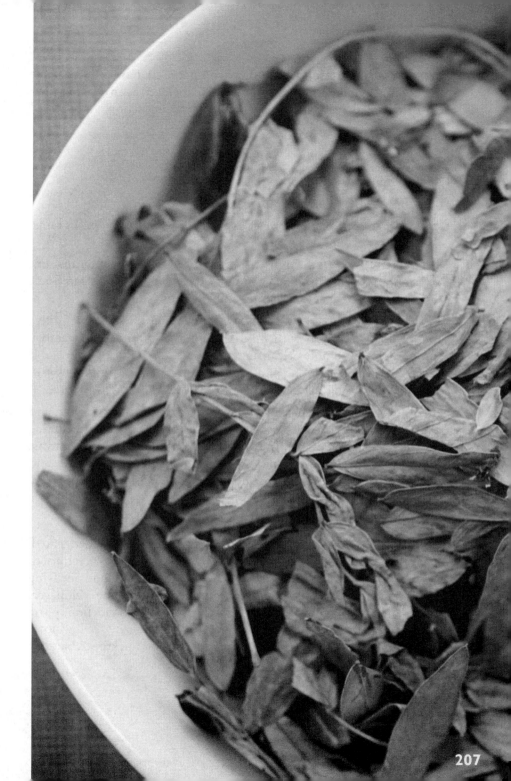

**SYNERGY WITH OTHER HERBS:** Use with oat bran, flax seed, vegetable acidophilus, guar gum, apple pectin and fennel seed as an effective fiber mix to regulate peristalsis and provide a cleansing action.

## Red Clover (Trifolium pratense)

**FAMILY:** Leguminosae

**MEDICINAL PARTS:** flower head.

**DOSAGE:** tincture: 5 – 30 drops, as needed; powder: 30 – 60 grains; infusion: 4 – 6 cups daily.

**NUTRITION PROFILE:** high in chromium, calcium, magnesium, phosphorus, potassium, and vitamins C, B1 and B3; contains significant amounts of manganese, selenium and vitamins A and B2.

**CLEANSING PROPERTIES & DETOX ACTIVITY:** Red clover is a definitive blood purifying herb with mild antibiotic and anti-inflammatory properties. It promotes cleansing and the elimination of toxins and deposits through diuretic and expectorant activity. It improves skin conditions through cleansing.

Red clover cleanses are used for cancer and tumors, arthritis, gout and rheumatism, heavy metal poisoning, all types of skin ailments, including eczema, all types of respiratory infections, including bronchitis, spasmodic coughing, asthma, swollen glands, and tuberculosis, and elimination system problems including constipation, urinary tract infections and diverticulitis.

**SAFETY PRECAUTIONS:** Dilute doses for older children.

**SYNERGY WITH OTHER HERBS:** Use with hawthorn lf. and flwr., pau d' arco, nettles, sage, alfalfa, horsetail, milk thistle seed, gotu kola, echinacea purpurea, blue malva, yerba santa and lemongrass for a blood purifying tea. Use with licorice rt., chaparral, burdock, pau d' arco, echinacea, ascorbate vit. C, goldenseal rt., garlic, kelp, alfalfa, dandelion, poria mushroom, American ginseng rt., sarsaparilla, astragalus, yellow dock, butternut, milk thistle seed, ginger, prickly ash and buckthorn bark for a detox formula.

## Rhubarb Root (Rheum palmatum)

**FAMILY:** Polygonaceae

**MEDICINAL PARTS:** root only

**DOSAGE:** Small dose: (astringing) tincture, 6 – 12 drops; Medium dose: (mild stimulating, laxative) tincture, 15 drops; Large dose: (purgative) tincture, 50 – 100 drops.

**NUTRITION PROFILE:** High in minerals like calcium, copper, iodine, iron, magnesium, manganese, phosphorus, potassium, silicon, sulphur and zinc, as well as vitamins A, C and B-complex. Oxalic and other acids help oxygen transport in the blood. Has an inhibiting effect on both cancerous tumors and bacteria, due to an antibiotic, antimicrobial and antitumor anthraquinone in the root.

**CLEANSING PROPERTIES & DETOX ACTIVITY:** Rhubarb root is effective for elimination problems: constipation, diarrhea and dysentery; for digestive problems: acute gastritis, food poisoning, swollen painful abdomen, duodenal and stomach ulcers, and gallstones; for skin conditions: jaundice, dermatitis, eczema, herpes and boils, and for cleansing the body of parasites. Rhubarb root acts as a stimulating tonic on the liver, gall ducts and mucous membranes to promote removal of toxic substances from the bowels and blood. It reduces liver congestion, infections and tumors. In large doses, it is a purgative.

**SAFETY PRECAUTIONS:** Not during pregnancy or with arthritis or gout. The leaves are poisonous.

**SYNERGY WITH OTHER HERBS:** Use with sheep sorrel, slippery elm and burdock rt. for the cancer fighting formula Essiac. Use with butternut, barberry, cascara, psyllium, fennel seed, licorice, ginger, Irish moss and capsicum to normalize bowels.

## Royal Jelly (Apis mellifea L.)

Medicinal Part: jelly

**DOSAGE:** 1 – 2 capsules daily; 1 tsp. daily.

**NUTRITION PROFILE:** Contains every nutrient necessary to support life. A powerhouse of B vitamins, the minerals calcium, iron, potassium and silicon, enzyme precursors, pure acetylcholine, sex hormones and the eight essential amino acids. A rich source of pantothenic acid to combat stress, fatigue and insomnia; nourishing for proper digestion and healthy, stronger skin and hair.

**CLEANSING PROPERTIES & DETOX ACTIVITY:** Royal jelly supplies key nutrients for energy, mental alertness and general well-being. Antibiotic properties stimulate the immune system, deep cellular health and longevity. Effective for gland and hormone imbalances that reflect in menstrual and prostate problems. It helps the endocrine glands, genital organs, the immune system, and increases better replication of DNA. Aids in liver disease, pancreatitis, insomnia, stomach ulcers, kidney disease, bone fractures and skin disorders such as acne.

**SAFETY PRECAUTIONS:** For those allergic to bees, it may cause asthma attacks and severe allergy reactions.

**SYNERGY WITH OTHER HERBS:** Use in a phyto-therapy skin gel, especially for blemishes, with extracts of licorice rt., burdock rt., rosemary, rose hips, sarsparilla, sage, chamomile, parsley, fennel sd., thyme, dandelion, propolis, bee pollen and Korean ginseng rt.

## Sage *(Salvia offficinalis)*

**FAMILY:** Labiatae

**MEDICINAL PARTS:** leaves and whole herb

**DOSAGE:** tea: 1 – 2 cups daily; tincture: 20 to 60 drops 3x daily; powder: 10 – 30 grains 3x daily.

**NUTRITION PROFILE:** Sage is high in zinc, calcium, magnesium, potassium, and vitamins A and B-1; contains significant iron, manganese, silicon and vitamins C, B2 and B3.

**CLEANSING PROPERTIES & DETOX ACTIVITY:** A good cleansing herb for colds, flu, fevers, sore throat, gas, indigestion, nerves, vertigo, depression and menopausal problems. Sage is a good memory aid.

**SAFETY PRECAUTIONS:** Not if there is epilepsy; only small doses during pregnancy.

**SYNERGY WITH OTHER HERBS:** Use with pau d'arco, kukicha, ginkgo biloba, hawthorn, sassafras, ginger, calendula, yellow dock, peppermint, butcher's broom, bilberry and licorice rt. to stimulate circulation and to deter cholesterol. Use with red clover, hawthorn, pau d' arco, nettles, alfalfa, horsetail, milk thistle seed, gotu kola, echinacea, blue malva, yerba santa and lemongrass for a cleansing and purifying tea. Use with peppermint, rosemary and wood betony for a headache remedy.

## Sarsaparilla *(Smilax officinalis)*

**FAMILY:** Liliacea

**MEDICINAL PARTS:** root

**DOSAGE:** tea: 2 cups daily; capsules: 2 to 6 daily with water at mealtime; extract: 2 – 4 tsp. daily or 20 – 40 drops 4x daily.

**NUTRITION PROFILE:** high in selenium, chromium, cobalt, iron, silicon and zinc; contains significant amounts of calcium, magnesium, manganese, phosphorus and potassium.

**CLEANSING PROPERTIES & DETOX ACTIVITY:** Sarsaparilla is an anti-inflammatory, cleansing herb that stimulates the kidneys to flush deposits and clear toxins, and promotes sweating to resolve fevers and release harmful pathogens. It binds to toxins in the gut and stops them from entering the bloodstream, it is a liver and blood restorer. Certain constituents act as natural hormone precursors, activating immunity, fighting infections, and benefiting the skin, muscle performance and female harmony.

Sarsaparilla is a primary herb for jaundice, hepatitis, gout, arthritis, rheumatism, psoriasis, herpes, acne, abcesses, boils, warts, burns, skin inflammations, venereal diseases, fevers, fatigue, anemia, impotence, bacterial infections, edema and other toxic blood conditions.

**SYNERGY WITH OTHER HERBS:** Use with yellow dock and sassafras for a spring tonic. Use with licorice, bladderwrack and Irish moss to stimulate and nourish exhausted adrenals. Use with Siberian eleuthero, fo-ti, licorice, Irish moss, barley grass, black cohosh, saw palmetto, dong quai, gotu kola, kelp, alfalfa, and ginger as a gland balancing compound.

## Sea Vegetables [Bladderwrack (Fucus vesiculosus); Dulse (Rhodymenia palmata); Kelp (Ascophyllum nodosum); Irish moss (Chondrus crispus)]

**MEDICINAL PARTS:** entire plant—dried root, bulbs, stem and leaves.

**DOSAGE:** 5 – 10 gm three times a day in capsules; to make an extract (70:30) using dried powdered herb: 1 part herb, 4 parts water and 2 parts alcohol. Seal and set overnight. Then, filter. Tea: pour a cup of boiling water onto 2 – 3 tsp. of dried plants; steep 10 minutes. Tincture: 4 – 8 ml three times a day for sluggish constitution. Infused oil for topical application: macerate equal parts dried sea plant and sunflower oil; heat it in warm water for two hours, then strain. As a salad or soup sprinkle, mineral drink or broth: 2 tbsp. daily of dried chopped sea vegetables are a therapeutic dose.

**NUTRITION PROFILE:** Sea vegetables have superior nutritional content. They transmit the energies and nutrients of the sea to us with easy absorption. They are nutritive tonics, containing over ninety elements essential to human well-being, including minerals and mineral salts, vitamins, amino acids, enzymes and trace elements. Their mineral balance is a natural tranquilizer for building sound nerve structure, and proper metabolism.

Ounce for ounce, along with herbs, they are higher in vitamins and minerals than any other food group. Some species contain over 30 minerals—rich in calcium, magnesium, iodine, manganese, potassium, selenium, chromium, silicon and zinc for human health. Sea vegetables are almost the only non-animal source of Vitamin B-12 for cell growth and nerve function. Sea plants are one of nature's richest sources of vegetable protein, and they provide full-spectrum concentrations of beta carotene, chlorophyll, enzymes and soluble fiber.

The distinctive salty taste is not just "salt," but a balanced, chelated combination of sodium, potassium, calcium, magnesium, phosphorus, iron and trace minerals. They convert inorganic ocean minerals into organic mineral usable nutrients for structural building blocks. In fact, sea vegetables contain all the necessary trace elements for life, many of which are depleted in the Earth's soil.

**CLEANSING PROPERTIES & DETOX ACTIVITY:** An important part of a cleansing program, sea vegetables alkalize the body, and reduce excess stores of fluid and fat. Sea plants bind radioactive strontium, barium, and cadmium, dangerous pollutants in the gastrointestinal tract, preventing their absorption into the body. They then transform the toxic metals in the system (including radiation), into harmless salts that the body can eliminate. They purify the blood from the acid effects of a modern diet, allowing for better absorption of nutrients. Natural iodine in sea plants stimulates the thyroid gland for help in weight control. Research indicates antiviral activity in tests against mumps and flu viruses.

Seaweed soothes irritated mucous membranes, dissolves abnormal tissue masses such as tumors, treats enlarged thyroid, lymph nodes and swollen painful testes, and reduces edema. It helps relieve rheumatoid arthritis when taken internally and topically applied to swollen areas. It is effective against bladder inflammation. It fights fatigue through alterative action on the glandular system.

**SAFETY PRECAUTIONS:** Sea plants can contain heavy metal pollutants if gathered from areas that are polluted with high levels of mercury, cadmium and other toxins. Some experts consider sea plants unsafe for people with sensitive thyroids if taken in large doses.

**SYNERGY WITH OTHER HERBS:** Use with plantain, fennel seed, licorice, marshmallow, burdock and hawthorn for weight loss and bloating. Use with uva ursi, dandelion, parsley, buchu, saw palmetto, bilberry and gentian for a nerve tonic and normalizing blood sugar. Use with extracts of alfalfa, ginger, dandelion, spearmint, capsicum, cinnamon, aloe vera gel, olive, rice bran, grapeseed oils and lecithin in an herbal wrap to increase enzyme and systol/diastole action in a cleansing program. Use with extracts of licorice root, sarsparilla and Irish moss as a gland cleansing tonic. Use with red raspberry as part of a prenatal combination to prevent cretinism. Use with wild cherry, plantain, goldenseal root, slippery elm and comfrey for bronchitis to overcome inflammation.

## Senna Lf. & Pods (Senna alexandrina)

**FAMILY:** Leguminosae

**MEDICINAL PARTS:** leaf and pod.

**DOSAGE:** tincture: 10 – 40 drops.

**NUTRITION PROFILE:** high in calcium, chromium, magnesium and vitamins A, C, B1 and B2; high in iron, manganese, selenium, silicon, sodium, zinc, vitamin B3; significant phosphorus.

**CLEANSING PROPERTIES & DETOX ACTIVITY:** Senna is a bitters, purging stimulant, acting mainly on the colon to encourage peristalsis. It is a highly valued cathartic for the lower bowel, with less intestinal griping than most laxatives. It is an effective vermifuge for intestinal worms and parasites.

**HERBAL HEALING ACTIONS:** laxative, purgative, bitter, stimulant.

**SAFETY PRECAUTIONS:** Not for use when pregnant—a uterine stimulant. Not for when inflammatory conditions of the alimentary canal exist or if there are hemorrhoids. Senna is slightly habit forming, especially in its over-the-counter drug form, and should be used sparingly.

**SYNERGY WITH OTHER HERBS:** With carminatives for best results, like ginger, cumin or fennel. With antispasmodics like cramp bark or lobelia to reduce cramps. With fennel seed, ginger, papaya, hibiscus, lemon balm, peppermint, parsley and calendula for a simple herbal laxative tea.

## Slippery Elm (Ulmus fulva)

**FAMILY:** Ulmaceae

**MEDICINAL PARTS:** inner bark

**DOSAGE:** tincture: 15 – 30 drops 3x daily, powder: 30 – 60 grains 3x daily; tea: 6 oz. 3 – 4x daily, syrup: 1 tbsp. as needed.

**NUTRITION PROFILE:** high in vitamin B3, calcium and vitamins B1 and B2, and contains significant amounts of chromium, magnesium, manganese, potassium, selenium, sodium and vitamin A.

**CLEANSING PROPERTIES & DETOX ACTIVITY:** Slippery elm soothes, nourishes, strengthens mucous membranes, especially in wasting diseases. Its mucilaginous properties aid the throat, stomach, bowels and colon helping to absorb toxins and regulate colonic bacteria. Slippery elm is a primary demulcent herb for diarrhea and constipation, colitis, irritable bowel syndrome, ulcers, indigestion, gastritis, nausea, bronchitis, congestion, coughs, asthma, croup, sore throat, inflammations, wounds, boils, burns, acne, abcesses, sores, and skin rashes. Expectorant action helps soothe respiratory ailments and discharge mucous.

**SAFETY PRECAUTIONS:** None in common use.

**SYNERGY WITH OTHER HERBS:** with peppermint/peppermint oil, comfrey rt., marshmallow rt., pau d' arco, ginger, aloe vera, wild yam and lobelia in a gentle bowel cleanser.

## Spirulina (Spirulina platensis)

**MEDICINAL PART:** dried powder

**DOSAGE:** 500 – 1500mg daily.

**NUTRITION PROFILE:** A chlorophyll-rich "superfood," spirulina supplies 21 amino acids including the top 8 essential for health. Research shows that spirulina alone could double the protein balance of the planet! Its protein composition is 60% more by weight than any other organic whole food. Acre for acre, spirulina yields 20 times more protein than soybeans, 40 times more protein than corn, and 400 times more protein than beef. It provides amino acids, and the entire B complex of vitamins, including vitamin B12, not commonly found in plants. It is rich in beta carotene, minerals, trace minerals and essential fatty acids. Extremely high in iron making it beneficial in ailments such as anemia. Digestibility is high, stimulating both immediate and long range energy.

**CLEANSING PROPERTIES & DETOX ACTIVITY:** Spirulina's chlorophyll content draws out toxins to cleanse and detoxify the body. Its alkaline properties directly help balance the effects of acidic foods like coffee, alcohol, sugar, and meat. Spirulina is easily digested providing quick energy and nourishment; helps malabsorption, especially in the elderly and the undernourished. It is a foundation nutrient for weight control and blood sugar support. Current research on spirulina identifies phytonutrients that enhance immunity. Spirulina's sulfolipids and glycolipids have amazing action on AIDS, preventing the HIV virus from attaching to or penetrating cells. It helps inhibit many viruses, like mumps, measles, even herpes viruses. Effective in stimulating an immune response that destroys malignant cells.

**SAFETY PRECAUTIONS:** None in common use.

**SYNERGY WITH OTHER HERBS:** In combination with bee pollen, alfalfa, hawthorn, chlorella, barley grass, Siberian eleuthero rt., carrot rt., sarsaparilla rt., red rasberry, kelp, wild cherry bk., rose hips ext., goldenseal rt., mullein for energy and to restore strength after exhaustion or illness. Use with garcinia gambogia, sida cordifolia extr., bancha lf., kukicha twig, guarana sd., capsicum fruit to balance thermogenesis. Use with a gentle effective herbal support program designed to re-establish friendly flora in the digestive tract combine with pau d' arco, black walnut hulls, vegetable acidophilus, garlic, barberry, cranberry juice, burdock rt., licorice rt., echinacea angustifolia and purpurea rt., dong quai, damiana, thyme, peppermint, rosemary, rose hips.

## St. John's Wort *(Hypericum perforatum)*

**FAMILY:** Hypericaceae

**MEDICINAL PARTS:** leaf, flower, buds

**DOSAGE:** tea: 1 – 2 tsp. herb to 1 cup hot water 3x daily; tincture: 15 – 30 drops 3x daily.

**NUTRITION PROFILE:** Contains choline. Contains hypericin (its MAO, anti-viral, and anti-cancer inhibitor ingredient), volatile oil such as carophyllene, and pseudohypericin and flavonoids.

**CLEANSING PROPERTIES & DETOX ACTIVITY:** St. John's wort is a potent antiviral, helping control viral infections of all types, including staph, strep, HPV, even HIV. It reduces congestion and tumor growth. It is immuno-modulating and lowers inflammatory reactions. It is an analgesic, anti-inflammatory, effective in compounds for colds, chest congestion, headaches, sciatica, neuralgia, rheumatism, skin sores and cancers. It is an anti-depressant for anxiety, insomnia and chronic fatigue syndrome. It acts as a nervine to curb nerve pain and rebuild strong nerve structure. It inhibits the brain chemical monoamine oxidase (MAO) which triggers depression. It is a serotonin modulator that helps as an appetite suppressant.

**SAFETY PRECAUTIONS:** Sun-sensitive people should avoid taking it. Very high doses may cause phototoxicity in humans, especially in those with fair skin.

**SYNERGY WITH OTHER HERBS:** With kirin ginseng, Chinese white ginseng, aralia, tienchi, suma, echinacea purpurea and angustifolia, pau d' arco bark, Siberian eleuthero, prince ginseng, astragalus bark, reishi mushrooms, ma huang and fennel seed for a purifying, restorative tea.

## Uña De Gato *(Uncaria tomentosa)*

**FAMILY:** Rubiacea

**MEDICINAL PARTS:** root and bark

**DOSAGE:** tea: 2 to 3 c. daily; capsules:1 – 2, 3x daily.

**NUTRITION PROFILE:** Contains six important oxindole alkaloids which enhance the process by which white blood cells and macrophages engulf and eliminate pathogens and cell debris. Rich phytochemicals like

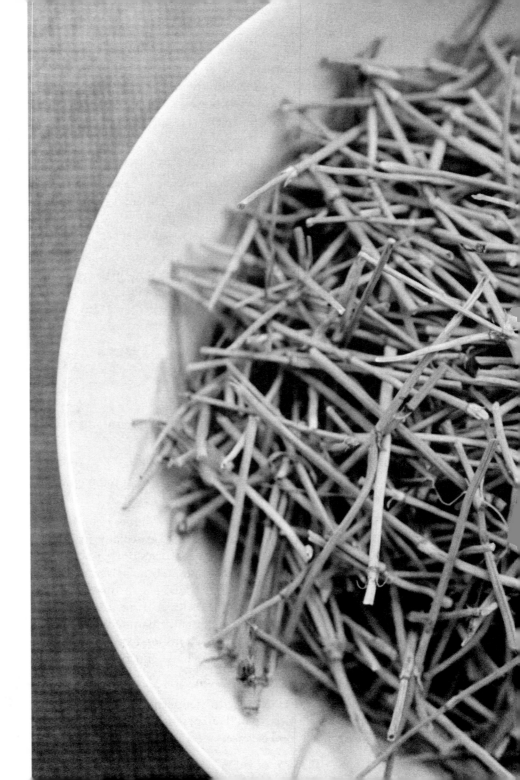

proanthocyanidins, triterpines, polyphenols, quinovic acid glycosides give it potent antioxidant properties.

**CLEANSING PROPERTIES & DETOX ACTIVITY:** An immunostimulating herb that benefits the entire gastrointestinal system, including disorders like gastritis and peptic ulcers. Because of its ability to cleanse the colon and reduce inflammation, una de gato is especially beneficial for colon problems like Crohn's disease, diverticulitis or leaky bowel syndrome. Some patients with I.B.S. (irritable bowel syndrome) have been relieved of all symptoms after just a week of taking una de gato! Una de gato has proven effective for T-Cell enhancement against the AIDS virus. New clinical trials show it delays, even sometimes prevents, progression into full-blown AIDS. Successful against cancer, (new studies show it both reduces and normalizes the side effects of chemotherapy in cancer treatment). Reduces viral infections like genital herpes.

**SAFETY PRECAUTIONS:** Avoid during pregnancy, when undergoing skin grafts or organ transplants, if you are hemophiliac or taking fresh blood plasma, if you're being administered certain vaccines, hormone therapies, thymus extracts, or insulin. Not for children under 3 years of age.

**SYNERGY WITH OTHER HERBS:** An immune restorative tonic with astragulus and reishi mushroom.

## Usnea (Usnea barbata)

**FAMILY:** Usneaceae

**MEDICINAL PARTS:** lichen.

**DOSAGE:** extract: 30 drops 3x daily; tea: 1 cup 3x daily.

**NUTRITION PROFILE:** part fungus, part algae, with significant Vitamin C amounts. Rich in usnic acid, said to be more effective against bacterial strains than penicillin. But most medicinally effective due to the polysaccharides and mucilage found in the inner cord of the plant.

**CLEANSING PROPERTIES & DETOX ACTIVITY:** Used for sore throats, colds and flu, for strep and staph infections, sinus infections, intestinal infections, impetigo, trichomonas and urinary tract infections, fungal infections, respiratory infections and for cuts, bites and stings.

**SAFETY PRECAUTIONS:** None in common use.

**SYNERGY WITH OTHER HERBS:** Use with licorice and ginger in a tea for colds and flu. Usnea tincture is mixed with water and used as a gargle or sinus spray.

## Uva Ursi (Arctostaphylos uva ursi)

**FAMILY:** Ericaceae

**MEDICINAL PARTS:** leaves

**DOSAGE:** tincture: 2ml 3x daily; tea: 3 cups daily.

**NUTRITION PROFILE:** rich in iron, manganese and vitamin A; high in calcium, selenium and silicon; significant amounts of chromium, magnesium, potassium, sodium, and vitamins C, B1 B2 and B3.

**CLEANSING PROPERTIES & DETOX ACTIVITY:** Uva ursi is a specific for bladder and kidney infections and irritations, like urethritis, acute cystitis, dysentery, mucous and blood in the urine, venereal infections, candida albicans, urinary stones and deposits, prostate irritation, hemorrhoids and bed wetting. It controls excess mucous discharge in the urine and bowels, and restores urogenital organs. It cleanses, strengthens and restores the liver, pancreas and spleen. Important as part of any cleansing formula for the skin.

**SAFETY PRECAUTIONS:** Avoid when pregnant. Do not use with fluid deficiency, wasting, or dryness, or with remedies which acidify the urine.

**SYNERGY WITH OTHER HERBS:** Use with nettles and buchu in a tea for bladder infections. Use with couchgrass, yarrow and horsetail to heal damaged mucous membranes.

## Watercress (Nasturtium officinale)

**FAMILY:** Cruciferea

**MEDICINAL PARTS:** leaves and root

**DOSAGE:** Fresh juice: 2 tsp. in water 3x daily.

**NUTRITION PROFILE:** One of the best herbal sources for vitamin E. Has high iron, calcium, phosphorus, potassium, iodine, magnesium, manganese, sulfur, zinc, B-complex vitamins and many amino acids.

**CLEANSING PROPERTIES & DETOX ACTIVITY:** A spring cleansing purifier, watercress is a chlorophyll-rich herb for conditions that need blood building along with cleansing, like anemia, eczema and other chronic skin eruptions. Watercress is a potassium-rich diuretic, effective as a liver and organ cleanser in a formula to stimulate better metabolic activity, increase bile production and dispel gas.

Watercress restores the endocrine, nervous and immune systems. It tonifies the blood, regulates metabolism and relieves fatigue. It stimulates digestion, removes mucous accumulations in the lymph and liver, promotes urination, and resolves blood toxins. Watercress helps remove respiratory congestion by dissolving viscous phlegm and promoting expectoration. Recent studies indicate that watercress is particularly potent against lung cancer.

**SAFETY PRECAUTIONS:** Don't take if there are gastric or duodenal ulcers, or inflamed kidneys.

**SYNERGY WITH OTHER HERBS:** Use with fresh nettle and dandelion for blood purification. Use with dandelion, yellow dock, pau d' arco, hyssop, parsley, Oregon grape, red sage, licorice, milk thistle seed and hibiscus for a liver flush tea. Use with kelp, dulse, barley grass, parsley and alfalfa, for naturally occurring, absorbable potassium to revitalize metabolic activity. Use with alfalfa, nettles, Irish moss, yellow dock, parsley, borage seed, dulse and barley grass for strong bones.

## Wheat Grass

**FAMILY:** Gramineae

**MEDICINAL PARTS:** grass

**DOSAGE:** 1 tsp. dehydrated juice to ½ cup water; 1 tbsp. whole grass powder to ½ cup of water; tablets: up to 10 grams daily. For external use: soak cloth in fresh juice, apply locally or make a poultice of crushed grass pulp. Retention enema: 1 to 4 oz. fresh juice. Taken with water before meals, wheat grass has the ability to purge candida yeasts from the body. Builds red blood cells and can treat anemia.

**NUTRITION PROFILE:** Highly nutritious—15 lbs of wheatgrass has the nutritional value of 350 pounds of vegetables! A rich source of vitamin A, C, B12, fiber, chlorophyll (over 70%), minerals, amino acids (including lysine, leucine, tryptophan, phenylalanine, threonine, valine and leucine.

High SOD contributes to wheat grass's ability to protect against free radical damage caused by chemicalized foods, pollution, radiation (from X-rays, cancer treatment or computers) and other toxins. An excellent vegetarian source of protein, laetrile (an anti-cancer compound) and mucopolysaccharides. High nutrient content aids in appetite suppression for weight loss. High chlorophyll in wheat grass detoxifies the liver and bloodstream and helps neutralize pollutants like carbon monoxide. Note: Wheat grass is NOT a source of the gluten responsible for much of wheat grain allergy today (OK for wheat-sensitive people.)

**CLEANSING PROPERTIES & DETOX ACTIVITY:** Wheat grass cleanses the blood and gastrointestinal tract. Abundant in alkaline minerals, wheat grass can reduce over-acidity in the blood making it useful for over-acid body conditions like arthritis, rheumatism, candida yeast overgrowth, chronic fatigue, AIDS and allergies. Wheat grass normalizes the thyroid gland, and is beneficial for thyroid-related obesity, fatigue and constipation. High chlorophyll and the fraction P4D1 in wheat grass also protects against damage from radiation exposure, and renews cellular DNA. Restores energy levels in people with chronic fatigue by improving the oxygenation of body tissues.

Used externally, wheat grass can successfully treat skin ulcers, impetigo or other allergic, itchy skin conditions. It is a powerful healing tool as a colon implant for colon cancer, bowel toxicity or chronic constipation. High chlorophyll in wheat grass attributes to its action as a natural body deodorizer.

**SAFETY PRECAUTIONS:** Large amounts of undiluted wheat grass juice may cause nausea and dizziness. Adding a small "shot" to other fresh vegetable juices is advised. Used therapeutically for detoxification, wheat grass juicing may induce a short "healing crisis" characterized by diarrhea or headaches and is usually a good indication that the body is beginning to detoxify. If symptoms continue, reduce dosage.

**SYNERGY WITH OTHER HERBS:** With spirulina or chlorella to cleanse the body of toxins.

## Wild Cherry Bark (*Prunus serotina*)

**FAMILY:** Rosaceae

**MEDICINAL PARTS:** bark and root

**DOSAGE:** tincture: 30 – 60 drops 3x daily; extract: ½ to 1 tsp. 3x daily; tea: 6 oz. 3 – 4x daily; syrup: ½ to 2 tsp. 3x daily.

**NUTRITION PROFILE:** the bark contains calcium, iron and potassium.

**CLEANSING PROPERTIES & DETOX ACTIVITY:** A specific for lung conditions such as tuberculosis, asthma, whooping cough, and colds with a cough. Its spring tonic qualities make it good for indigestion problems such as loss of appetite, diarrhea, gastritis and heartburn. Works as a restorative for nerves, lungs, heart and intestines helping to calm the nerves and heart, to relieve irritation of mucous membranes, stimulate and tonify digestion, and generate strength. The tea is especially helpful for children's coughs, colds, diarrhea and colic. Helps inflammations of the eye.

**SAFETY PRECAUTIONS:** Not for use during pregnancy.

**SYNERGY WITH OTHER HERBS:** Use with elecampane, cramp bark and ¼ part lobelia and ginger in honey for an effective cough syrup. Use with beet, milk thistle seed, Oregon grape, dandelion, wild yam, yellow dock, licorice, ginkgo biloba, barberry, gotu kola, ginger, for a liver cleansing capsule combination.

## Wormwood (*Artemisia absinthium*)

**FAMILY:** Compositae

**MEDICINAL PARTS:** leaves and tops

**PREPARATION FORMS:** tincture, capsules, tea, wash, compress oil (externally).

**DOSAGE:** tincture: 10 – 30 drops 3x daily; powder: 15 – 20 grains 3x daily; tea: 2 cups daily.

**NUTRITION PROFILE:** vitamins A and C, a bitters herb for bile stimulation and cholesterol reduction.

**HERBAL HEALING ACTIONS:** vermifuge, alterative, astringent, stimulant, antiseptic, diuretic and tonic.

**CLEANSING PROPERTIES & DETOX ACTIVITY:** Wormwood's main use today is in formulas to expel intestinal worms and parasite infestations (both in people and animals), and as a poison antidote, especially for food poisoning. Small amounts may be used during acute illness to reduce fever and inflammation. As a bitters herb in small amounts, it stimulates enzyme secretions for better bile flow, reduces liver congestion and stimulates bowel peristalsis. Bitters herbs also encourage urination and drain fluid congestion. As a body cleanser, wormwood promotes menstruation, clears toxins and benefits the skin.

Wormwood may be used as a compress to relieve headaches, fevers, skin rashes, swellings, sprains and bruises, and to neutralize poisons from insect bites.

**SAFETY PRECAUTIONS:** Not for use when pregnant or breast feeding as it is a uterine stimulant.

**SYNERGY WITH OTHER HERBS:** With caraway seeds, peppermint and frangula bark for a bitters tea with laxative and carminative action.

## Yarrow (*Achillea millefolium*)

**FAMILY:** Compositae

**MEDICINAL PARTS:** the whole herb

**DOSAGE:** tincture: 5 – 20 drops 3x daily, tea: 6 oz. 3 – 4x daily, powder: 30 – 60 grains 3x daily.

**NUTRITION PROFILE:** Yarrow is high in chromium and potassium, selenium, vitamin B1 and C, and contains significant amounts of calcium, magnesium, manganese, phosphorus and silicon. Its amino acids include alanine, glutamic acid, histidine, leucine, and lysine.

**CLEANSING PROPERTIES & DETOX ACTIVITY:** Yarrow is used today as a hemostatic, antiseptic poultice to stop bleeding and reduce wound pain. Its cleansing properties restore the liver, stomach and spleen, reducing inflammation, clearing congestion, resolving intestinal mucous, stimulating liver activity and scouring the kidneys. It is effective as a urinary antiseptic for cystitis, urinary stones and bladder infections; its diuretic qualities help lower blood pressure. It has hormone stimulating properties for hormone imbalances, promoting cleansing, encouraging menstruation and removing pelvic congestion.

Yarrow is a powerful diaphoretic and antiseptic to induce sweating and lower fever during colds and flu. A good herb for childhood diseases like measles, chickenpox and diarrhea. Effective in cleansing for arthritis and rheumatism, gastroenteritis and colitis. Use externally for skin sores and hemorrhoids, it promotes tissue repair. Also effective as a compress for toothaches.

**SAFETY PRECAUTIONS:** Not for use during pregnancy—strong astringent action may be abortive.

**SYNERGY WITH OTHER HERBS:** With yucca, alfalfa, devil's claw, guggul resin, buckthorn bk., black cohosh, St. John's wort, burdock rt., licorice rt., dandelion, parsley, hydrangea, slippery elm, bilberry, ligusticum, poria mushroom, tumeric, rose hips, hawthorn to neutralize acids and increase mobility against arthritis.

## Yellow Dock Root (*Rumex crispus*)

**FAMILY:** Polygonaceae

**MEDICINAL PARTS:** root

**DOSAGE:** tincture: 5 – 30 drops 3x daily; powder: 30 – 60 grains 3x daily.

**NUTRITION PROFILE:** A rich source of herbal iron. High in phosphorus and vitamin A, vitamin C, B1 and B2; high in calcium, iron, magnesium, selenium; contains significant amounts of manganese, potassium, silicon, sodium, and vitamin B3, as well as trace amounts of chromium and zinc.

**CLEANSING PROPERTIES & DETOX ACTIVITY:** Yellow dock is especially effective for liver congestion, gallbladder and spleen. Yellow dock increases liver ability to filter and purify the blood and promotes production of bile. A specific in treating anemia—blood building against iron deficiency. A lymphatic cleanser for swollen glands. Helpful in dissolving cancerous growths and tumors. A mild astringent for hemorrhoids and ulcers. A mild purgative for constipation and ridding the body of intestinal parasites. Specific ailments that benefit from yellow dock's detox properties include breast and uterine fibroids and vaginal infections. Helps reduce the pain and inflammation of gout, rheumatism and arthritis. Helps relieve and dissolve urinary stones, and gravel in the kidney and urethral areas. Important in herbal skin formulas for eczema, psoriasis and other inflammatory skin conditions.

**SAFETY PRECAUTIONS:** Do not take during pregnancy or while breast-feeding. Not recommended for prolonged use (60 days) as it may cause laxative dependence.

**SYNERGY WITH OTHER HERBS:** With dandelion, watercress, pau d'arco, hyssop, parsley, Oregon grape rt., red sage, licorice, milk thistle seed and hibiscus for a liver flush tea. With beet, milk thistle seed, Oregon grape, dandelion, wild yam, licorice, ginkgo biloba, barberry, gotu kola, ginger, wild cherry for a liver cleansing capsule. With beet, alfalfa, dandelion, Siberian ginseng, parsley, nettles, burdock, dulse, bilberry and capsicum for spleen and liver activity, blood building, mental clarity and disease resistance.

## Yerba Santa (*Eriodictyon californicum*)

**FAMILY:** Hydrophyllaceae

**MEDICINAL PARTS:** leaves

**DOSAGE:** tincture: 10 – 30 drops 3x daily; powder: 15 – 60 grains 3x daily; tea: 2 – 3 oz. 3x daily.

**NUTRITION PROFILE:** Contains free formic acid and glycerides of fatty acids, phytosterols, resins, tannins that work on the bronchials, mucous membranes (useful in respiratory tract ailments), and urogenital areas. Also contains a mild amount of caffeine.

**CLEANSING PROPERTIES & DETOX ACTIVITY:** An expectorant herb with digestive cleansing properties. Used as part of a "spring cleansing" combination, especially for bladder and kidney. Used externally as an astringent antidote for poison oak rashes. Releases bronchitis phlegm and relieves coughing. Stimulates digestion and promotes the appetite. Reduces infection and opens the sinuses.

**SAFETY PRECAUTIONS:** None in common use.

**SYNERGY WITH OTHER HERBS:** With grindelia flowers for an expectorant. With red clover, hawthorn, pau d'arco, nettles, sage, alfalfa, horsetail, milk thistle seed, gotu kola, echinacea purpurea, blue malva and lemon grass in a spring cleansing tea.

# bibliography

Anderson, Dr. Richard, N.D., N.M.D. Cleanse & Purify Thyself. 1994

Anderson, Nina & Dr. Howard Peiper. Crystalloid Electrolytes: Our Body's Energy Source for the New Millennium. 1997

Arvigo, Rosita & Michael Balick. Rainforest Remedies: 100 Healing Herbs of Belize. Lotus Press, 1993

Baker, Elizabeth & Dr. Elton. The Uncook Book. 1983

Baranowski, Zane, C.N. Living Ecology. 1997

Bauman, Edward, Ph. D. "Immune Boosting Foods and Herbal Tonics." 1994

Bennett, Peter, ND, RAc, DHANP, "Working Up the Toxic Patient: Practical Intervention and Treatment Strategies," 13th International Symposium of The Institute for Functional Medicine. 2006

Bragg, Patricia, N.D., Ph.D. Vegetarian Health Recipes. Health Science 2008

Bubny, Paul, "Digestive Health: The Art and Science of Untoxification," Vitamin Retailer, Jan. 2007

Buchman, Dian Dincin, Herbal Medicine. Gramercy Publishing Company, 1980

Calbom, Cherie, MS, CN; Keane, Maureen, MS, CN. Juicing For Life. Avery Publishing Group, 1992

Carper, Jean, Food: Your Miracle Medicine. Harper Collins Publishers, 1993

Cass, Hyla, M.D. and Kathleen Barnes. 8 Weeks to Vibrant Health: A Woman's Take-Charge Program to Correct Imbalances, Reclaim Energy and Restore Energy. McGraw Hill 2005

Cass, Hyla, M.D. "Environmental Imbalances," Total Health Volume 28, No. 1

Chen, Ze-lin, M.D. and Mei-fang Chen, M.D. A Comprehensive Guide to Chinese Herbal Medicine. Ojai Press, 1992

Cichoke, Anthony J., D.C. Enzymes & Enzyme Therapy: How To Jump Start Your Way To Lifelong Good Health. 1994

"Coffee, Exercise Fight Skin Cancer," NewsMax Health Alerts, 8/11/07

"Consumer Bulletin: The Road to Detox," Whole Foods, July 2007

Davis, F. A. Taber's Cyclopedic Medical Dictionary. 1989

"Detoxification," Let's Live, July 1999

DiPasquale, Anthony. "Detox Products: Helping Your Customers Survive The Chemical Revolution," Whole Foods. Jan. 1996

Duke, James, PhD. Handbook of Medicinal Herbs. CRC Press, 1985

Duke, James, PhD. Handbook of Northeastern Indian Medicinal Plants. Quaterman Publications, 1986

"Exercise Slows Muscle Aging," Life Extension, Sept. 2007

Foster, Steven, Herbal Renaissance. Gibbs-Smith Publisher, 1984

Gates, Donna. The Body Ecology Diet. 1996

"Get the Lead Out," Taste for Life, Nov. 2006

Grieve, Mrs. M. A Modern Herbal. Dover Publications, 1971

Haas, Elson M., M.D. The Detox Diet. 1996

Harrison, Lewis. 30 Day Body Purification. How To Cleanse Your Inner Body & Experience the Joys of Toxin-Free Health. 1995

"Health and Longevity: The Probiotic Revolution", Health Sciences Institute. 1997

Hoffman, David. The Herbal Handbook. Healing Arts Press, 1988

Holmes, Peter. The Energetics of Western Herbs Vol. I & II. NatTrop Publshing, 1993

Howard, Judy. Bach Flower Remedies for Women. 1992

Howard, Judy. The Bach Flower Remedies Step By Step. 1994

Hsu, Hong-Yen Dr. How to Treat Yourself With Chinese Herbs. Keats Publishing, 1993

Hsu, Hong-Yen Dr. Oriental Materia Medica. Oriental Healing Arts Institute, 1986

Hughes, Aimee, N.D. "Choose the World's Best Spring Cleanse." Herbs for Health, April 2007

Hutchens, Alma R. Indian Herbology of North America. Shambhala Publications, 1973

Jensen, Bernard, D.C. Tissue Cleansing Through Bowel Management. 1981

Jensen, Bernard, Ph. D. Chlorella, Jewel Of The Far East. 1992

Kaminski, Patricia and Richard Katz. Flower Essence Repertory. 1994

Kapoor, L.D. CRC Handbook of Ayurvedic Medicinal Plants. CRC Press. 1990

Keith, Velma J.; Gordon, Monteen, The How To Herb Book. Mayfield Publishing, 1987

Kennedy, David C. DDS, June, 18, 1998 Letter & Paper (Addressing Fluoride's relationship to Dental Fluorosis, Hip Fracture, Cancer, & Tooth Decay Costs Savings).

Keuneke, Robin. Total Breast Health: The Power Food Solution for Protection & Wellness. 1998

Kircheimer, Sid, "Toxins in 20% of US Food Supply," WebMD Medical News Oct. 14, 2002

Levine, Stephen A., Ph.D. "Food Addiction, Food Allergy and Overweight", Bestways. Nov. 1988

Levine, Stephen A., Ph.D. "More About Allergy and Addiction." April 1988

Lewallen, Eleanor and John. Sea Vegetable Gourmet Cookbook & Wildcrafter's Guild. 1996

"Life Expectancy in U.S. Rises to Nearly 78 Years," Foxnews.com, Sept.12, 2007

Martlew, Gillian, N.D. Electrolytes The Spark Of Life: The Key To Longevity & Quality of Life.1998

Markowitz, Elysa. Living With Green Power - A Gourmet Collection of Living Food Recipes.1997

Millspaugh, Charles F. American Medicinal Plants. Dover Publications, 1974

Mindell, Earl, Ph.D. and Hester Mundis, "How to Avoid Common Toxins in Your Food," Natural Health May/June 2003

Mowrey, Daniel B., Ph.D. Next Generation Herbal Medicine. Keats Publishing, 1990

Mowrey, Daniel B., Ph.D., The Scientific Validation of Herbal Medicine. Keats Publishing, Inc. 1986

Murray, Michael, N.D. and Joseph Pizzorno, N.D. Encyclopedia of Natural Medicine. Prima Publishing, 1998

Nadkarni, K.M., DR., Indian Materia Medica. Popular Prakashan, 1982

Ody, Penelope, The Complete Medicinal Herbal, Dorling Kindersley, 1993

Olarsch, I. Gerald, N.D. Electrolytes - Your Body's Strongest Health Link! 1998

Page, Linda, Ph.D. Healthy Healing: A Guide To Self-Healing For Everyone 12th Edition. 2006

Page, Linda, Ph.D. How To Be Your Own Herbal Pharmacist. 1997

Pedersen, Mark, Nutritional Herbology Vol. I & II. Pedersen Publishing, 1987

Pitchford, Paul. Healing with Whole Foods. 1993

Price, Shirley. Practical Aromatherapy - How to Use Essential Oils to Restore Vitality. 1987

**"Probiotics = Proactive Health Care",** Whole Foods. Dec. 1997

**Rose, Jeanne,** Herbs & Things. Perigee Books, 1972

**Royal, Penny C.** Herbally Yours. Sound Nutrition, 1982

**Salome, Richard.** Hippocrates Health Institute Health Manual. 1993

**Santillo, Humbart, B.S., M.H.,** Natural Healing with Herbs. Holm Press, 1991

**Schauss, Alexander G., Ph.D.** "An analysis of colloidal mineral claims." Health Counselor. Feb/Mar 1997

**Scheer, James F.,** "Acidophilus Nature's Antibiotic", Better Nutrition. Aug. 1993

**Schroeder, Henry A., M.D.** The Trace Elements and Man. 1973

**Steenblock, Dr. David, B.S., M.Sc., D.O.** Chlorella: Natural Medicinal Algae. 1987

**Studer, William H.** American Ginseng In America. American Ginseng Society, 1993

**Swann, Denise.** Light Vegetarian Recipes for Higher Energy. 1993

**Tart Jensen, Ellen,** Ph.D. Health is Your Birthright: How to Create the Health You Deserve. Celestial Arts. 2007

**Tenney, Louise.** Today's Herbal Health. Woodland Books, 1992

**"Tests reveal high chemical levels in kids' bodies,"** Cnn.com 10/22/07

**Tierra, Dr. Michael, C.A., N.D.,** O.M.D. Planetary Herbology. Lotus Press. 1988

**Tierra, Dr. Michael, C.A., N.D.** The Way of Herbs Pocket Books. 1990

**Tisserand, Robert.** Aromatherapy: To Heal and Tend the Body. 1988

**Transformation Enterprise Corporation.** Enzymes - The Life Force Within Us. 1991

**Trattler, Ross,** Dr. Better Health Through Natural Healing. McGraw-Hill Book Company, 1985

**Tunella, Kim, C.D.C.** "Changing American Dietary Patterns." 1994

**Turner, Kristina.** The Self-Healing Cookbook. 1989

**Turner, Lisa.** Probiotics - "The Good, The Bad and The Friendly," Health Foods Business. Feb. 1997

**Valnet, Jean, M.D.** The Practice of Aromatherapy: A Classic Compendium of Plant Medicines & Their Healing Properties. 1990

**Walker, N.W. D. Sci.** Raw Vegetable Juices. Jove Books, 1987

**Weiss, Rudolf Fritz, M.D.** Herbal Medicine. Beaconsfield Publishers LTD, 1988

**Wigmore, Ann.** Recipes for Longer Life. 1978

**Wren, R.C., F.L.S.** Potter's New Cyclopaedia of Botanical Drugs and Preparations, 1989

# product resources

## Where you can get what we recommend...

The following list is for your convenience and assistance in obtaining further information about the products I recommend in *Healthy Healing's Detoxification*. The list is unsolicited by the companies named. Each company has a solid history of testing and corroborative data that is invaluable to me and my staff, as well as empirical confirmation by the stores that carry these products who have shared their experiences with us. I realize there are many other fine companies and products who are not listed here, but you can rely on the companies below for their high quality products and good results.

**Alacer Corp.,** 19631 Pauling, Foothill Ranch, CA 92610, 800-854-0249

**All One,** 719 East Haley St., Santa Barbara, CA 93103, 800-235-5727

**Aloe Life International,** P.O. Box 710759, Santee, CA 92072, 800-414-2563

**American Health,** 2100 Smithtown Avenue, Ronkonkoma, NY 11779, 800-445-7137

**Anabol Naturals,** 1550 Mansfield Street, Santa Cruz, CA 95062, 800-426-2265

**Arise & Shine,** P.O. Box 400, Medford, OR 97501, 800-688-2444

**Ark Naturals Products for Pets,** 6166 Taylor Rd. #105, Naples, FL 34109, 800-926-5100

**Barleans Organic Oils,** 4936 Lake Terrell Rd., Ferndale, WA 98248, 800-445-3529

**Baywood Intl.,** 14950 N. 83rd Pl., Ste.1, Scottsdale, AZ 85260, 800-481-7169

**Beehive Botanicals,** Route 8, Box 8257, Hayward, WI 54843, 800-233-4483

**BHI (Heel Inc.)** P.O. Box 11280, Albuquerque, NM 87192, 800-621-7644

**Biostrath,** 75 Commerce Drive, Hauppauge, NY, 11788-3943, 800-439-2324

**Body Ecology,** 218 Laredo Drive, Decatur, GA 30030, 800-511-2660

**Bodyonics (Pinnacle),** 140 Lauman Lane, Hicksville, NY 11801, 800-899-2749

**Boericke & Tafel Inc.,**(B & T) 2381 Circadian Way, Santa Rosa, CA 95407, 707-571-8202

**Bragg/Live Food Products, Inc.,** 7340 Hollister Ave., Santa Barbara, CA 93102, 805-968-1028

**CC Pollen Co.,** 3627 East Indian School Rd., Suite 209, Phoenix, AZ 85018-5126, 800-875-0096

**Clear Products,** 4320 Vandever Ave Suite A, San Diego, CA 92120, 888-257-2532

**Country Life,** 180 Vanderbilt Motor Pkwy, Hauppauge NY, 11788, 800-645-5768

**Crystal Star Herbs,** 121-B Calle Del Oaks, Del Rey Oaks, CA 93940, 800-736-6015

**Designing Health,** 28410 Witherspoon Parkway, Valencia, CA 91355, 800-774 -7387

**Diamond/Herpanacine Ass,** 145 Willow Grove Ave. #1 Dept. #WP 5, Glenside, PA 19038, 888-467-4200

**Dr. Rath's Vitamins,** 1260 Memorex Drive, Suite 200, Santa Clara, CA 95050, 800-624-2442

**Earth Mama Angel Baby,** 9866 SE Empire Court, Clackamas, OR 97015, 503-607-0607

**East Park Research, Inc.,** 2709 Horseshoe Drive, Las Vegas, NV 89120, 800-345-8367

Eidon Mineral Products,12330 Stowe Drive, Poway, CA 92060, 800-700-1169

Enzymedica, 752 Tamiami Trail, Port Charlotte, FL 33954, 888-918-1118

Earth's Bounty/Matrix Health Products, 1101 N.E. 144th St. #109, Vancouver, WA 98685, 800-736-5609

Esteem Products Ltd.,1800 136th Pl. NE Suite 5, Bellevue, WA 98005, 800-954-5515

Ethical Nutrients/Unipro, 971 Calle Negocio, San Clemente, CA 92673, 800-668-8743

Fit for You, Intl., 971 S Bundy Dr., Brentwood CA 90049-5828, 800-521-5867

Flora, Inc., 805 East Badger Road, P.O. Box 73, Lynden, WA 98264, 800-446-2110, (Info.) 604-451-8232

Futurebiotics, 70 Commerce Drive, Hauppauge, NY 11788, 800-645-1721

Gaia Herbs, Inc., 108 Island Ford Road, Brevard, NC 28712, 888-917-8269

Golden Pride, 1501 Northpoint Pkwy., Suite 100, West Palm Beach, FL 33407, 561-640-5700

Green Foods Corp., 320 North Graves Ave., Oxnard, CA 93030 800-777-4430

Grifron/Maitake Products, Inc., 1 Madison St. Bldg. F, East Rutherford, NJ 07073, 800-747-7418

Health from the Sun/Arkopharma, P.O. Box 179, Newport, NH 03773, 800-447-2229

Heather's Tummy Care, 80 S. Washington St., Suite 304 Seattle, WA 98104

Herbal Answers, Inc., P.O. Box 1110, Saratoga Springs, New York 12866, 888-256-3367

Herbal Magic, Inc., P.O. Box 70, Forest Knolls, CA 94933, 800-684-3722

Herbal Products & Development, P.O. Box 1084, Aptos, CA 95001, 831-688-4200

Herbs Etc.,1340 Rufina Circle, Santa Fe, NM 87507, 888-433-1212

Home Health, 2100 Smithtown Avenue, Ronkonkoma, NY 11779, 800-445-7137

Immudyne, 7453 Empire Drive, Suite 300, Florence, Kentucky 41042, 888-246-6839

Imperial Elixir, P.O. Box 970, Simi Valley, CA 93062, 800-284-2598

Jagulana Herbal Products, Inc., P.O. Box 45, Badger, CA 93603, 888-465-3686

Jarrow Formulas, 1824 South Robertson Blvd., Los Angeles, CA 90035, 800-726-0886

Jason Natural/Earth's Best, 4600 Sleepytime Dr., Boulder, CO 80301, 800-434-4246

Lane Labs, 25 Commerce Drive, Allendale, NJ 07401, 800-526-3005

Lane Labs TOKI, 1-888-AGELESS, Please mention code #6404

MagneLyfe/Encore Technology, Inc., 115 W 29th Street Ste 1100-B, New York, NY 10001, 877-624-6353

Maine Coast Sea Vegetables, 3 Georges Pond Road, Franklin, Maine 04634, 207-565-2907

Maitake Products, Inc., 1 Madison St. Bldg. F, East Rutherford, NJ 07073, 800-747-7418

Mendocino Sea Vegetable Co., P.O. Box 1265, Mendocino, CA 95460, 707-937-2050

Merix Health Care Products, 18 E. Dundee Rd. #3-204, Barrington, IL 60010, 847-277-1111

Metabolic Response Modifiers, 236 Calle Pintoresco, San Clemente, CA 92672, 800-948-6296

Moon Maid Botanicals, 535 Tall Poplar Road, Cosby, TN 37722, 877-253-7853

MRI (Medical Research Institute), 444 De Haro St. Suite 209, San Francisco CA 94107, 888-448-4246

Mychelle Dermaceuticals, Box 1, Frisco, CO 80443, 800-447-2076

Natural Balance, 3130 N. Commerce Ct., Castle Rock, CO 80104-8002, 303-688-6633

Natural Labs Corporation (Deva Flowers), P.O. Box 20037, Sedona, AZ 86341-0037, 800-233-0810

Nature's Apothecary/NOW Foods, 395 S. Glen Ellyn Rd., Bloomingdale, IL 60108, 888-669-3663

Nature's Path Supplements, PO Box 7862, North Port, FL 34286, 800-326-5772

Nature's Secret/Irwin Naturals, 5310 Beethoven St., Los Angeles, CA 90066, 800-297-3273

Nature's Way, 1375 N. Mountain Springs Parkway, Springville, UT 84663, 800-962-8873

Nelson Bach, Wilmington Technology Park, 100 Research Dr., Wilmington, MA 01887, 800-319-9151

New Chapter, 90 Technology Dr., Brattleboro, VT 05301, 800-543-7279

Nordic Naturals, 94 Hangar Way, Wastonville, CA 95076, 800-662-2544

NOW, 395 S. Glen Ellyn Rd., Bloomingdale, IL 60108, 888-669-3663

NutriCology /Allergy Research Group, 2300 North Loop Rd., Alameda, CA 94507, 800-545-9960

Oshadhi, 1340 G Industrial Ave., Petaluma, CA 94952, 888-674-2344

Pacific BioLogic, P.O. Box 520, Clayton, CA 94517-0520, 800-869-8783

Penta Water, 2091 Rutherford Rd., Carlsbad, CA 92008, 800-531-5088

Planetary Formulas, P.O. Box 533, Soquel, CA 95073, 800-606-6226

Prince of Peace, 3536 Arden Road, Hayward, CA 94545, 800-732-2328

PSP Marketing, 23241 Areco Ct., Laguna Nigel, CA 92677, 866-777-5050

Pure Essence Laboratories, Inc., P.O. Box 95397, Las Vegas, NV 89193, 888-254-8000

Pure Form, 3240 West Desert Inn Rd., Las Vegas, NV 89103, 888-363-9817

Pure Planet, 1542 Seabright Ave., Long Beach, CA 90813, 562-951-1124

Rainbow Light, 125 McPherson St., Santa Cruz, CA 95060, 800-571-4701

Rainforest Remedies, Box 325, Twin Lakes, WI 53181, 800-824-6396

Real Life Research, Inc., 14631 Best Ave., Norwalk, CA 90650, 800-423-8837

Rejuvenative Foods, P.O. Box 8464, Santa Cruz, CA 95061, 800-805-7957

Solaray, Inc., 1400 Kearns Boulevard, Park City, UT 84060, 800-669-8877

Source Naturals Inc., 19 Janis Way, Scotts Valley, CA 95066, 800-815-2333

Spectrum Naturals, 5341 Old Redwood Hwy., Suite 400, Petaluma, CA 94954, 707-778-8900

Springlife Inc., 4630 N. Paseo De Los Cerritos, Tucson, AZ 85745, 888-633-9233

Starwest Botanicals, 11253 Trade Center Drive, Rancho Cordova, CA 95742, 800-800-4372

Sun Wellness (Sun Chlorella), 3305 Kashiwa Street, Torrance, CA 90505, 800-829-2828

Superior Trading, 835 Washington Street, San Francisco, CA 94108, 415-495-7988

Transformation Enzyme Corporation, 2900 Wilcrest, Suite 220, Houston, TX 77042, 800-777-1474

Trimedica International, Inc., 1895 South Los Feliz Drive, Tempe, AZ 85281-6023, 800-800-8849

UAS Laboratories, 9953 Valleyview Rd., Eden Prairie, MN 55344, 800-422-3371

Wakunaga of America / Kyolic, 23501 Madero, Mission Viejo, CA 92691, 800-421-2998 / 800-825-7888

Yoanna Skin Care, P.O. Box 610072, Redwood City, CA 94061, 800-366-4617

Y.S. Royal Jelly and Organic Bee Farm, 2774 N. 4351 Rd., Sheridan, IL 60551, 800-654-4593

Zand Herbal Formulas, 1441 West Smith Road, Ferndale, WA 98248, 800-232-4005

Zia Natural Skincare, 4600 Sleepytime Drive, Boulder, CO 80301, 800-334-7546

# index